A Colour Atlas of
Tropical Medicine and Parasitology

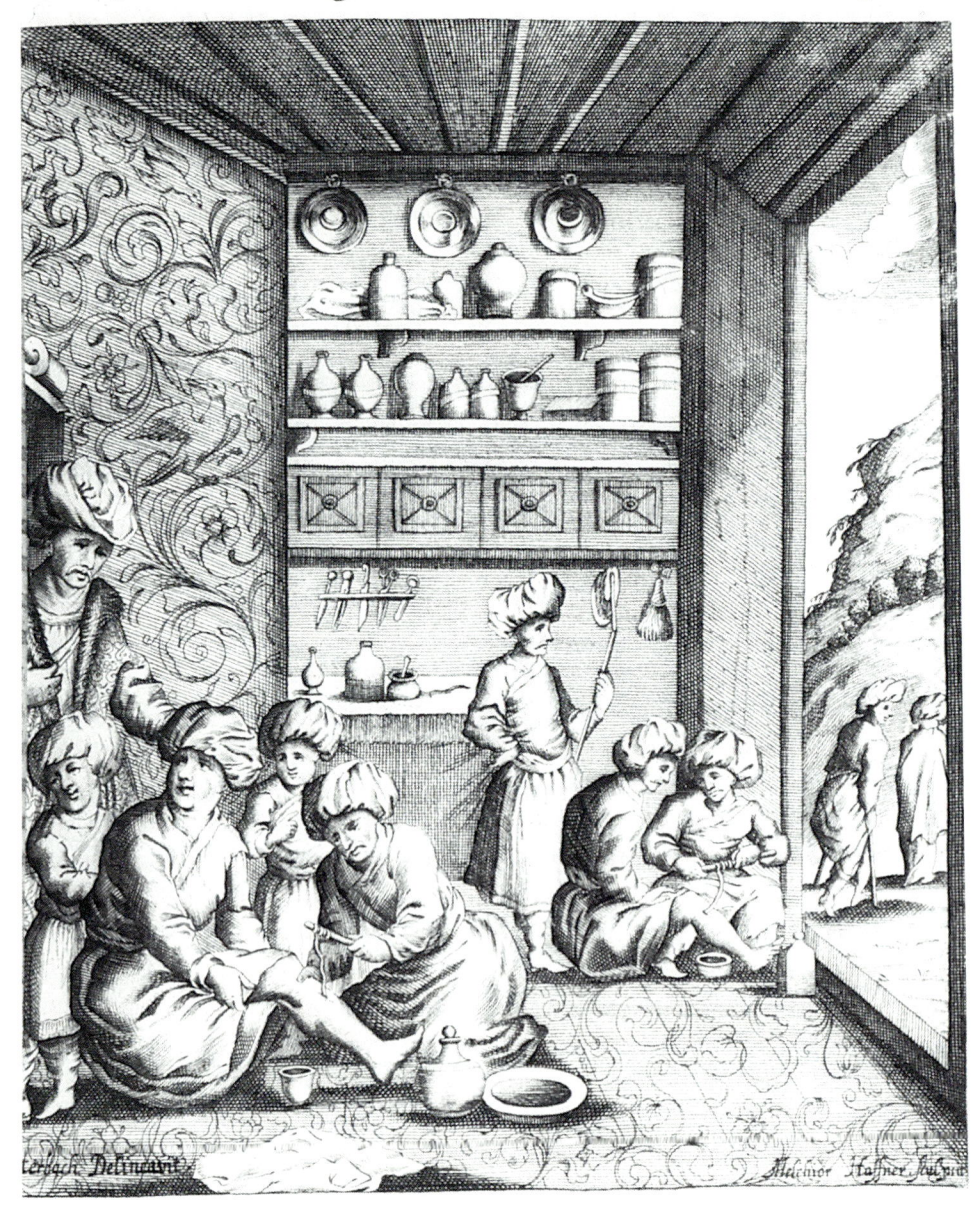

Guinea or 'Medina' worms (*Dracunculus medinensis*) being extracted from the legs of patients in Persia, using a simple technique that is still widely employed. (From *Exercitationes de Vena Medinensis et de Vermiculis Capillaribus Infantium* by G H Velschius, published in Augsburg, 1674—reproduced by permission of The British Library.)

A *Colour Atlas* of
TROPICAL MEDICINE & PARASITOLOGY
Third Edition

WALLACE PETERS
MD (London), DSc (London), FRCP (England), DTM&H
Professor of Medical Protozoology
London School of Hygiene and Tropical Medicine

HERBERT M GILLES
KOSJ, MSc (Oxon), MD (Malta), DSc (Hon Causa, Malta),
DMedSc (Hon Causa, Karolinska Institute, Stockholm),
FRCP (England), FFCM (London), FMCPH (Nigeria), DTM&H
Emeritus Professor of Tropical Medicine, University of Liverpool
and Senior Research Fellow, Department of Pharmacology and
Therapeutics, University of Liverpool.

Wolfe Medical Publications Ltd

Copyright © Wallace Peters & Herbert M Gilles, 1977, 1981 & 1989
Published by Wolfe Medical Publications Ltd, 1977, 1981 & 1989
Printed by Royal Smeets Offset, Weert, Netherlands
ISBN 0 7234 1534 X Cased edition
ISBN 0 7234 1535 8 Paperback edition
First published 1977
Second edition 1981, Reprinted 1985
Third edition 1989, Reprinted 1991

All rights reserved. No reproduction, copy or transmission of this
publication may be made without written permission.

No part of this publication may be reproduced, copied or
transmitted save with written permission or in accordance with the
provisions of the Copyright Act 1956 (as amended), or under the terms of
any licence permitting limited copying issued by the Copyright Licensing
Agency, 33–34 Alfred Place, London, WC1E 7DP.

Any person who does any unauthorised act in relation to this publication
may be liable to criminal prosecution and civil claims for damages.

A CIP catalogue record for this book is available from the British Library.

This book is one of the titles in the series of Wolfe Medical Atlases, a series
that brings together the world's largest systematic published collection of
diagnostic colour photographs.

For a full list of Atlases in the series, plus forthcoming titles and details of
our surgical, dental and veterinary Atlases, please write to Wolfe Medical
Publications Ltd, Brook House, 2–16 Torrington Place, London WC1E 7LT,
England.

Contents

Acknowledgements	7
Preface and Introduction	9

Part I: Arthropod-borne Infections — 11
Arboviruses	12
Rickettsioses	18
Bacterial Infections	21
Protozoal Infections	25
Trypanosomiasis	41
Leishmaniasis	52
Nematodes—the Filariases	63

Part II: Soil-mediated Helminthiases — 83
The Hookworm Infections	84
Infection with *Ascaris* and Related Nematodes	93
Trichuriasis	97

Part III: Snail-mediated Helminthiases — 98
Schistosomiasis	99
The Intestinal Flukes	112
Liver Fluke Infections	115
Paragonimiasis	121
Angiostrongyliasis	124

Part IV: Infections Acquired through the Gastrointestinal Tract — 126
Viral Infections	127
Bacterial Infections	129
Protozoal Infections	134
Helminthiases—Nematodes	146
Helminthiases—Cestodes	152
Pentastomiasis	163

Part V: Infections Acquired through the Skin and Mucous Membranes — 166
Viral Infections	167
Bacterial Infections	171
Protozoal Infections	179
The Superficial Mycoses	180
The Systemic Mycoses	181
Ectoparasitic Arthropods	186

Part VI: Airborne Infections — 190
    Measles — 190
    Cytomegalovirus — 191
    Meningococcal Meningitis — 192
    Tuberculosis — 193
    Whooping Cough — 194

Part VII: Nutritional Disorders — 195
    Kwashiorkor and Marasmus — 196
    Nutritional Marasmus — 197
    Avitaminoses — 197

Part VIII: Miscellaneous Disorders — 202
    Zoonotic Viral Infections — 202
    Pneumocystosis — 205
    Neoplastic Conditions — 206
    Genetic Blood Dyscrasias — 207
    Venomous Bites and Stings — 209
    Diseases of Uncertain Aetiology or Epidemiology — 211

List of Tables — 214
Bibliography — 233
Index — 234

Acknowledgements

Professor H de Oliveira Almeida, **163**; Dr J Almeida, **17**; Professor D Alves Meira, **640**; Drs J Anderson and H Fuglsang, **270, 282, 292, 294, 296, 297**; Dr Kemal Arab, **589**; Armed Forces Institute of Pathology, **340, 496, 597**; Professor V S Arean, **371**; Dr O P Arya, **293, 717, 803**; Dr E Åsbrink, **53**; Dr R W Ashford, **174, 175, 177, 352, 561, 569**; Professor N H Ashton, **369**; Dr D A T Baldry, **135, 142, 278**; Dr G Barr, **518**; Mr N R Barrett CBE, **653**; Dr D Baxby, **673**; Dr F Beltran, **377**; Professor E Bengtsson, **651**; Dr R Ben-Ismail, **198**; Professor J K A Beverley* and Royal Sheffield Hospitals, **571, 575**; Dr A E Bianco, **264**; Dr R G Bird*, **26, 35**; Dr A Björkman, **683**; The British Library, Frontispiece; Dr S G Browne*, **696, 698, 707**; Professor C F A Bruijning, **381**; Dr A Bryceson, **32, 34, 136, 137, 164, 295, 507, 512, 514, 649, 685, 690, 722, 723, 764, 766, 780, 790, 801, 849**; Dr A Buck, **725**; Dr C Bullough, **807**; Professor E Canning, **579**; Dr J L Champalimaud, **143, 144**; Mr A R Chandler and Smith Kline & French Laboratories, **148**; Dr M L Chance, **15, 172**; Professor Shiu-Nan Chen, **445, 456, 471, 485, 491, 493**; Professor M J Clarkson, **368**; Dr R Cooke, **31, 88, 520, 576, 635, 637, 716, 742, 752, 773, 776, 785, 826, 842**; Cooper, McDougall & Robertson Ltd., **33**; Col G Cowan, **786**; Col J C Crook, Royal Army Medical College, **496, 597**; Dr J H Cross, **261**; Professor J-P Dedet, **216**; Dr D T Dennis, **261**; Professor W O Dobbins III and Dr W M Weinstein, **580**; Dr C C Draper, **430**; Dr B Duke, **283**; Professor J Eckert, **657**; Professor G Edington*, **503**; Dr D S Ellis, **228, 229, 566, 681, 777, 813, 819**; Dr D W Ellis-Jones, **671**; Professor A El Rooby, **404, 405**; Professor R T D Emond and Dr H A K Rowland, **505, 774**; Professor Z Even-Paz, **203**; Mr M G Falcon, **730**; Mr J Ferguson, **257, 372**; Professor J K Frenkel, **573**; Mr H Furse, **408**; Dr P J Gardener, **173**; Professor J D Gillett, **58**; Dr J M Goldsmid, **354, 365, 639**; Dr B M Greenwood, **147, 608, 782**; Dr D Greenwood, **355, 356, 397, 464, 585, 643, 644**; Dr A Griffiths, **199**; Mr M Guy, **182**; Professor D R W Haddock*, **19**; Professor P Hamilton*, **120, 830**; Professor T Harinasuta, **453, 467, 487, 522, 554**; Dr R Hay, **749**; Dr A Heller-Haupt, **490**; Professor R Hendrickse, **501, 509, 688, 775, 788, 794, 798, 831, 832, 845**; Dr R H Heptinstall and Department of Pathology, Johns Hopkins University, **596**; Dr B Heyworth, **511, 594, 595, 674, 779**; Dr P R Hira, **650, 656**; Dr Holliman, **341**; Professor M Hommel, **195**; Dr H Hoogstraal*, **406**; Professor R E Howells, **329, 386-393, 441, 469, 659, 665**; Professor Hung Tao, **816, 817**; Dr M P Hutchinson, **141**; Professor W M Hutchinson, **568**; Professor M S R Hutt, **121, 122, 546, 689, 824, 825, 843**; Dr A G Ironside, **787**; Dr H Jackson, **818**; Professor P G Janssens, **138**; Dr P Jayanetra, **521**; Dr J M Jewsbury, **433-440**; Dr G J Kane, Wellcome Reagents Ltd., **578, 590**; Dr J F Kassel, **241, 242**; Professor D Katamine, **247**; Professor B H Kean, **246**; Dr G Khalil and Professor J F Schacher, **661, 662**; Professor F Köberle*, **161, 162, 165**; Dr W A Krotoski and *American Journal of Tropical Medicine and Hygiene*, **65**; Professor R E Kuntz, **188**; Professor R Lainson, **214**; Professor Y Larsson, **712**; Dr R Lindley, **828**; Dr R Lindner, **291**; Dr S Lucas, **89, 90, 145, 159, 245, 284, 312, 345, 349, 370, 398, 399, 407, 409, 416, 432, 459, 488, 539, 540, 547, 555, 556, 564, 565, 574, 577, 581, 582, 593, 617, 618, 638, 654, 658, 682, 750, 756, 811, 820, 821**; Dr Lily Ma, **460**; Mr S N McDermott, **168, 191**; Professor W W MacDonald, **49, 232**; Dr C D Mackenzie, **286-289** (and University of Chicago Press), **285**; Dr I Maddocks and the Medical Learning Resources Unit, University of Papua New Guinea, **519, 550, 714**; Professor B G Maegraith, **447**; Professor El Sheikh Mahgoub, **738-741**; Professor R A Marcial-Rojas, **351**; Dr K Markwalder, **636**; Professor P Marsden, **55, 848**; Dr B E Matthews (reprinted with permission from the *Journal of Nematology*), **330-334, 362**; Dr S Migasena, **603**; Dr M Miles, **158**; Dr A Mindel, **755, 827, 828**; Professor I Miyazaki, **602**; Mr P Montague, **512**; Professor H Morgan, **761**; Major General R J G Morrison, **139**; Dr M F Muhlemann, **52**; Dr R Muller, Frontispiece, **264, 268, 298, 305, 309, 431, 474, 495, 606, 652**; Dr F A Murphy, **809**; Dr M Murray, **175, 477**; Dr P Myak, **524, 525**; Dr H Nakajima, **619**; Dr B M Nelson, **573**; Professor G S Nelson, **641**; Professor B Ochoa, **366, 367**; Dr T O Ogunlesi, **410**; Dr G F Otto, **596**; Dr R Owen, **642**; Professor H E Parry, **505**; Professor F M Paul, **23**; Dr P L Perine, **27, 28, 679**; Dr W Petana, **129, 154**; Dr E H Pike, **628**; Dr Prentice, **277**; Professor M Quilici, **124, 668**; Professor A J Radford, **84, 604, 708, 709, 720, 760, 784, 788, 800**; Dr G Rapeport, **554**; Dr H A Reid*,

834-839; Professor J A Rioux, **205**; Dr R Ross, **783**; Ms S Ryall, **534**; Mr P Sargeaunt, **533, 535, 541**; Dr G D Scarrow, **310, 797, 799, 833**; Professor H Schenone, **153, 841**; Dr C W Schraft Jr, **548**; Dr A Schrank, **715**; Dr D Scott, **141**; Professor J T Self, **666, 667**; Professor V Sery, **197**; Shell International Chemical Co. Ltd., **395, 412, 423**; Dr A J Shelley, **772**; Professor D I H Simpson, **813, 814**; Dr R Sinden, **62**; Dr J A Smith and Ibadan University, **669**; Dr M Smith, **33**; Professor S Sornmani and the Applied Malacology Centre, Faculty of Tropical Medicine, Mahidol University, **432**; Air Vice Marshall W Stamm*, **551**; Dr H Striebel, **383**; Dr R Sturrock, **384**; Professor M Suzuki, **455, 457, 599**; Dr Y Suzuki, **394**; Dr J S Tatz, **559**; Dr A C Templeton, **660**; Dr D Theakston, **117**; Dr H Townson, **230, 231**; Mr G Tovey, **67**; Dr B Thylfors, **306**; Dr Tin Chua Kian, **21**; Dr S Vajasthira, **444, 450, 454, 461, 462, 465, 480, 482**; Dr F L Vichii, **160**; Professor K Vickerman, **128**; Dr A Voller, **167**; Dr J Walters, **183, 189, 304, 350, 572, 610, 737, 804, 850, 851**; Dr D C Warhurst, **92, 536, 727, 729, 731**; Professor D Warrell, **83, 86, 87, 685, 686, 811**; Professor J Waterlow, **793, 794, 802, 808**; Wellcome Museum of Medical Science and Dr A J Duggan, **605, 823**; Dr R R Willcox, **680**; Mr J Williams, **149, 567**; Dr A Wisdom, **680, 728**; Professor M Wittner, **258, 428, 483**; Dr D J M Wright, **33**; World Health Organization, **25, 46, 47, 298, 347, 357, 443, 622, 672, 676-678,** **840**; Professor Y Yoshida, **481**; Professor H Yoshimura, **600**; Dr H Zaiman, **374, 375, 648**; Professor A J Zuckerman, **17, 497, 499, 500**.

[* Now deceased]

The copyright of the following figures is held by those named:
Professor R G Hendrickse, **501, 509, 688, 775, 788, 796, 798, 831, 832, 845**; Professor Y Larrson, **712**; MEDDIA, Amsterdam, **57, 126, 151, 170, 233, 267, 274, 335, 346, 360, 373, 378, 452, 583, 630, 646, 692, 693, 704-706**; Dr A Mindel, **755, 827, 828**; Professor A J Radford, **84, 604, 708, 709, 720, 760, 784, 788, 800**; the late Dr H A Reid, **834-838**.

In addition to those whose assistance we acknowledged in the second edition of this work, we wish to thank Mrs T Sargeaunt for secretarial and Mr J Williams for technical help. Drs V Southgate and D Brown kindly advised us on the terminology in Tables XI and XII and Dr R Hay on Table XV. The maps were skilfully redrafted by Mr Alick Newman. Our thanks go again to the publishers for their guidance in the preparation of this new edition. We deeply regret that the late Mr Peter Wolfe, who gave us constant encouragement, could not have shared in its completion. Finally we would like to acknowledge the constructive comments made by reviewers of the first two editions of this Atlas, all of which we have taken into account in the present work as far as possible.

Preface and Introduction

In the decade since the first edition of this Atlas appeared, a number of previously unknown parasitic and viral infections have been described, while several of those already known have taken on a quite unexpectedly serious significance. In part these innovations are attributable to the emergence, since 1981, of a new pandemic viral infection, the Acquired Immune Deficiency Syndrome (AIDS) which we now see to be caused not only by the Human Immunodeficiency Virus (HIV, LAV, HTLV III), but also by several related viruses. These have unleashed a number of other infections, particularly of bacterial, fungal and protozoal origin. Some of these are otherwise relatively innocuous and are retained in the body as chronic, virtually commensal infections. Others probably invade the organs as opportunistic infections that would, in individuals with a normally responsive immune defence, never gain a foothold. It is currently believed that AIDS arose in the relatively recent past, in some unknown manner, in Central Africa where it threatens to ravage large indigenous populations. Be that as it may, because AIDS has since spread almost universally, the disease and its concomitant manifestations fully merit a prominent place in the pages of this new edition. The World Health Organization estimated in late 1986 that up to 10 million people could be infected with HIV and that this figure could rise to 100 million within five years. The estimate of 100,000 overt AIDS cases could rise to between a half and three million of whom, on present experience, one half would die. In Africa this means that in 1990 as many may die of AIDS as are currently believed could die of malaria, namely one million.

Other viral pathogens have been identified recently, Hantaan virus, for example, which causes a haemorrhagic syndrome, often with renal involvement (HFRS), both in the tropics and elsewhere. This virus is now seen, in retrospect, to have been the agent responsible for a fatal form of haemorrhagic fever during the Korean war, when some 3000 cases were seen. Globally at least 12,000 people develop HFRS each year. Lassa fever, as well as Ebola and Marburg fevers (which figured in our second edition) have, for the time being at least, taken a back seat, but not without obliging health authorities in a number of non-endemic countries to establish a strict system for the quarantine of suspect cases inside elaborate, futuristic-looking, plastic isolation units. Viral hepatitis, on the contrary, is ubiquitous and a newly discovered pathogen, the Delta agent, has been shown to cause fulminating hepatitis in individuals who are already infected with hepatitis B. A new, tick-borne, *Borrelia* infection, Lyme disease, has been found to occur commonly both in the New and Old Worlds. It is responsible for a syndrome of fever, erythema, arthritis and transitory motor neurone disorders, the high level of incidence of which is only just becoming apparent.

On the positive side, during the four years that elapsed between the publication of the first and second editions of this Atlas, the eradication of one of the world's greatest scourges, smallpox, was heralded. Since then, major advances in immunology and molecular biology have begun to open up a new era of diagnostic procedures which make use of monoclonal antibodies and of more specific antigens than have ever been available up to now. DNA probes which are increasingly in the news, may soon find a place especially in epidemiological studies, supplementing standard serology and microscopy. Modern medical imaging techniques, computerised tomography, scintillography, nuclear magnetic resonance spectrometry, etc. are being applied in the diagnosis of parasitic infections, at least in those more sophisticated centres that can afford to establish them. Genetically engineered vaccines against the major infectious and parasitic diseases are emerging, or are in a relatively advanced state of development.

A word of caution, however, in the light of all these promising novelties. The grim statistics of infection in the world as set out in the preface to our first edition remain, today, little changed. If anything the situation looks worse and, apart from the shining example of the eradication of smallpox, it does not seem likely that radical improvements will be made in the near future. To start with, the world's population has risen from the 3.8 billion quoted in 1977 to 4.75 billion, with all that implies in terms of undernutrition and land pressure. In its latest estimates the World Health Organization gave the following figures: *Malaria* 54.3 per cent of the world's inhabitants at risk of infection, 200 million chronically infected in tropical Africa and at least 7.8 million new cases elsewhere each year; *Schistosomiasis* 600 million exposed to infection in 74 countries, 200 million actually infected; *Lymphatic filariases* 905 million at risk, 90 million infected; *Onchocerciasis* 40 million affected; *African trypanosomiases* 50 million at risk, at least 20,000 cases a year; *Chagas' disease* 65 million at risk, 15 to 20 million infected; *Leprosy* over 10.6 million cases with an increasing incidence of drug resistance. Many of the sophisticated new diagnostic tools will still not help a great majority of the sick people in the poor, developing countries of the tropics and subtropics, nor will such people readily have access to the more expensive of the newer vaccines. It will still be necessary to exercise the old diagnostic skills and to treat those who have access to primary health care services with the most basic, and cheapest, drugs. At the same time, the ever-increasing mobility of the human population both within national borders and internationally, will continue to disseminate many 'exotic' conditions and the need for a simple guide to their recognition will remain.

While the second edition was updated and contained, unlike its predecessor, illustrations of parasite life cycles, the production of the present version in an entirely new format has provided the opportunity to revise the subject matter in its entirety. As well as replacing many figures with those of a better quality, we have added new ones that increase both the depth and breadth of the Atlas and have brought the zoological terminology as up to date as possible in this dynamic field. We hope, therefore, that it will serve its readers as well as the earlier editions appear to have done.

Part I
Arthropod-borne Infections

Numerically speaking mosquitoes are probably responsible for more disease than any other group of arthropods but other insects too are of great importance. While *Anopheles* mosquitoes carry malaria, various viral infections and some types of filariasis, other viruses and filarias are transmitted by culicines. Other biting flies transmit African trypanosomiasis, leishmaniasis, bartonellosis and several other kinds of filariasis. Fleas carry a species of typhus and plague, lice carry epidemic typhus, and mites and ticks other varieties of typhus. Ticks are also responsible for transmission of the haemorrhagic and the relapsing fevers. The arthropod vectors of disease are classified in **Table I**.

The important arthropod-borne (arbo) viruses considered here are yellow fever, SE Asian haemorrhagic fever and Japanese B encephalitis. These are representative of the arbovirus diseases which include many other infections of man in the tropics (*see* **Table II**). Of the rickettsioses, louse-borne typhus due to *R. prowazeki* is potentially the most important, but tick typhus is fairly common in some areas (e.g. East Africa) and mite-borne scrub typhus (tsutsugamushi disease) in Southeast Asia and the Southwest Pacific.

Plague is still endemic in certain tropical and subtropical areas, and localised outbreaks are not uncommon, especially in the disrupted social and ecological situations brought about by wars. Relapsing fever in Africa and bartonellosis (Carrión's disease) are geographically limited in extent.

Among the protozoal infections, African trypanosomiasis is increasing both in West and East Africa but, in numerical terms, is still mainly of importance for its effect on domestic animals. South American trypanosomiasis (Chagas' disease) extends through much of the subcontinent and is responsible for considerable ill health in parts of its distribution. Malaria and the leishmaniases are widespread; malaria, in particular, causes severe morbidity and mortality in many countries.

Of the tissue filariases, those due to *Wuchereria bancrofti* and *Brugia malayi* may produce serious deformity, while infection with the skin-dwelling parasite, *Onchocerca volvulus*, is a serious cause of blindness in parts of tropical Africa and Central America.

Whereas the diagnosis of the viral and bacterial infections must be confirmed by appropriate serological and cultural techniques, most protozoal and helminthic infections are readily recognised, if not on clinical grounds alone, then by fairly simple techniques designed to demonstrate the presence of the causative parasites.

ARBOVIRUSES
Yellow Fever

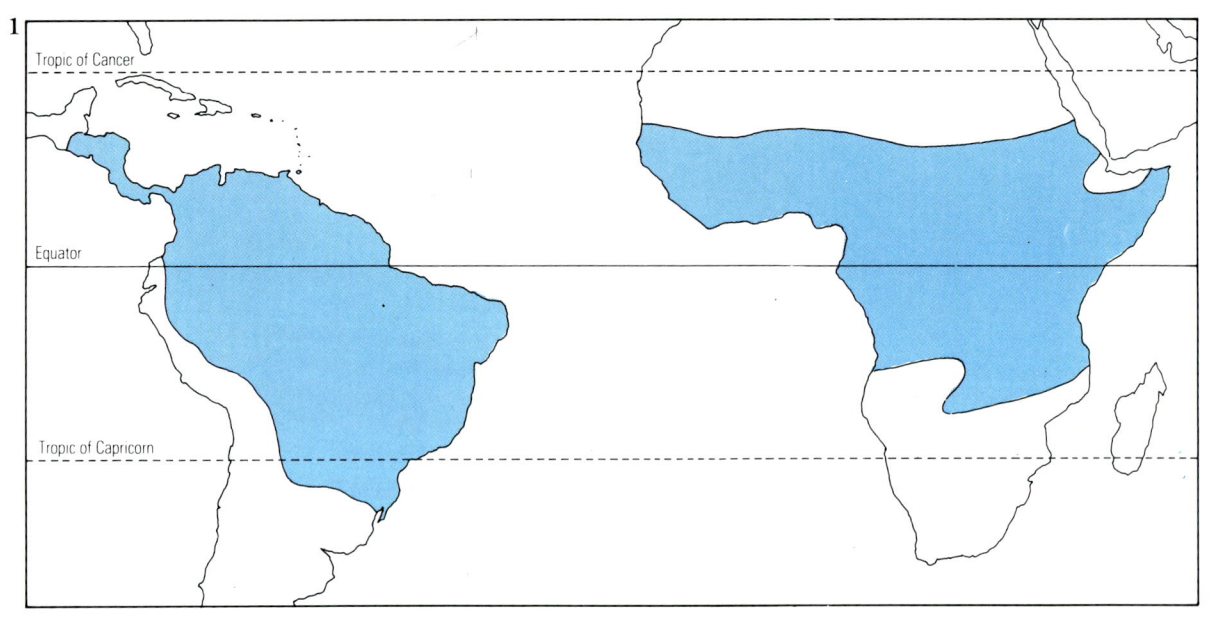

1 Distribution map of yellow fever virus Focal outbreaks of mosquito-borne yellow fever still occur in South America and tropical Africa where the disease is seriously underdiagnosed. Vaccination provides a high level of protection for 10 years and is a legal requirement for travellers entering endemic countries. The virus is transmitted by mosquitoes of the genus *Aedes*. It is now accepted that the main reservoirs are the susceptible mosquitoes in which the virus is transmitted from generation to generation by transovarial infection. The main differential characters of the principal families of mosquito vectors of disease are shown in the next figures (*see also* **59, 224-232, 234**).

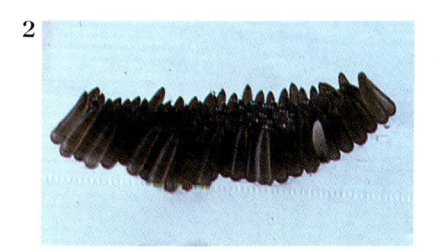

2-4 Mosquito eggs *Culex* eggs (**2**) are deposited on the water surface in 'rafts' (× 40); *Aedes* (**3**) are laid singly. They often have a conspicuously sculptured surface. *Anopheles* (**4**) eggs have lateral floats. They tend to aggregate on the water surface forming 'Chinese figure' patterns. (× 55)

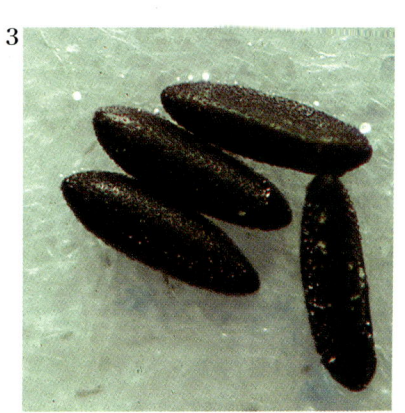

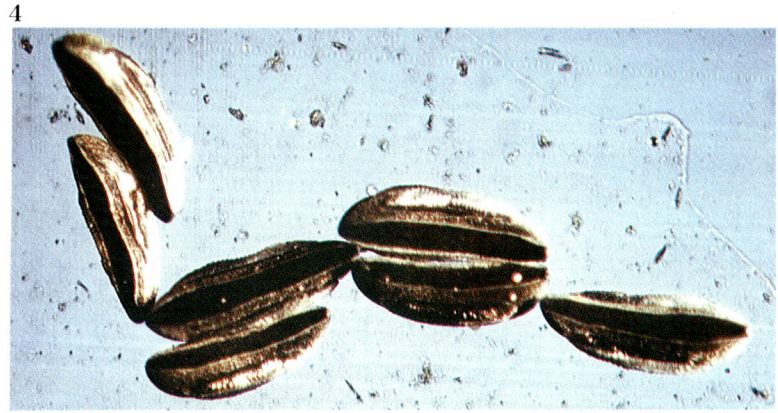

5 & 6 Mosquito larvae The larvae of *Culex* and *Aedes* (**5**) are suspended under the air-water interface by their siphons. Those of *Anopheles* (**6**) lie parallel to the surface. ($\times 10$)

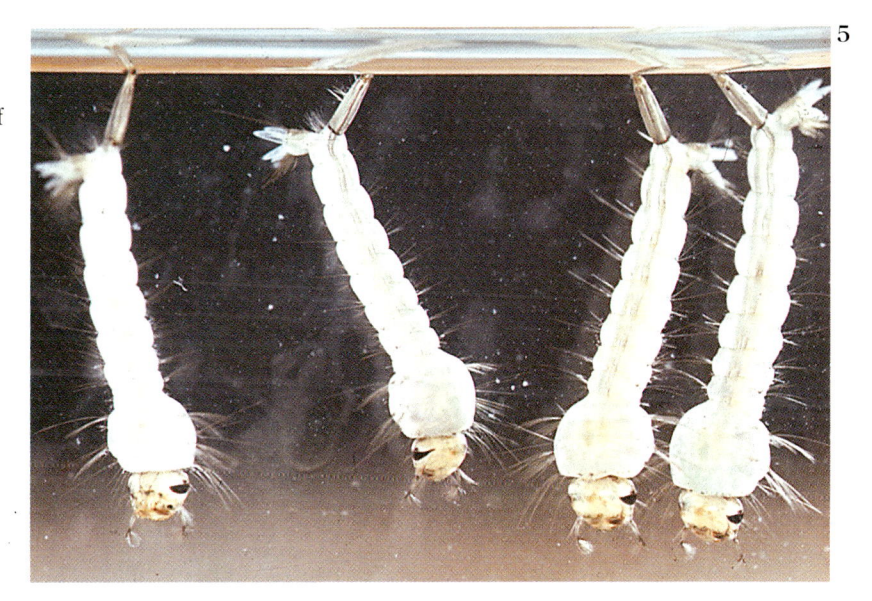

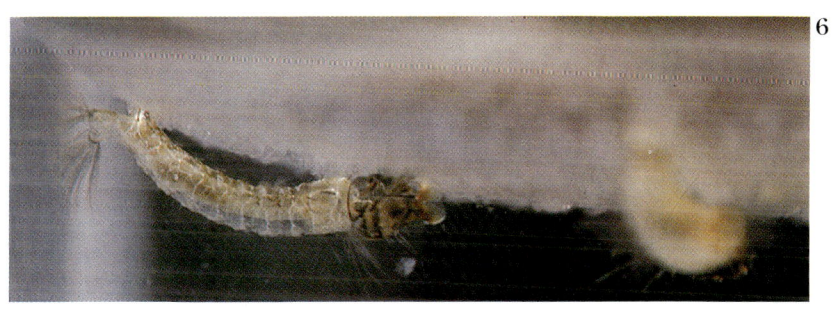

7 Mosquito pupae Pupae of *Culex*, *Aedes* and *Anopheles* are very similar. They obtain air through siphons on the cephalothorax. ($\times 12$)

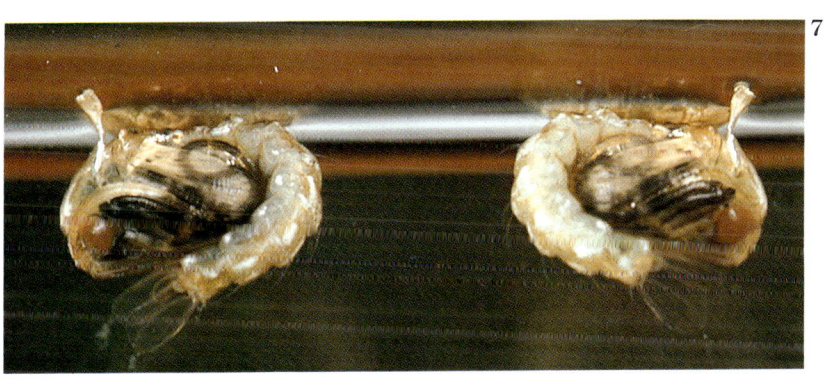

8 & 9 Adult mosquitoes hatching from pupae Mature pupa (**8**); newly emerged *Anopheles* female (**9**). ($\times 8$)

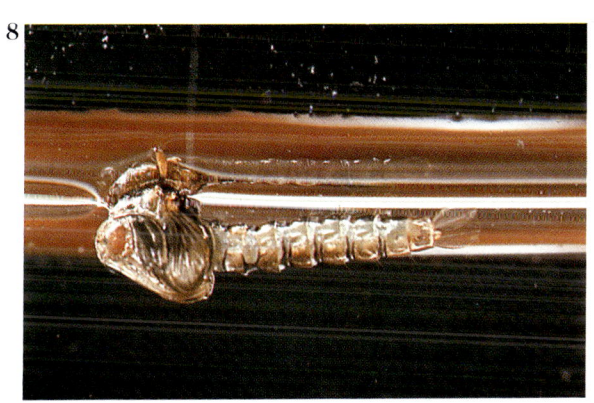

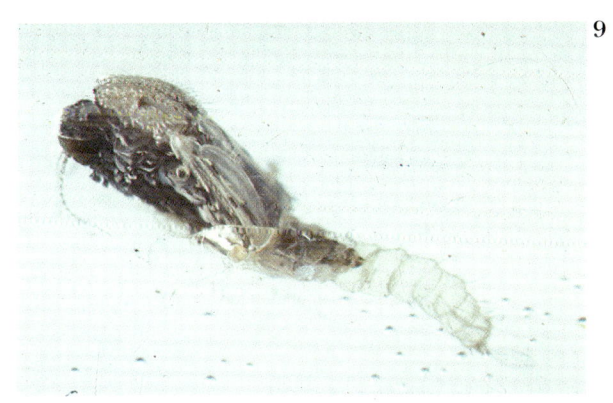

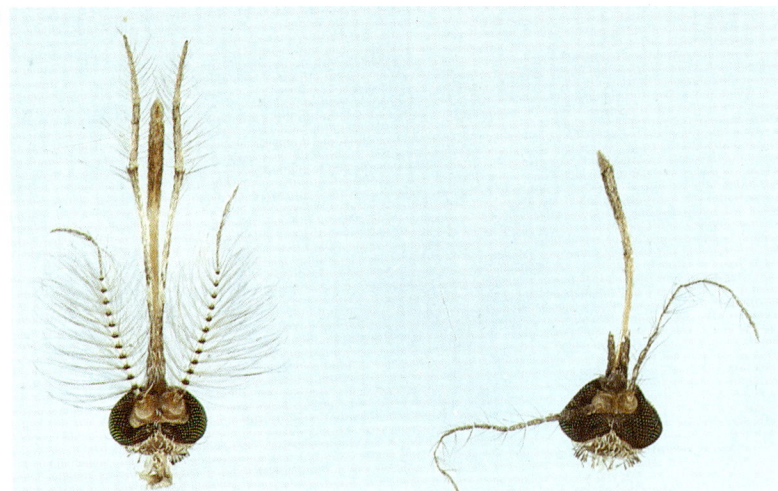

10 & 11 Heads of adult culicine and anopheline mosquitoes The adults are distinguished by the form of the antennae and palps. *Culex* ♂ (left) ♀ (right) (**10**); *Anopheles* ♂ (left) ♀ (right) (**11**). (× 50). *Aedes* ♂ and ♀ are similar to those of *Culex*. Compare the short palps of the ♀ *Culex* with the long ones of the ♀ *Anopheles*.

12 *Aedes* biting Photograph taken at midday in rain forest near Belém at the mouth of the River Amazon. Mosquitoes of the genera *Aedes* (*Stegomyia*) and *Haemagogus* transmit yellow fever virus to forest monkeys in which there is a sylvatic reservoir, from monkeys to man, and subsequently from man to man. Viraemia in monkeys, as in man, is short-lived.

13 Water containers near houses—typical vector breeding sites *Aedes aegypti*, which breeds in fairly clean water in domestic containers, as well as in old tyres, tin cans and other rubbish, is responsible for urban epidemics of yellow fever as well as other arbovirus infections such as dengue haemorrhagic fever.

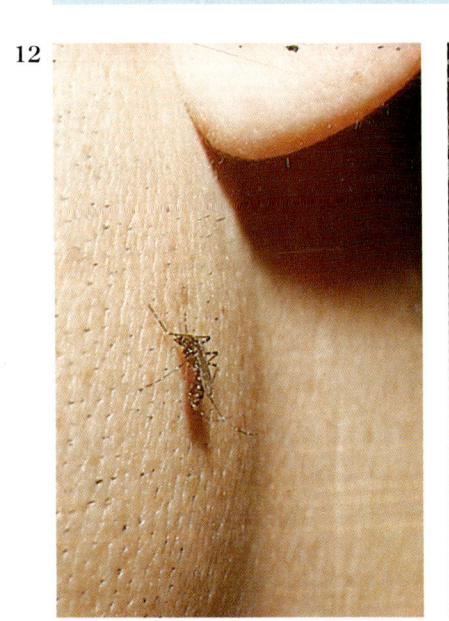

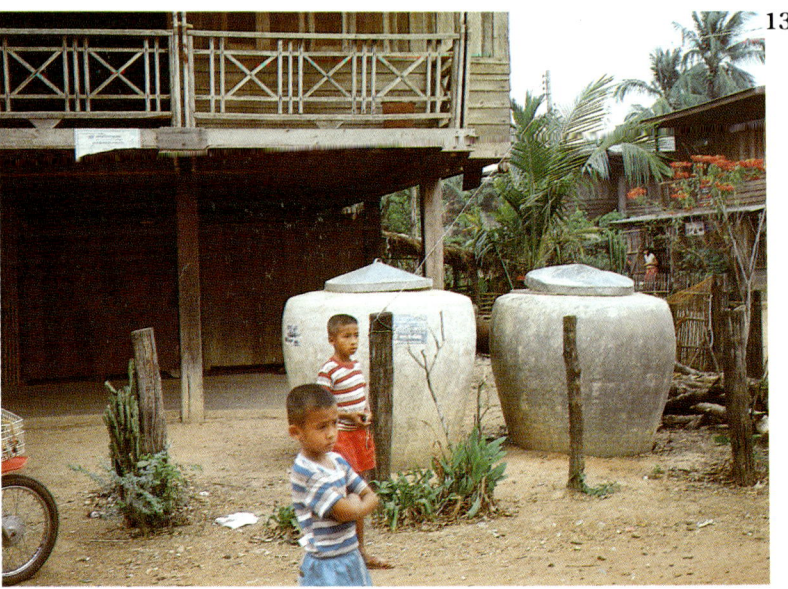

14 Temperature chart of yellow fever case The increasing slowness of the pulse relative to the temperature (Faget's sign) is of clinical diagnostic value. D refers to day of illness, P to pulse and T to temperature °C.

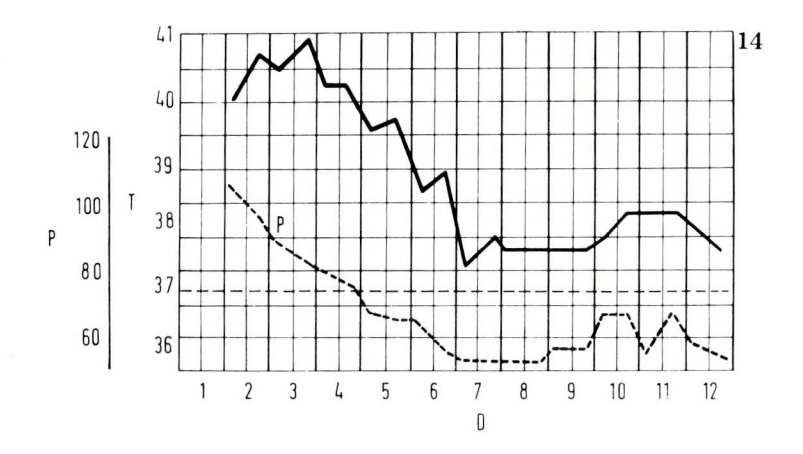

15 'Black vomit' of yellow fever Despite the name, jaundice is usually not marked in yellow fever. Bleeding from the gut is a grave portent, and vomiting may occur of material resembling coffee grounds, such as that shown here.

16 Section of liver from fatal yellow fever case Midzonal necrosis and eosinophilic, intranuclear inclusions (Councilman bodies) are characteristic histological features. (*H&E* × *470*)

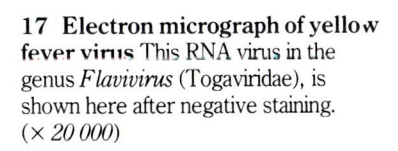

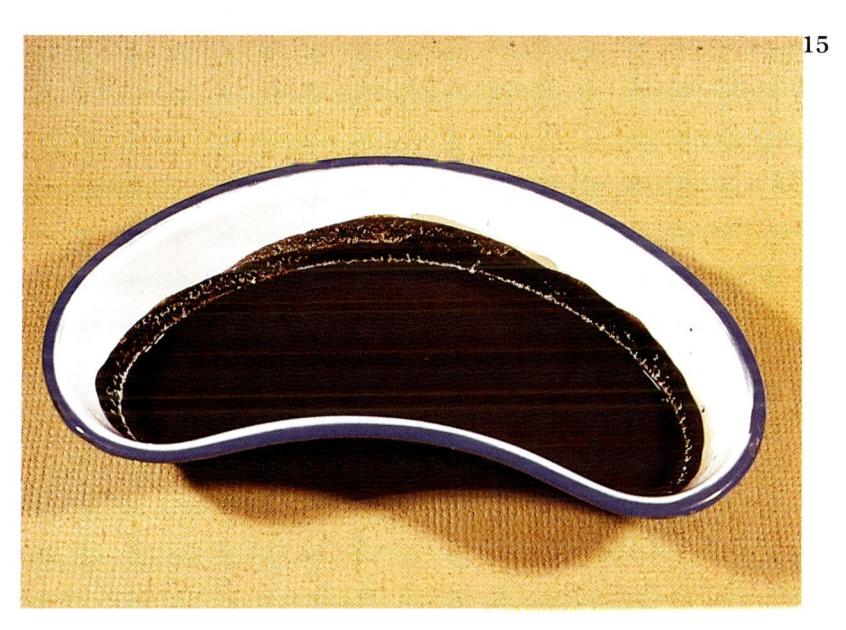

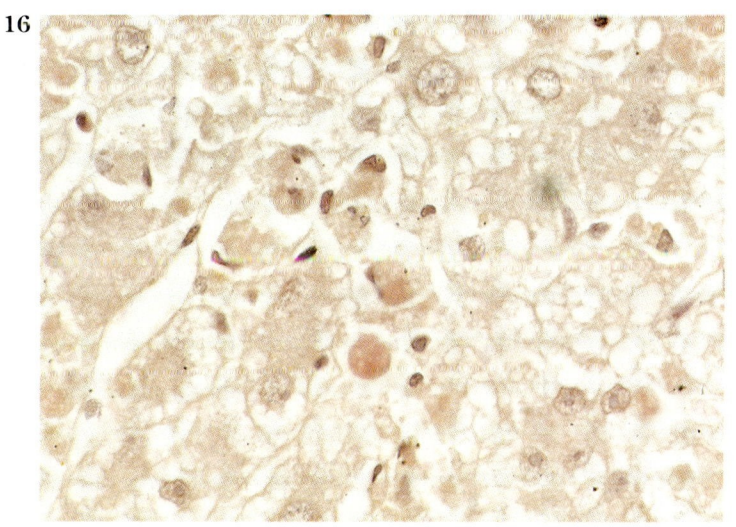

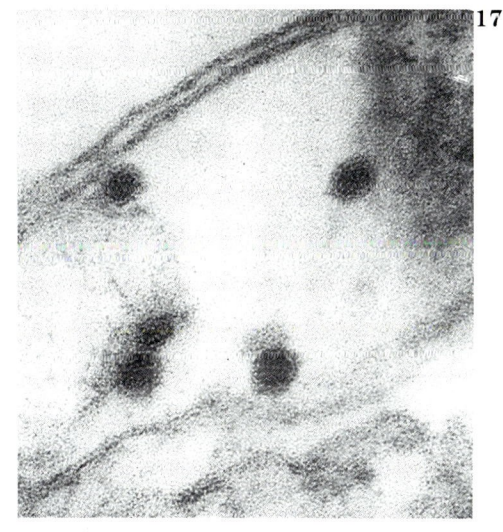

17 Electron micrograph of yellow fever virus This RNA virus in the genus *Flavivirus* (Togaviridae), is shown here after negative staining. (× *20 000*)

Dengue

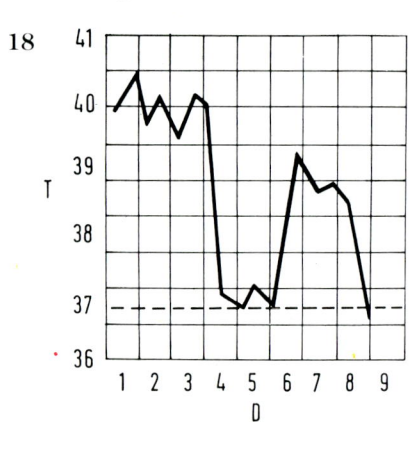

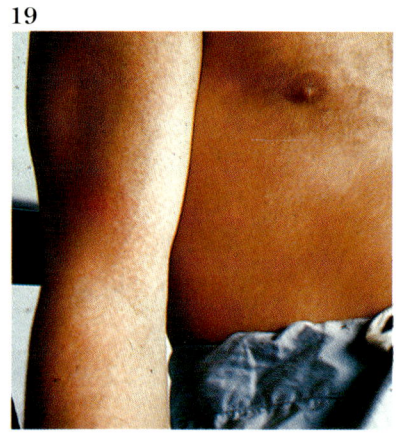

18 Dengue temperature chart
Dengue is an *Aedes*-borne disease of wide distribution in the tropics and subtropics, caused by several flaviviruses. It is often of short duration with a characteristic 'saddle-back' fever.

19 Rash of dengue An erythematous generalised rash appears in uncomplicated dengue, usually during the second bout of fever.

Dengue Haemorrhagic Fever

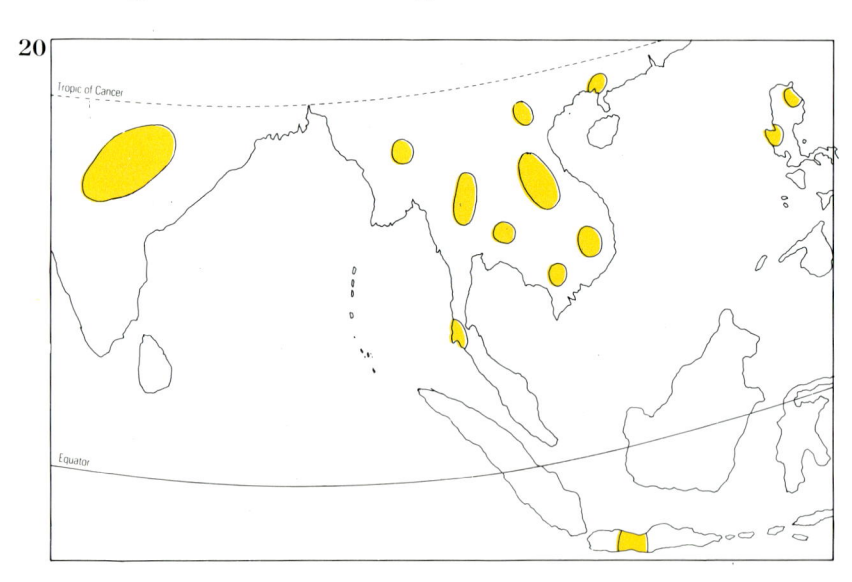

20 Distribution map of dengue haemorrhagic fever During the last two decades, epidemics of dengue haemorrhagic fever (DHF) have occurred in SE Asia. All four known types of dengue virus have been isolated in almost all the countries involved and *Aedes aegypti* has been identified as the main vector. Its peridomestic habits ensure intimate man-vector contact. Monkeys may serve as amplifier hosts.

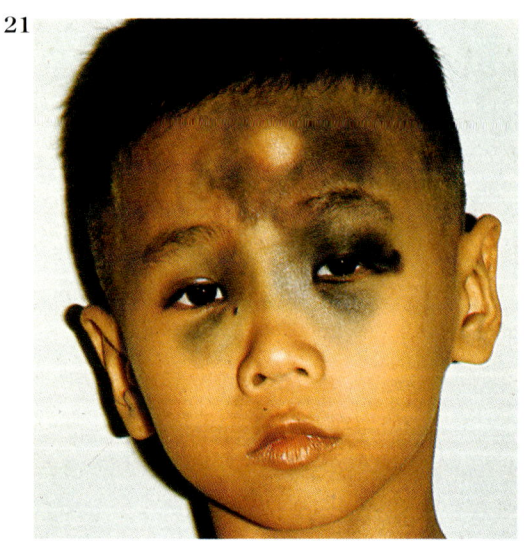

21 Marked ecchymoses in a Chinese boy Cutaneous haemorrhagic manifestations ranging from petechiae to gross ecchymoses characterise the infection, especially in children. Over 200 were admitted daily in an outbreak in Vientiane in 1987. The peak age-specific prevalence was four to nine years and the severity of cases ranged from Grade I (fever and positive tourniquet test) to Grade IV (undetectable blood pressure and pulse—dengue shock syndrome). Rapid restoration of plasma volume is mandatory.

Congo-Crimea haemorrhagic fever

22 Congo-Crimea haemorrhagic fever This condition is also often accompanied by severe ecchymoses.

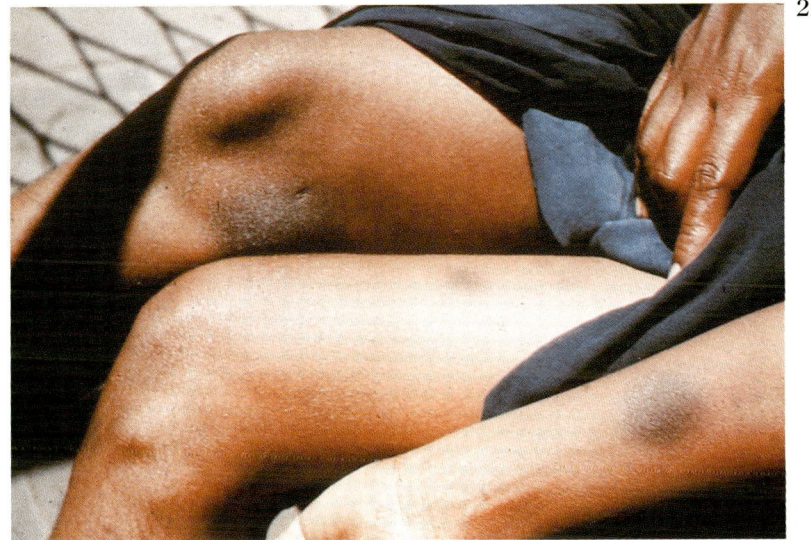

Japanese B Encephalitis

The distribution of Japanese B encephalitis, which is also caused by a flavivirus, is similar to that shown in **20**. The virus is spread through birds, and transmitted by various species of *Culex* and *Anopheles* mosquitoes. These are commonly found breeding in surface water such as flooded paddy fields. Birds form a reservoir for the virus which is amplified in infected pigs.

23 Encephalitis due to Japanese B virus Encephalitis is severe and results in serious sequelae such as mental retardation. This former Sri Lankan school teacher survived the infection but she was only able to lead a 'vegetable' existence thereafter. In Nepal, where a large outbreak occurred in 1986, this condition is referred to as 'the visitation of the Goddess of the forest'.

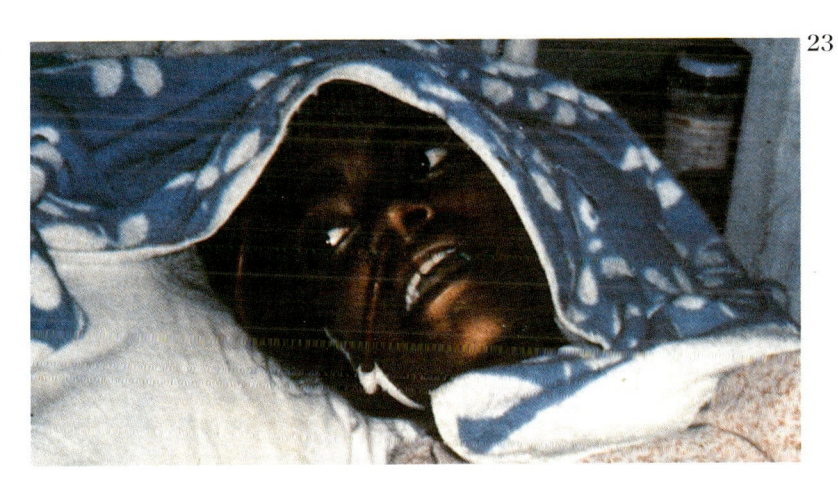

24 Section of brain showing neuronal damage Neuronal degeneration and necrosis are commonly seen in many parts of the brain. A striking change is destruction of the Purkinje cells in the cerebrum. ($\times 400$)

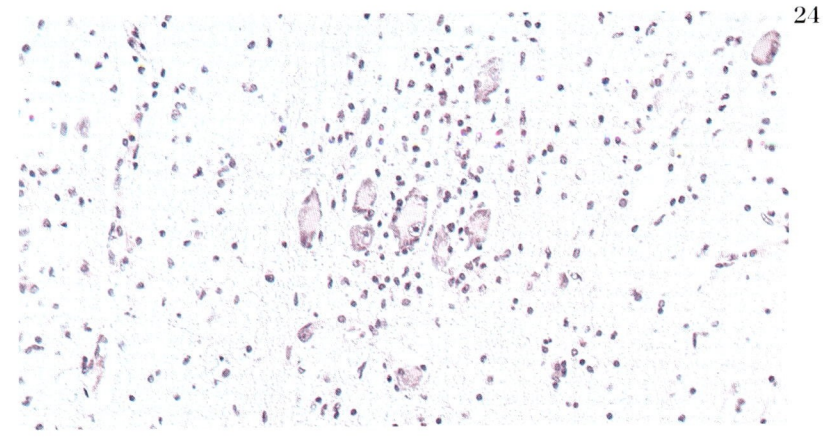

THE RICKETTSIOSES (*see* **Table III**)
Louse-borne Typhus

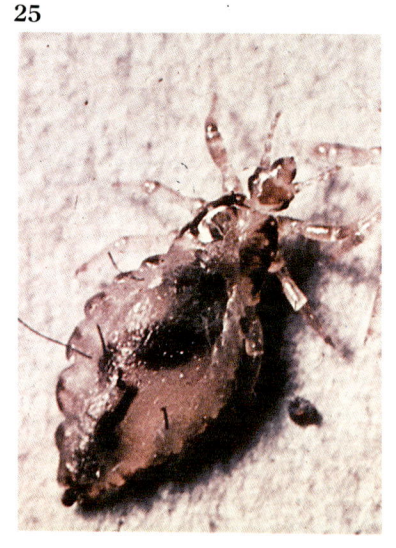

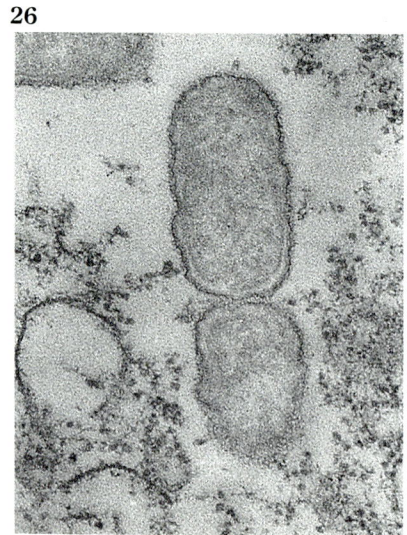

25 Body louse The body louse *Pediculus humanus* transmits typical epidemic typhus due to *Rickettsia prowazeki*, and trench fever. Rickettsial infection is cosmopolitan. The use of DDT for disinfestation of louse-infested communities is a primary control measure in epidemic situations. (Recent studies suggest that a zoonotic reservoir of *R. prowazeki* may exist in flying squirrels in North America.) (× *10*)

26 Ultrastructure of *R. prowazeki* Electron micrographs show that the rickettsial organisms have structural affinities to the bacteria. (× *55 000*)

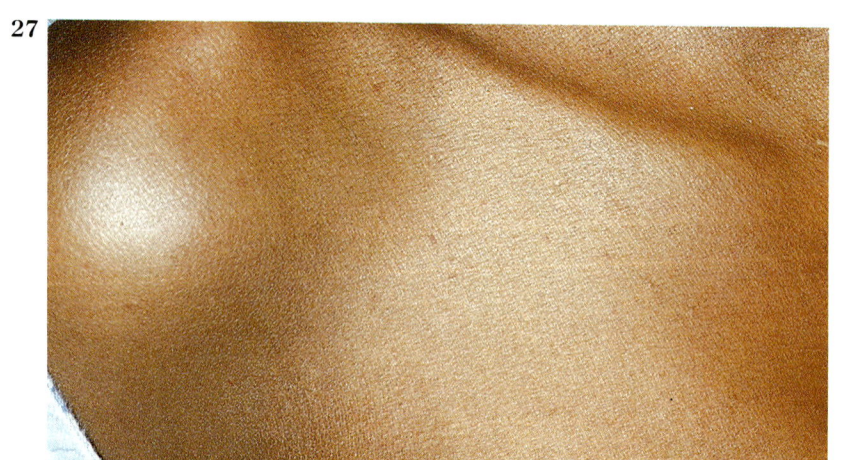

27 Rash of typhus in an Ethiopian The generalised macular or maculopapular rash is similar in all types of rickettsial infections. The discrete rash shown here has a typical purplish colour.

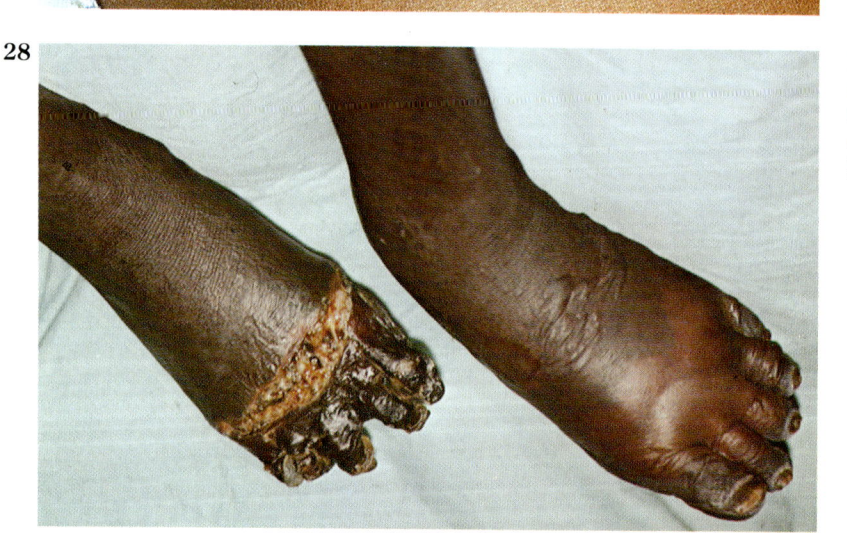

28 Peripheral gangrene in severe typhus One of the characteristic features of typhus is the severe toxicity of the infection. Gangrene of feet and hands occasionally occurs.

Scrub Typhus

29 Distribution map of scrub typhus Scrub typhus occurs in the Indian subcontinent, SE Asia, the Far East and parts of the Southwest Pacific. *R. tsutsugamushi* is present in trombiculid-infested rodents in specialised ecological niches known as mite islands, particularly in SE Asia and islands of the Western Pacific. Not far from Kuala Lumpur, for example, *Leptotrombidium deliensis* is found in the forest, and *L. akamushi* in the grass ('lalang').

30 Larva of *Leptotrombidium* Larval mites transmit the infection from rodent to man when he comes into accidental association with mite-infested terrain. The mites act as reservoirs since transovarial transmission of the *Rickettsia* occurs. ($\times 125$)

31 Eschar of mite bite A typical 'eschar' forms at the site of the trombiculid bite and precedes the fever.

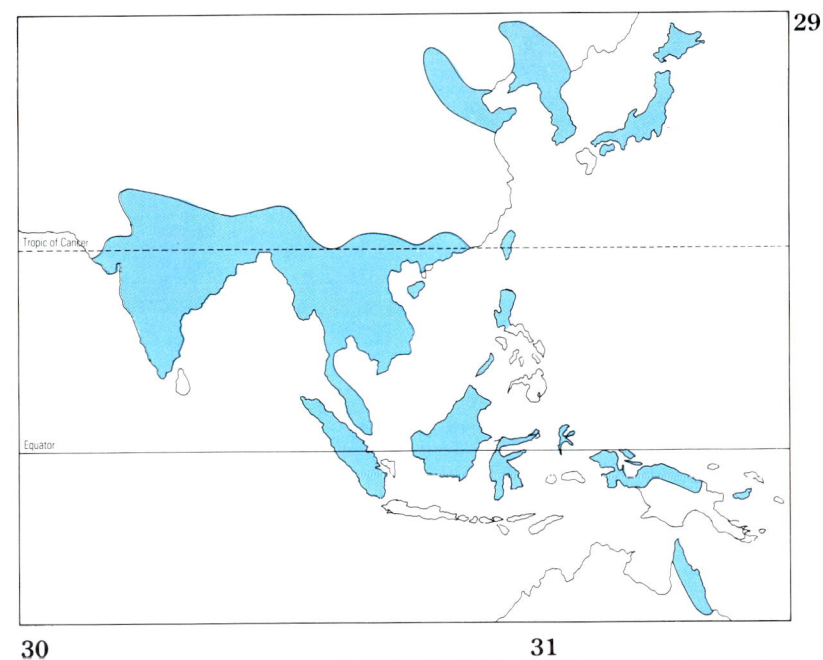

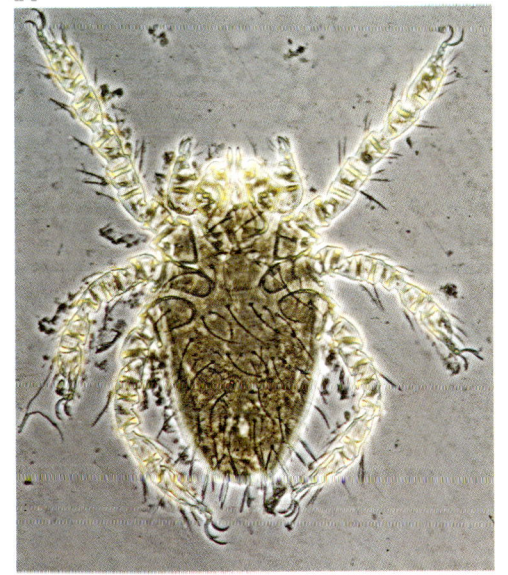

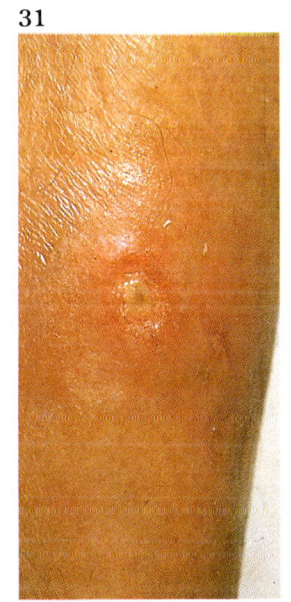

32 Scrub typhus rash The maculopapular eruption, which appears on about the sixth or seventh day of the illness, lasts three or four days. While seen mainly on the trunk, upper arms and thighs, it may also appear on the face, hands (as shown here) and feet.

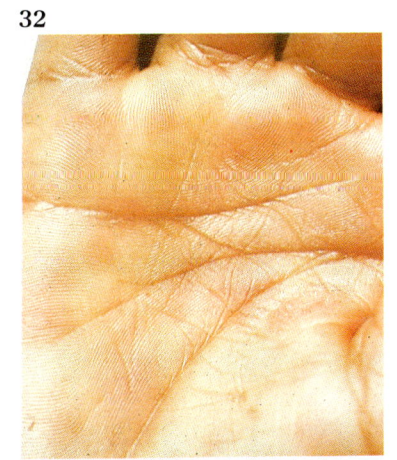

Tick Typhus

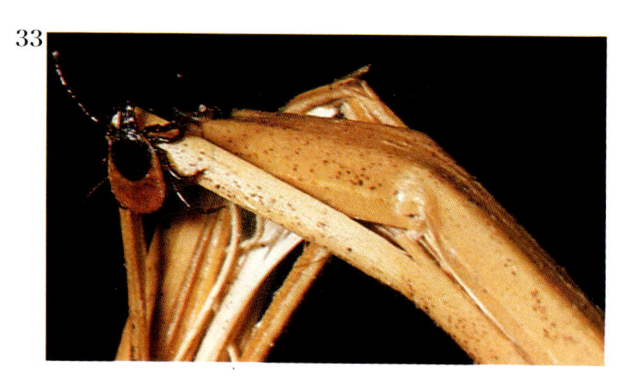

33 Adult female hard tick Various species of hard ticks transmit a variety of *Rickettsia* species, e.g. *R. conori* var. *pijperi* in Africa. (× 4)

34 Eschar at site of tick bite As with mite-borne typhus, an 'eschar' forms at the site of the infective tick bite. The distribution of the rash is also seen clearly on the back of this individual infected in South Africa.

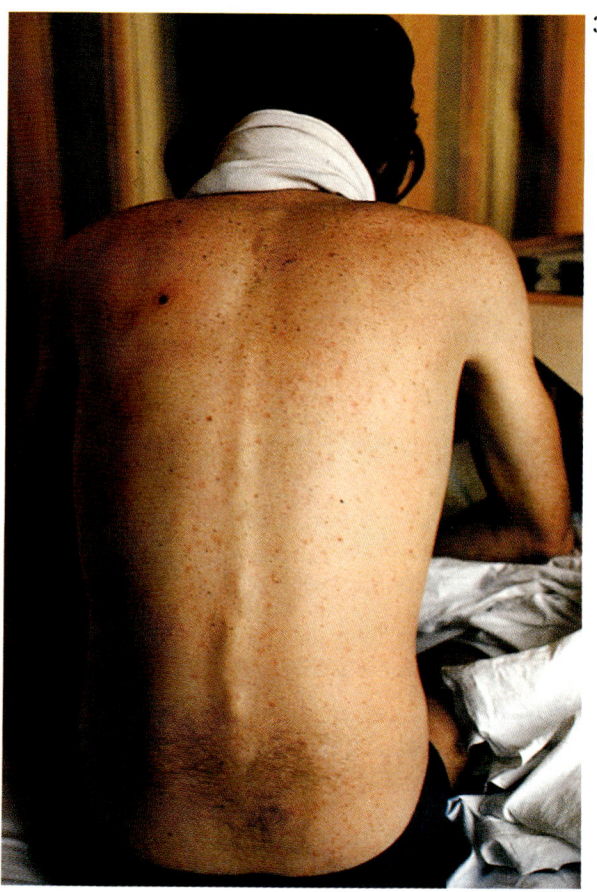

Q Fever

35 Cross-section of *Coxiella burnetii* Q fever due to *C. burnetii* of ruminants is cosmopolitan. It may be spread to man by ticks, but is mainly acquired by direct contact with milk. (× 57 000)

Murine typhus may be acquired when fleas from *Rickettsia*-infected rodents harboured, for example, in deserted buildings in the countryside, transmit infection to newcomers who take up residence there.

BACTERIAL INFECTIONS
Plague

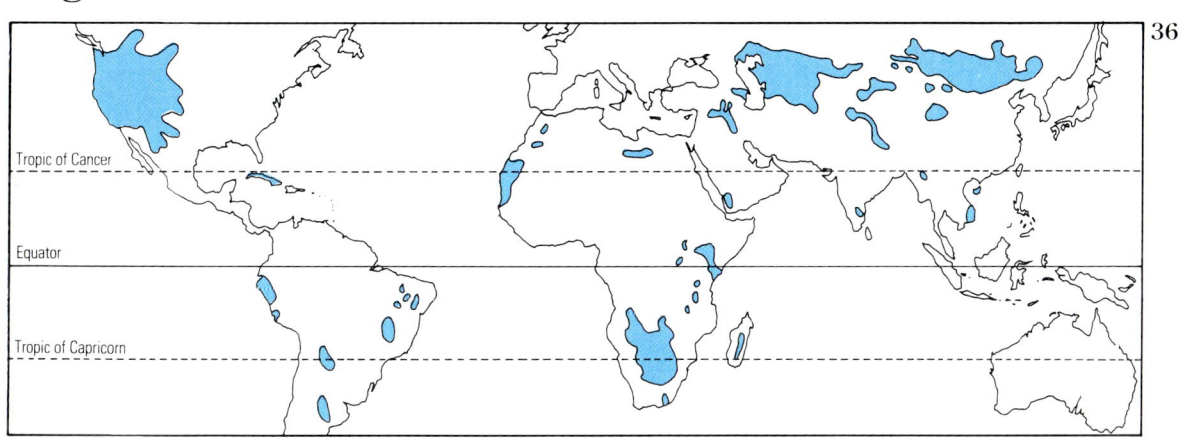

36 Known and probable foci of plague Plague is now largely focal in distribution. It spreads rapidly in conditions of war and other catastrophes, e.g. earthquakes. Epidemics still occur from time to time.

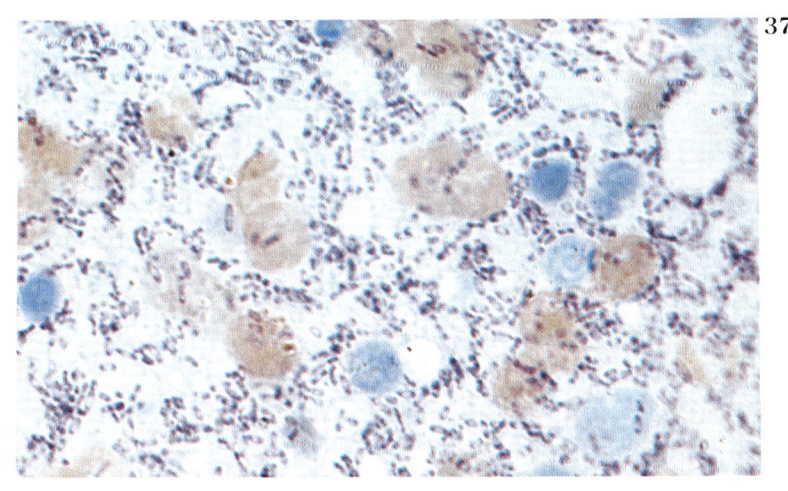

37 *Yersinia pestis* in liver smear *Y. pestis* (syn. *Pasteurella pestis*) is a Gram-negative coccobacillus with bipolar staining. It is normally enzootic in rats. ($\times 1\,250$)

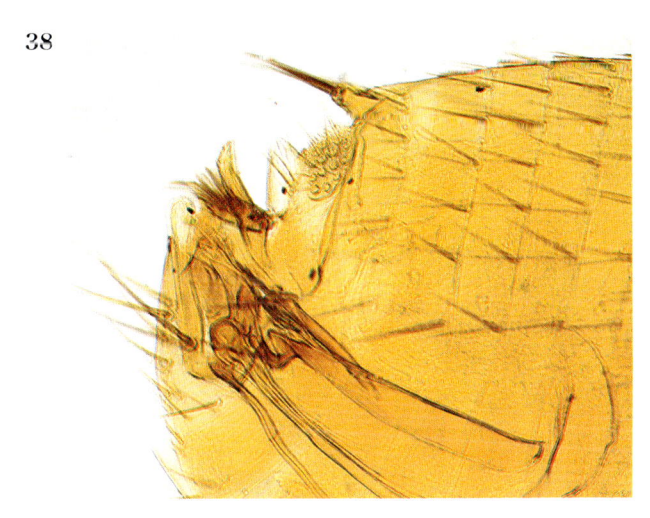

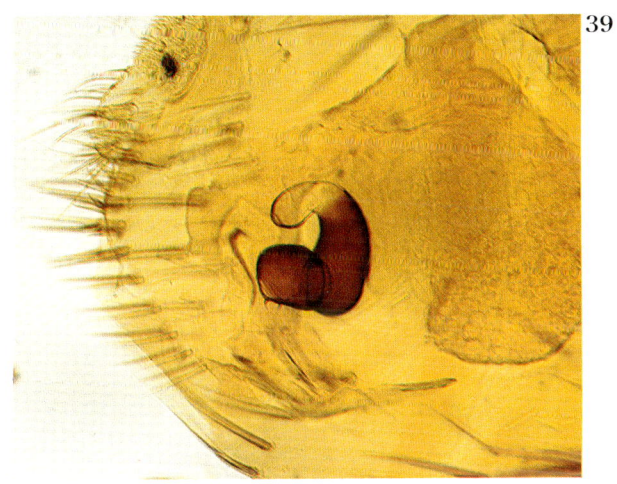

38-43 Male and female *Xenopsylla* fleas compared Plague is transmitted by fleas of the genus *Xenopsylla*. *X. cheopis* ♂ ♀ (**38 & 39**); *X. astia* ♂ ♀ (**40 & 41**); *X. brasiliensis* ♂ ♀ (**42 & 43**). The rat flea *X. cheopis* is the main vector. ($\times 120$)

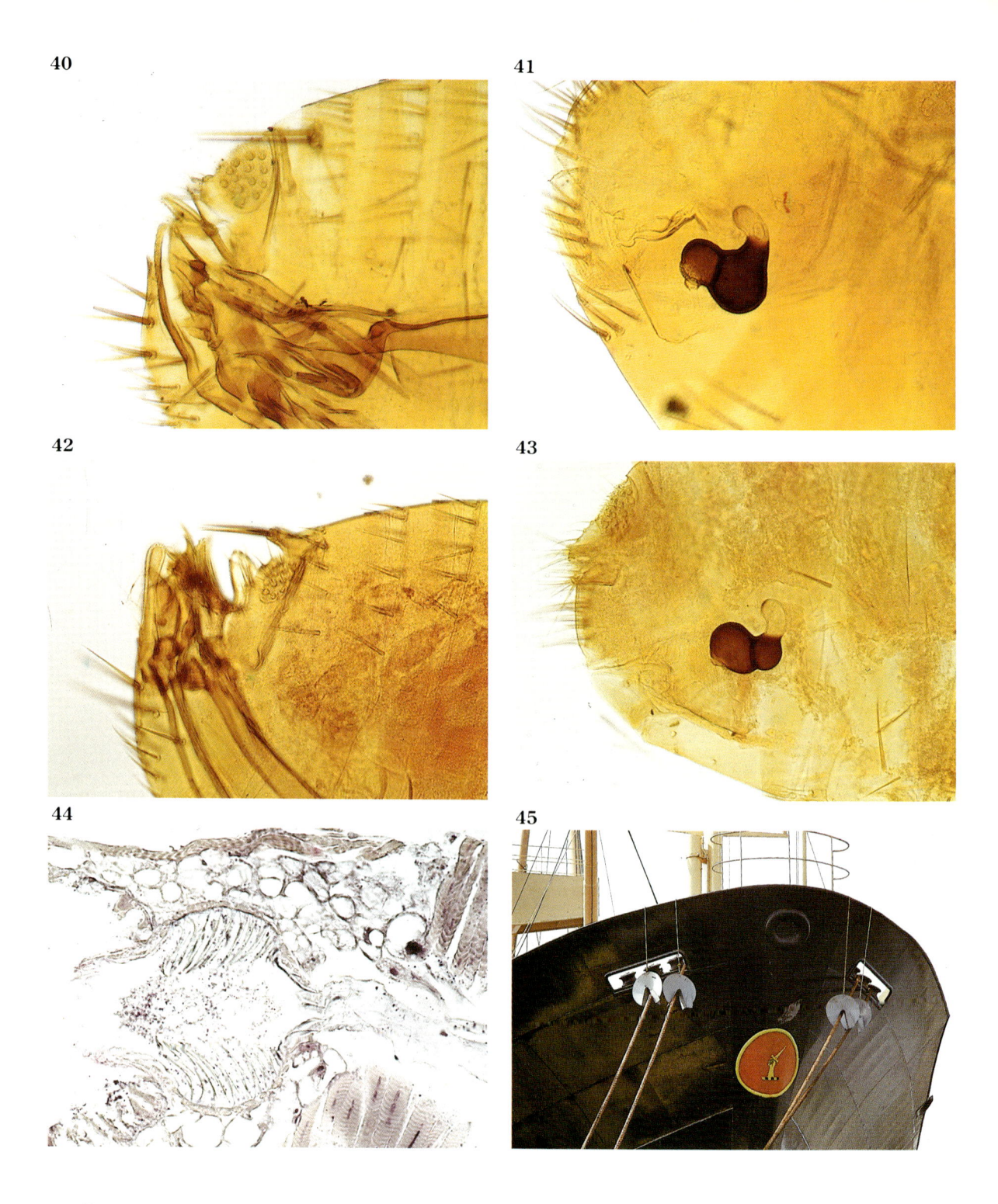

44 Proventriculus of *X. cheopis* blocked by plague bacilli Hungry fleas abandon dying domestic rats (*R. norvegicus, R. rattus*), often with their foreguts blocked by bacilli. In this condition they will attempt to feed on any animal. If they bite man they transmit the disease. (× *240*)

45 Metal guards preventing access of rats along ships' hawsers Plague control demands strictly enforced rodent control measures and international quarantine regulations, particularly for shipping.

46 Bubonic plague One of the most characteristic clinical features is lymphadenopathy with suppuration, especially in the inguinal and axillary regions.

47 Pneumonic plague Pneumonic infection allows direct spread of bacteria from man to man. The X-ray shows infection in the left lower lobe on the second day of the illness.

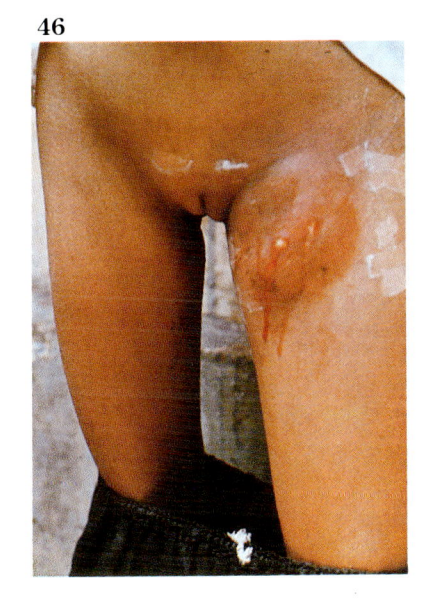

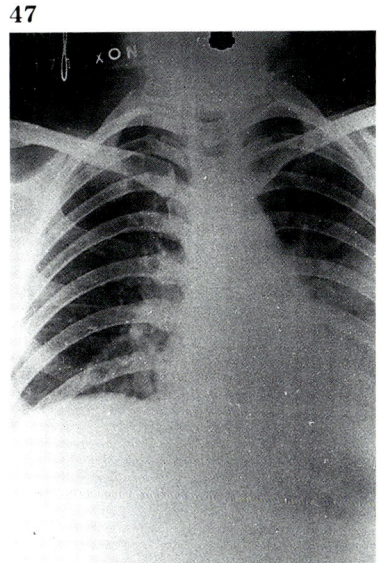

The Relapsing Fevers (See **Table IV**)

48 *Borrelia duttoni* **in human blood film from Tanzania** Endemic relapsing fever, a cosmopolitan disease caused by *B. duttoni*, occurs in rodents and man. First described from Africa, it occurs also in the Middle East, Mediterranean basin, and the New World including the US. (*Giemsa—phase contrast × 900*)

49 Soft tick with coxal fluid Soft ticks such as *Ornithodoros moubata* transmit *B. duttoni* from rodents to man, and from man to man through infected coxal fluid which enters skin abrasions. As the organism passes from tick to tick by transovarial transmission, the arthropod is itself a reservoir host. (× 4). In East Africa *O. moubata* lives in soft earth at the base of mud-lined walls.

50 Temperature chart of tick-borne relapsing fever The infection acquires its name from the typical relapsing nature of the fever. *B. duttoni* only appears in the blood during the febrile episodes which are numerous and of short duration. (P = parasitaemia).

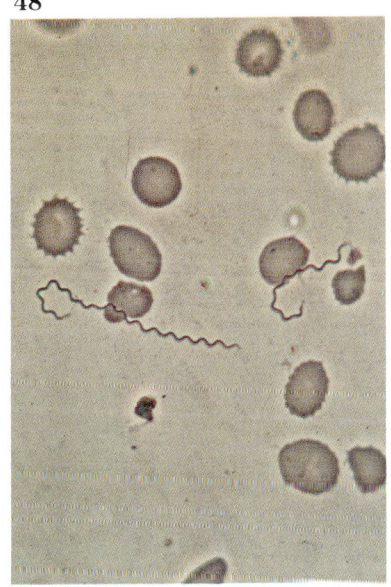

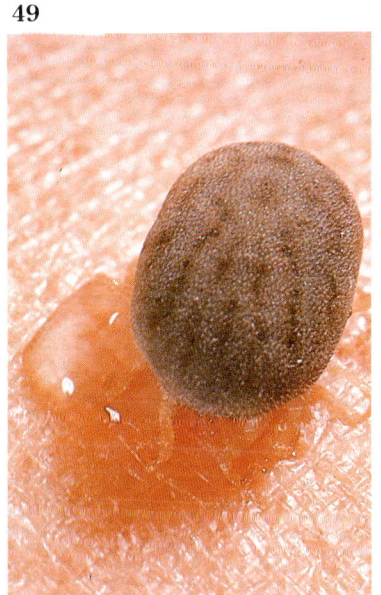

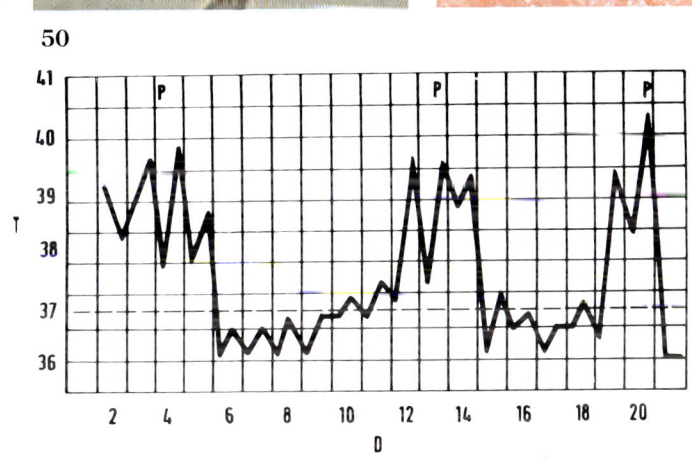

23

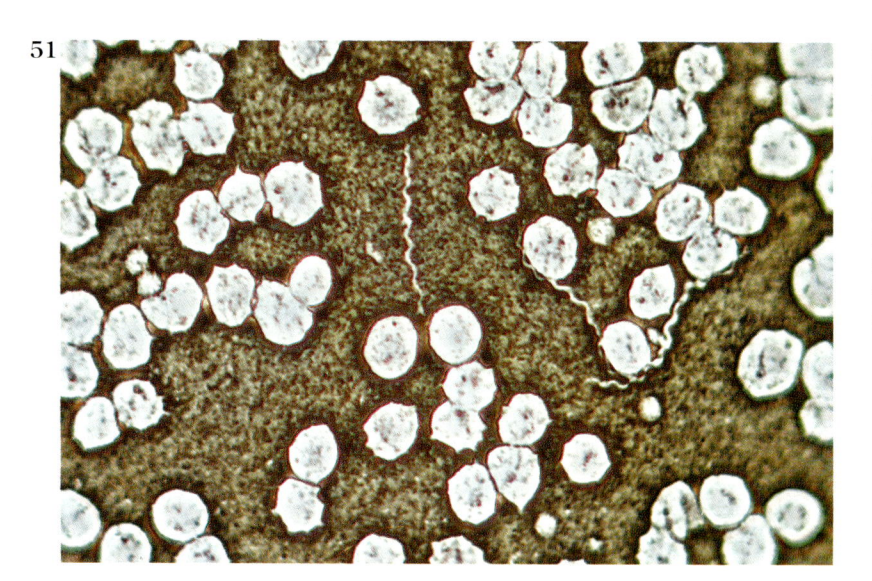

51 *Borrelia recurrentis* in blood film *B. recurrentis* transmitted by body lice occurs in epidemic form in Ethiopia and Eritrea. The febrile periods recur on one or two occasions only, but mortality can be high. Infection is acquired from the body fluids of lice crushed on the skin during scratching. The organisms are readily seen in this Indian ink preparation. ($\times$ *1 200*)

Lyme Disease

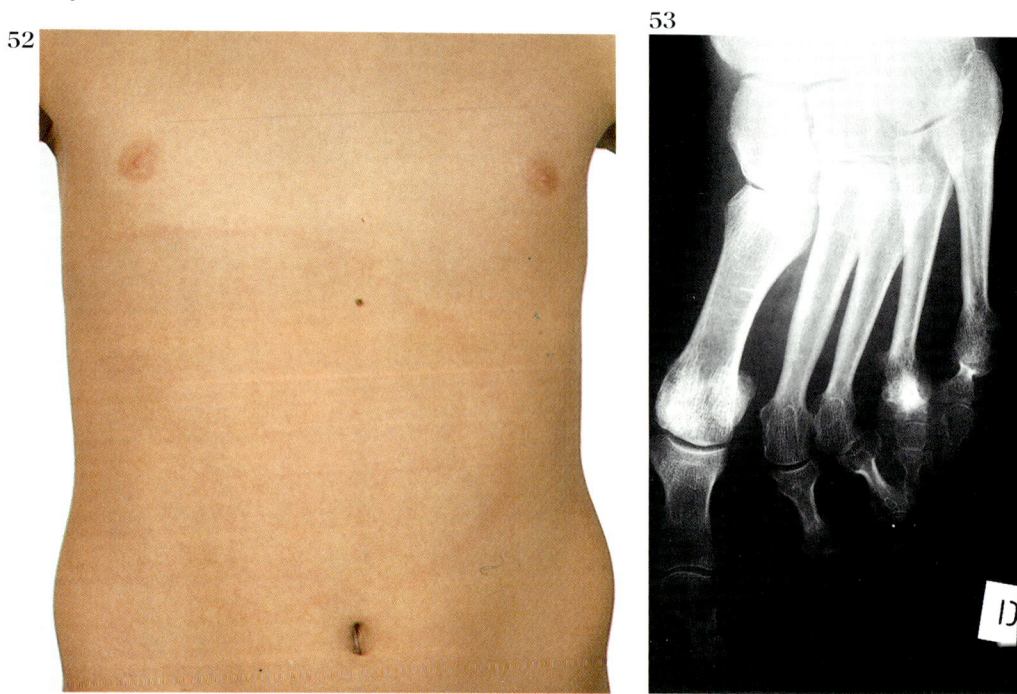

52 Erythema chronicum migrans This unusual type of chronic rash is associated with a recently identified, tick-borne infection caused by *Borrelia burgdorferi*, which is widely distributed in Europe and North America. Its presence is also suspected in parts of Africa. There is little doubt that this infection will be recognised on an increasing scale.

53 Bone changes and deformity of the foot associated with *B. burgdorferi* infection Both acute and chronic, disabling arthritic lesions, usually associated with skin lesions, appear to be common late sequelae of Lyme disease. This patient had a history of acrodermatitis chronica atrophicans of more than 10 years' duration. Neurological changes such as meningo-encephalitis, sometimes with cranial or peripheral radiculopathy, are also being reported increasingly. The infection, in fact, can produce protean manifestations and the diagnosis is probably missed in many cases. If the diagnosis, which may be confirmed by culturing the organisms from skin or other tissues and by serology, is made sufficiently early, the disease is usually cured rapidly by chemotherapy.

Bartonellosis (Carrión's Disease, Oroya Fever)

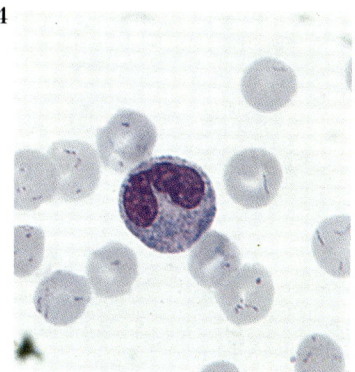

54 Blood film showing *Bartonella bacilliformis* *B. bacilliformis* is a Gram-negative, intra-erythrocytic bacillus which produces fever and acute haemolytic anaemia (Oroya fever), associated with severe bone and joint pains. The infection is fatal in 10 to 40 per cent of cases within two or three weeks. The bacilli also invade reticuloendothelial cells. This disease occurs in Bolivia, Peru, Colombia and Ecuador. (Giemsa × 950)

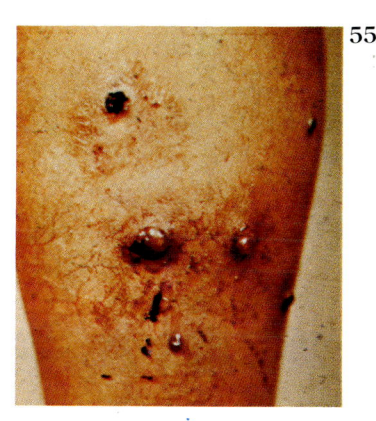

55 'Verruga Peruviana' The infection may persist for several months to produce a generalised verrucous eruption, sometimes becoming haemorrhagic in late cases. Organisms can be cultured from the cutaneous nodules. This condition is usually self-healing after two or three months. The disease is transmitted by the sandfly *Lutzomyia verrucarum* at altitudes of 800 to 3000 m.

PROTOZOAL INFECTIONS (*See* Table V)
Malaria

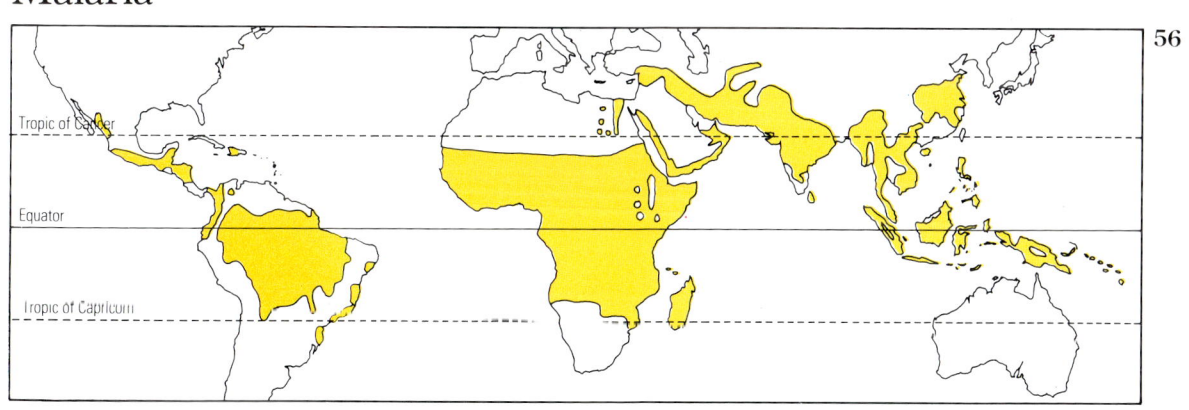

56 Distribution map of malaria In spite of intensive control measures over the last 30 years, malaria is still widely distributed in the tropics and subtropics.

57 Generalised life cycle of malaria parasites The figure is based on the life cycle of *Plasmodium vivax* and *P. ovale*. Sporozoites (2) injected by the mosquito enter liver parenchyma cells where they grow into the first generation of pre-erythrocytic schizonts (3). These give rise to merozoites which invade red blood cells, to develop into the asexual erythrocytic cycle (4). Some sporozoites in the hepatocytes stay dormant to mature after an interval of weeks or months into secondary exo-erythrocytic schizonts (3a, b). The successive waves of merozoites emerging from these give rise to relapse infections in the blood after months or years. Some blood stages mature to form sexual forms, the macro- and microgametocytes (5). These enter the mosquito where the males exflagellate to fertilise the females (6). The ookinete thus produced forms oöcysts on the outside of the midgut (7). Sporozoites (8 & 9) develop in the oöcysts. The sporozoites enter the mosquito salivary glands (2) where they are ready to infect a new host. (In *P. falciparum* and *P. malariae* stages 3a, b do not exist and true relapses do not occur.) (*See also* **60-67, 94-98, 102.**)

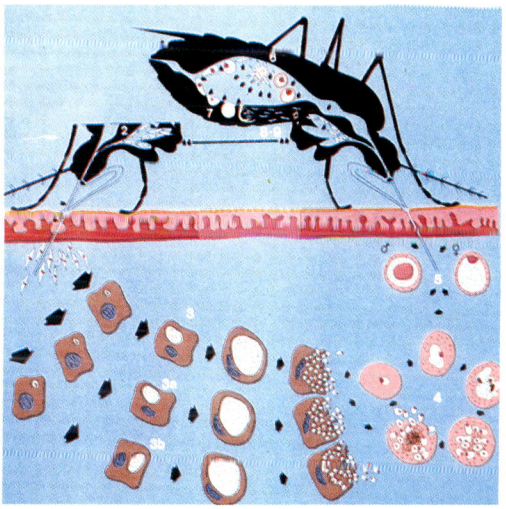

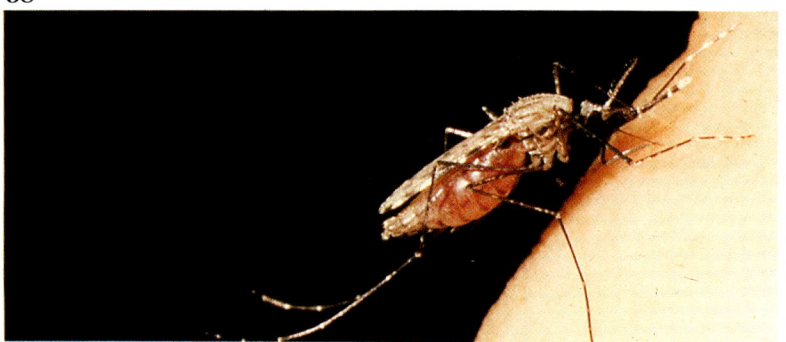

58 *Anopheles gambiae* biting
Malaria is transmitted by female *Anopheles* mosquitoes. Most species bite indoors at night but some are outdoor feeding. The adults are recognised by the antennae and palps. (*See also* **9 & 11**). (× 4)

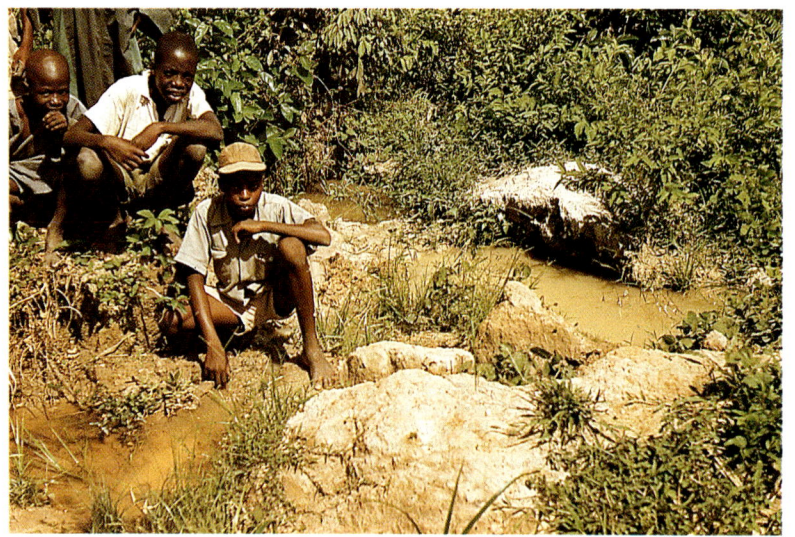

59 Breeding site of *Anopheles gambiae* in West Africa *A. gambiae* and closely related species are the most dangerous malaria vectors in tropical Africa. *A. gambiae* breeds in small temporary collections of fresh surface water exposed to sunlight and in such sites as residual pools in drying river beds. The majority of important vectors in other parts of the world are also surface water breeders. The most successful malaria control operations since the early 1950s have been based largely on the destruction of house-haunting anopheline vectors by DDT or other insecticides sprayed on the interior walls where mosquitoes usually rest before and/or after feeding. Some South American vectors of the subgenus *Anopheles* (*Kerteszia*) breed in bromeliads. The adults bite outdoors rather than inside houses. Consequently, the control of these larvae by insecticides is extremely difficult.

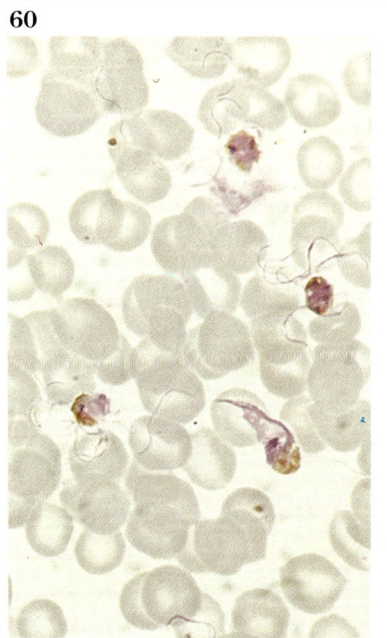

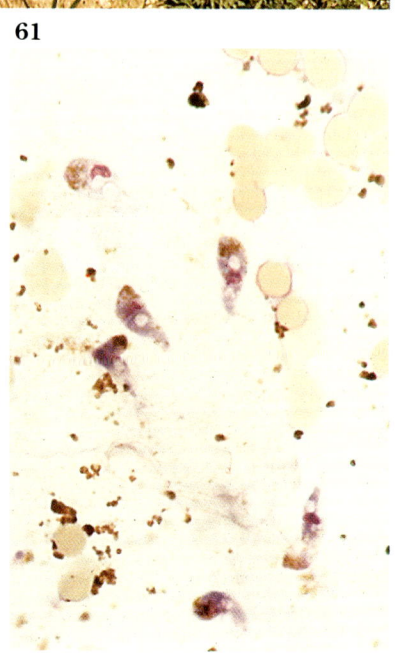

60 Development of male gametes Male gametes develop by exflagellation from microgametocytes contained in a blood meal in the midgut of the female anopheline. (× *950*)

61 Oökinete in midgut Male and female gametes fuse to produce motile oökinetes which enter midgut epithelial cells. (× *950*)

62 Scanning electron micrograph of oöcysts outside anopheline midgut Infective stages (sporozoites) develop in oöcysts which lie on the outside of the mosquito midgut. (× 125)

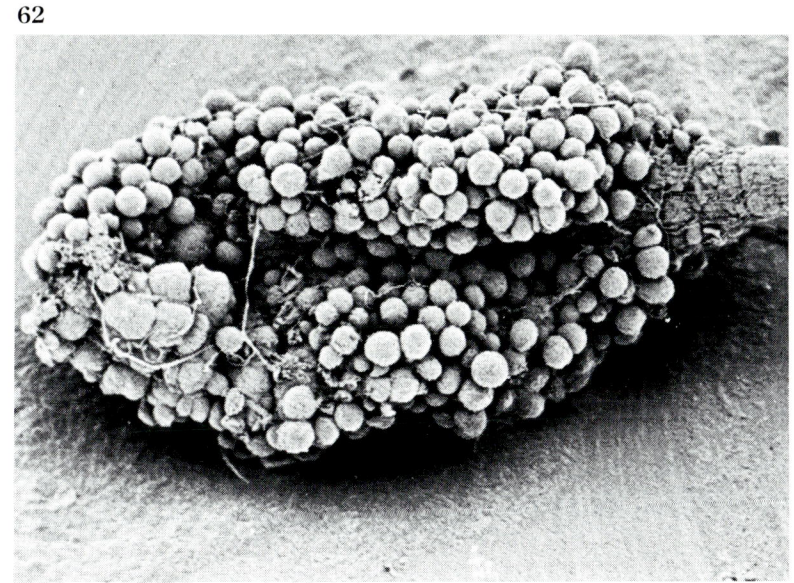

63 Living infective sporozoites Bow-shaped sporozoites emerge from the oöcysts and enter the insect's salivary glands. They are passed into the skin with saliva when the mosquito next takes a blood meal. (× 350)

64 Exo-erythrocytic schizont of *P. malariae* in liver Within 30 minutes the sporozoites enter the parenchymal cells of the host's liver where they may form large pre-erythrocytic (PE) 'tissue' schizonts or, in *P. vivax* and *P. ovale*, hypnozoites (see **65 & 66**). The PE schizonts mature in six to 14 days according to the species, liberating daughter cells called merozoites. (*Giemsa colophonium technique* × 350)

65 Hypnozoite and pre-erythrocytic schizont in liver biopsy The unicellular, dormant hypnozoite (arrow) stands in sharp contrast to the maturing PE schizont in this fluorescent antibody-stained section of rhesus monkey liver containing *P. cynomolgi* (a relapsing species with the same life cycle as *P. vivax*). (× 350)

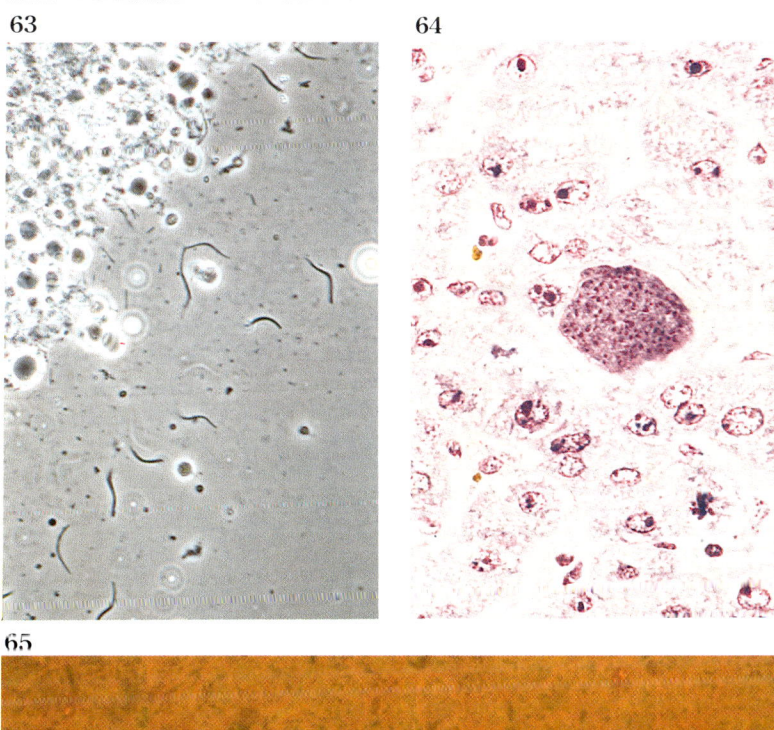

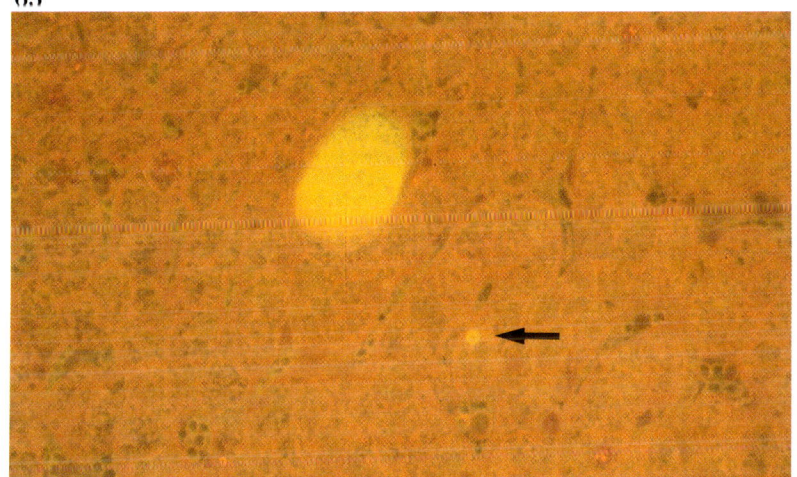

27

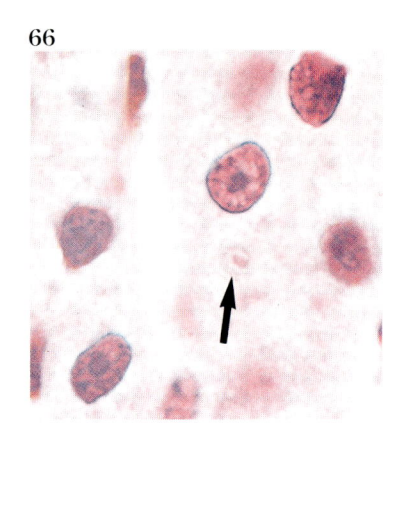

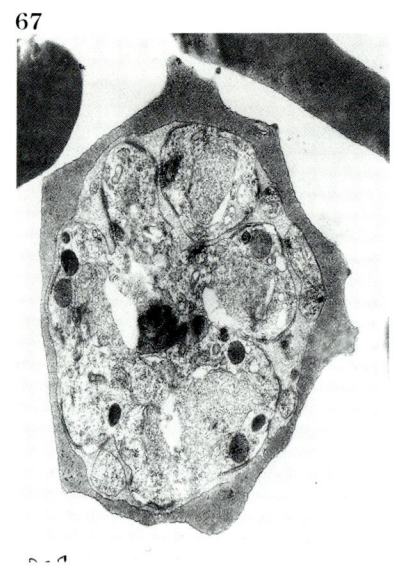

66 Hypnozoite of *P. cynomolgi* Enlarged view of a single hypnozoite. (*Giemsa—colophonium technique* × 2 000)

67 Electron-micrograph of mature *P. falciparum* schizont in red cell The merozoites form asexual parasites which grow inside erythrocytes to form the trophozoites. These feed on red cell contents producing insoluble pigment (haemozoin) as a waste product. When growth is complete the parasites undergo cell division (schizogony) and the daughter cells, after rupture of the host, invade new red cells. Note the small protrusions ('knobs') on the surface of the host cell. (× 11 000)

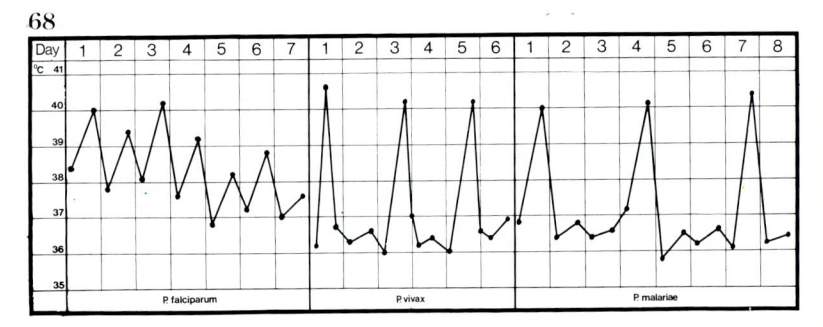

68 Tertian and quartan fever patterns The asexual blood stages of *P. falciparum, P. vivax* and *P. ovale* require 48 hours to complete their schizogony. Fever is produced when the schizonts mature, i.e. at 48-hour intervals. This gives the classical tertian periodicity which is, however, uncommon in a primary attack of *P. falciparum* malaria. *P. malariae* requires 72 hours and is associated with quartan fever, i.e. 72 hours between paroxysms.

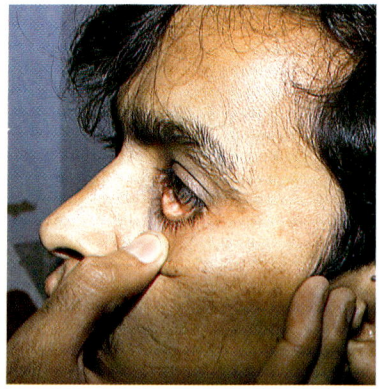

69 Malarial anaemia The growth of intra-erythrocytic parasites leads to disruption of the host cells. This (and possibly also autoimmunity) results in severe haemolytic anaemia. Jaundice can also occur. *P. falciparum* cannot develop normally in erythrocytes that contain haemoglobin S. (See **829**)

70 New Guinea child with grossly enlarged liver and spleen Haemolysed red cells and parasite debris are phagocytosed by macrophages, particularly of the spleen and liver, which become enlarged. This child was seen on a field survey.

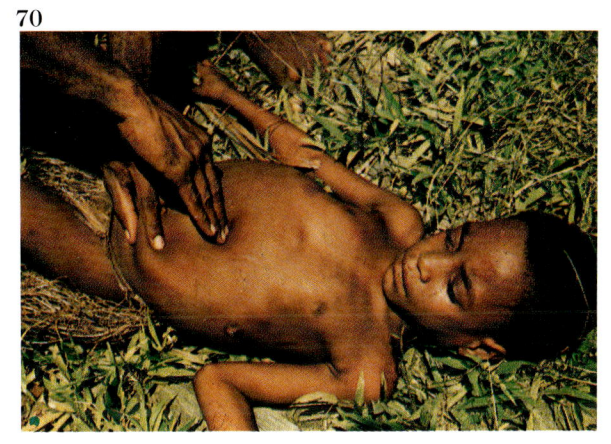

71 IgG increase in malaria The characteristic immunological response is an increase in the IgG level. However, cellular immunity also plays a vital role in protecting the host. Vaccines are currently being developed against three stages: the sporozoite, the intra-erythrocytic merozoites and the gametes. The response to them may prove to be mainly the production of antibodies.

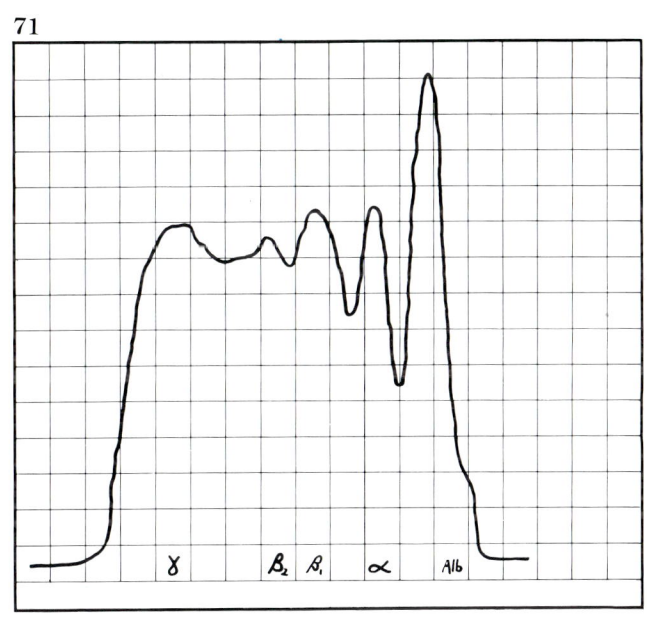

72-75 Preparation of blood film The diagnosis of malaria is based primarily on the recognition of parasites in well-prepared thick and thin blood films stained with a Romanowsky stain (Giemsa, Leishman, Field, etc.) at pH 7.2 to 7.4. A small drop of blood from a finger or ear is placed on a clean slide (**72**). The thin film is made by pulling a second slide away from the drop (**73**). The drop is spread for a thick film (**74**). Comparative thicknesses of thin and thick films are shown in **75**. Sophisticated diagnostic tools such as *Plasmodium*-specific DNA probes are of value mainly for epidemiological surveys and are of little use in diagnosing malaria in individual patients.

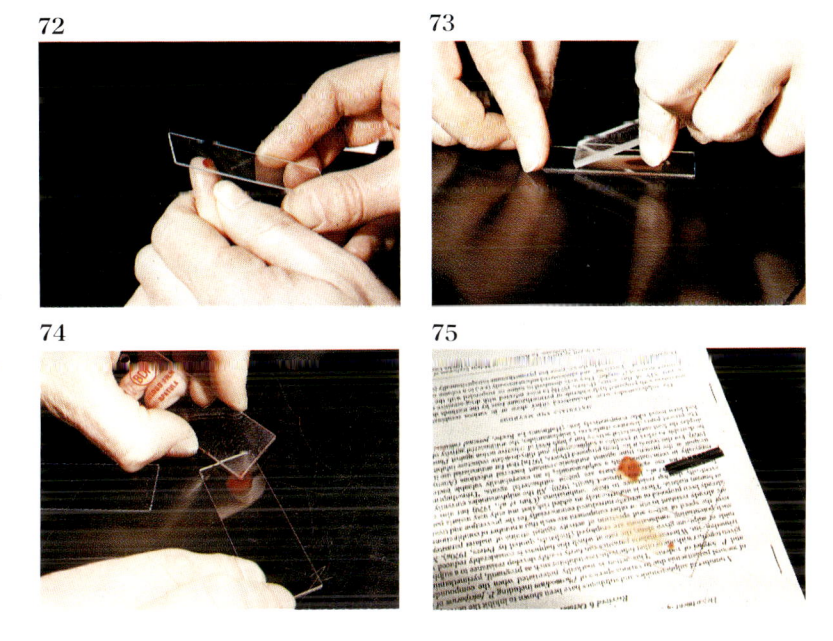

P. falciparum

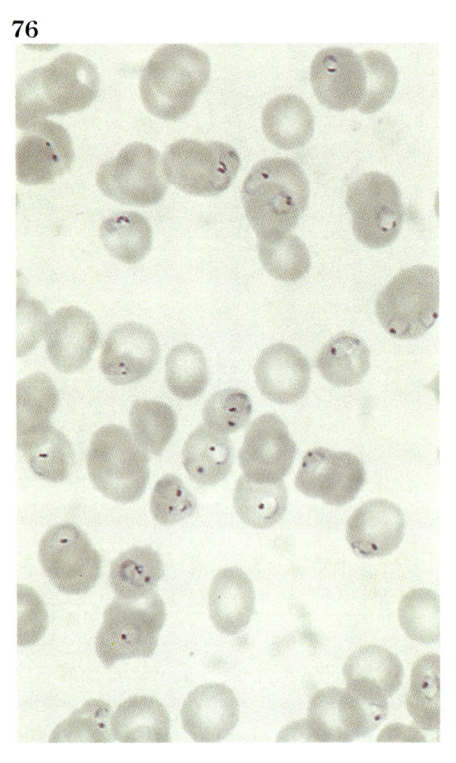

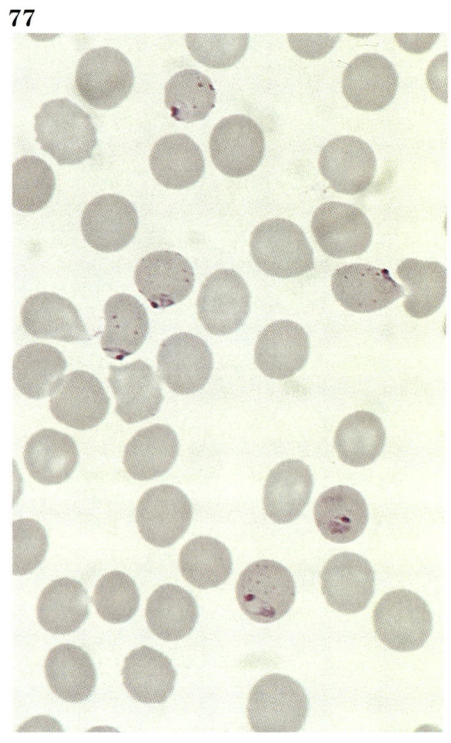

76-79 Life cycle of the blood stages Fine rings (**76**) predominate, mature trophozoites and schizonts (**78**) appearing uncommonly in the peripheral circulation because parasites mature in capillaries of the internal organs. Host cells are not enlarged. Spots of irregular shape and size (Maurer's dots) may be seen in older rings (**77**). Crescent-shaped gametocytes (**79**) are diagnostic. Infection with *P. falciparum* gives rise to 'malignant tertian malaria', so-called because severe, often lethal, complications such as those figured below can develop and such cases must be treated as medical emergencies. (*Giemsa × 900*)

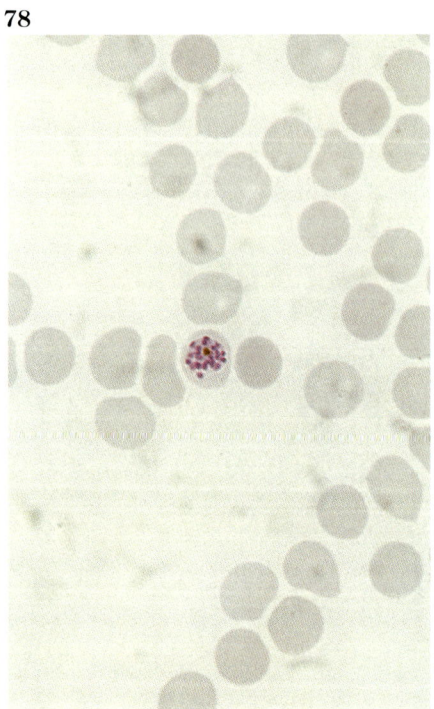

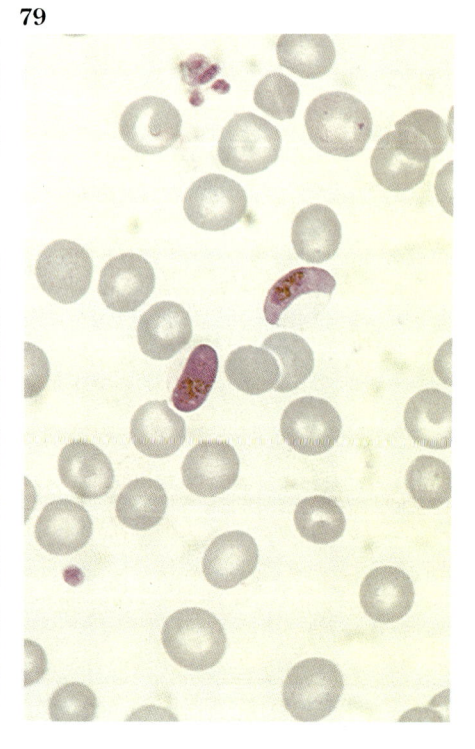

80 & 81 Thick blood films Usually only young rings (**80**) are seen in acute infections, sometimes in very large numbers. Heavy parasitaemia leads to severe haemolytic anaemia. Gametocytes (**81**) appear about a week after the onset of the illness. (*Field × 900*)

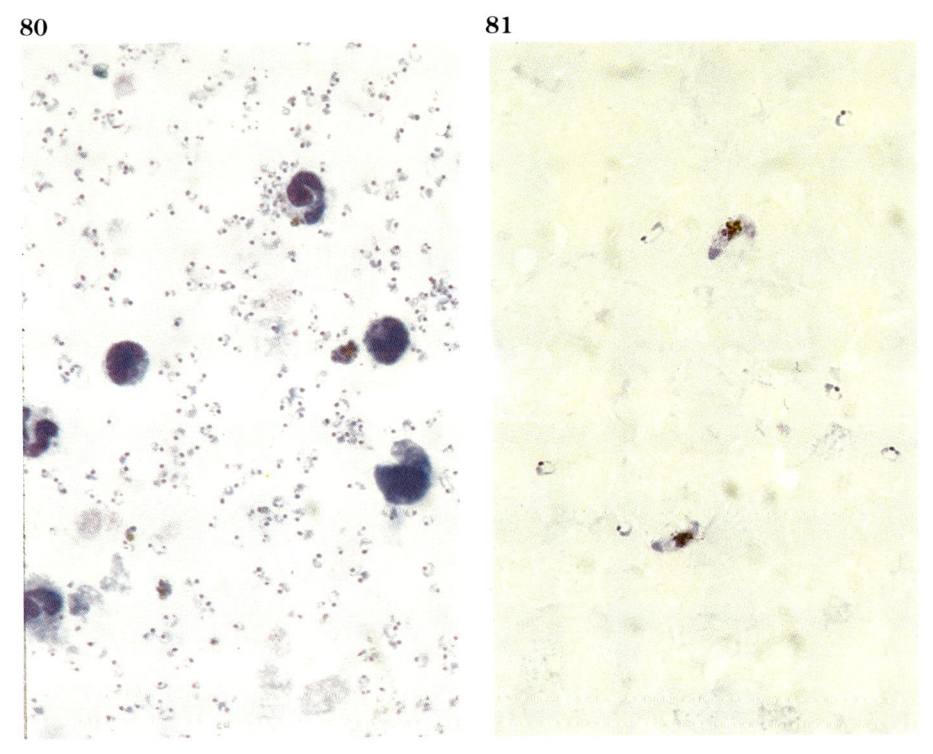

82 Temperature chart In first infections the fever is usually irregular rather than tertian. No relapses occur after adequate treatment with blood schizontocides since there are no hypnozoites, hence no secondary tissue schizogony (cf. *P. vivax* and *P. ovale*).

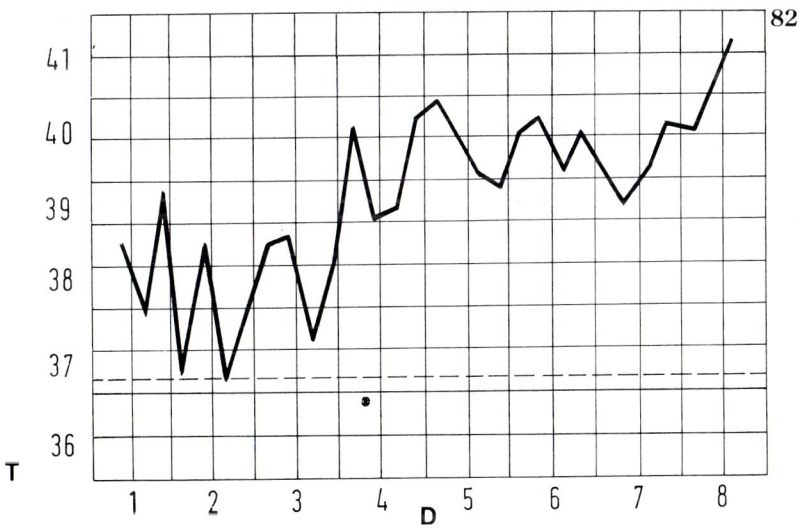

83 Retinal haemorrhage in severe falciparum malaria Examination of the fundus is a very important part of the physical examination of a patient with severe malaria because the presence of retinal haemorrhages in a *non-comatose* patient usually indicates that the person is likely to develop cerebral malaria within hours. In this Thai patient with cerebral malaria the haemorrhage is near the macula. Such haemorrhages have been found in as many as 18 to 30 per cent of patients with cerebral malaria and are an indication for parenteral therapy.

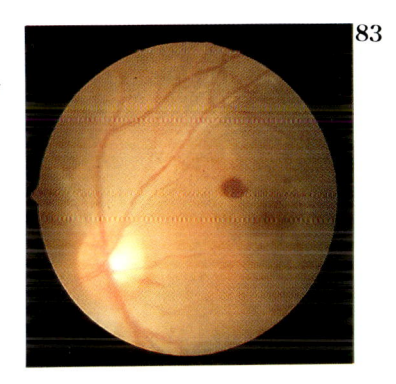

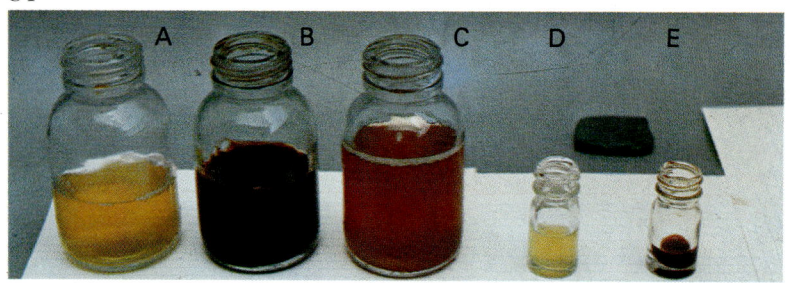

84 Blackwater urine and serum taken during course of illness An acute haemolytic crisis resulting in malarial haemoglobinuria occasionally occurs in severe attacks (Blackwater fever). Haemoglobinuria can also be drug induced in patients deficient in the enzyme glucose 6-phosphate dehydrogenase (G-6-PD). A = normal urine; B = patient's urine; C = patient's urine, diluted; D = normal serum; E = patient's serum.

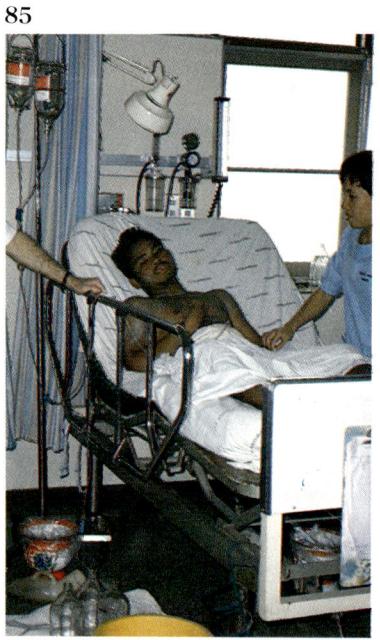

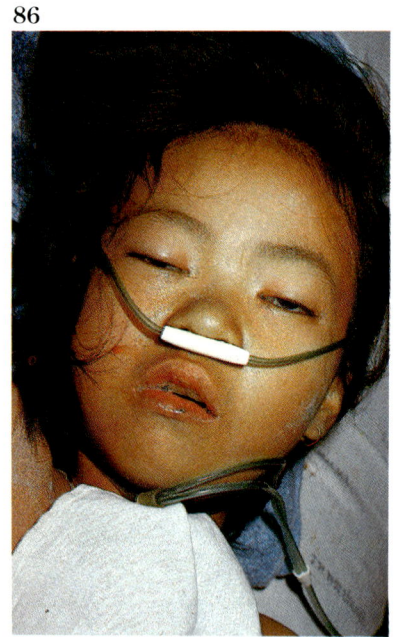

85 Multiorgan failure in cerebral malaria This Thai patient developed acute renal failure which responded to peritoneal dialysis. In addition, the patient was severely anaemic and developed Gram-negative septicaemia with severe hypotension ('Algid malaria').

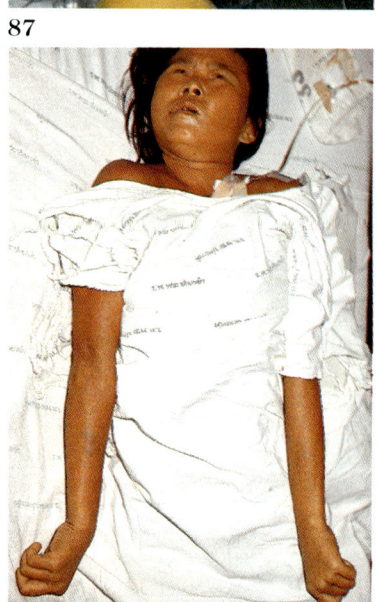

86 Acute pulmonary oedema Two types of pulmonary oedema occur in severe falciparum malaria. The first, due to overhydration, is preventable with good management of the patient. The second occurs during the fourth or fifth day of the illness, when the patient appears to be improving, and its causation is not clearly understood.

87 Classical decerebrate rigidity complicated by hypoglycaemia This Thai woman with cerebral malaria displays classical decerebrate rigidity which, in her case, is complicated by quinine-induced hypoglycaemia. The latter is more common during pregnancy when the warning signs are fits, abnormal behaviour and a change in the level of consciousness.

88 Gross section of brain in cerebral malaria Cerebral malaria results when cerebral capillaries are blocked by 'knobby' erythrocytes containing developing falciparum schizonts (*see also* **67**). This condition is a medical emergency which demands immediate treatment by intravenous administration of suitable antimalarials, e.g. quinine. Rehydration is also often needed, but overhydration may result in pulmonary oedema.

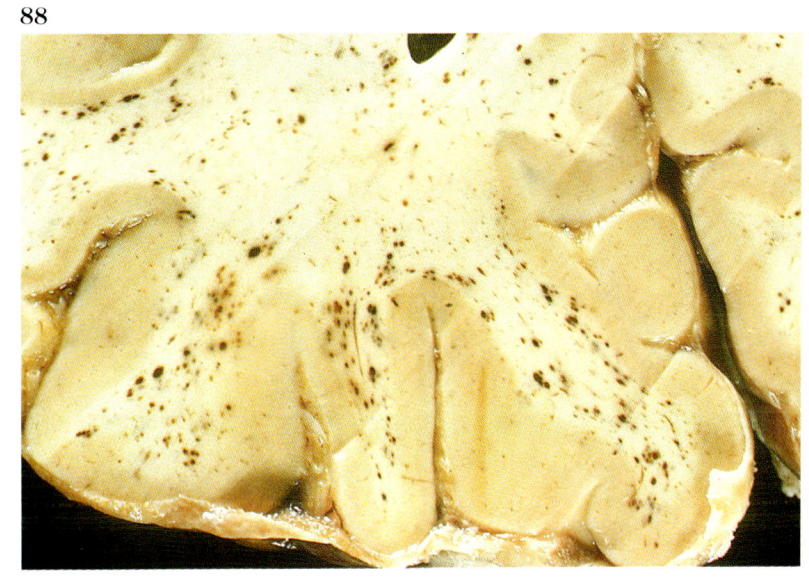

89 Microscopic section of brain The blockage of a capillary has led to its disruption and the formation of a microhaemorrhage. (*H&E × 200*)

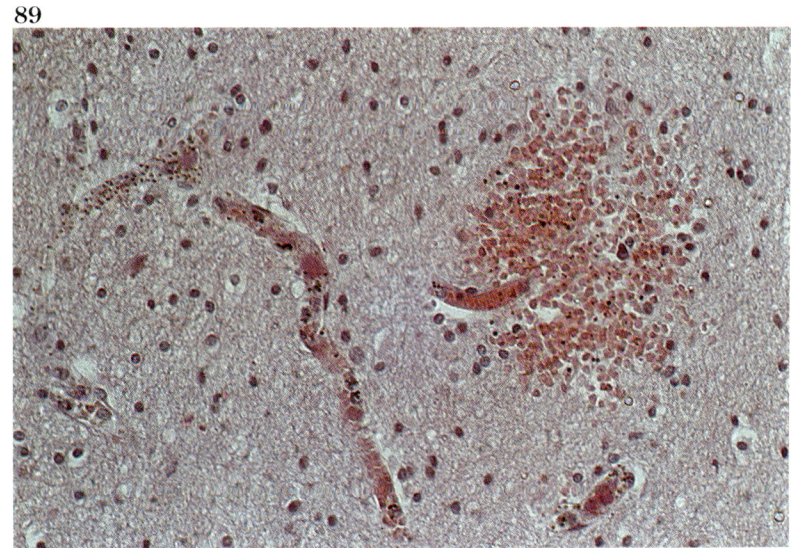

90 Liver in chronic malaria In chronic infection accumulation of malaria pigment (haemozoin) produces a dark brown coloration of liver and spleen.

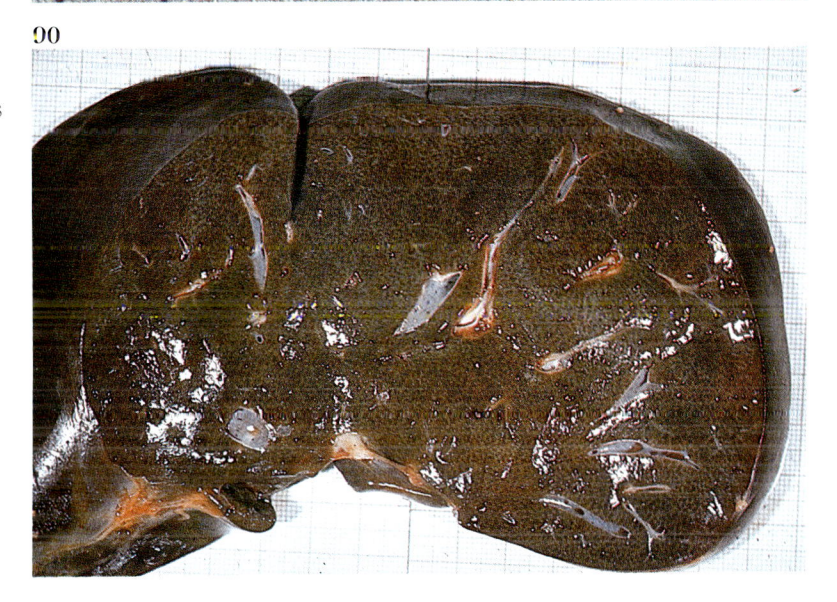

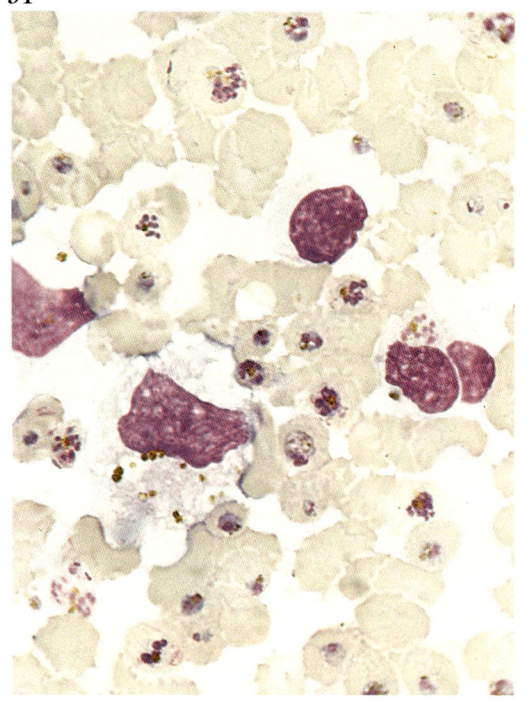

91 Placental smear with falciparum schizonts and macrophage The accumulation of falciparum schizonts in the maternal side of the placental circulation may result in the delivery of underweight infants, especially in primigravidae. True congenital malaria is very rare. (*Giemsa × 900*)

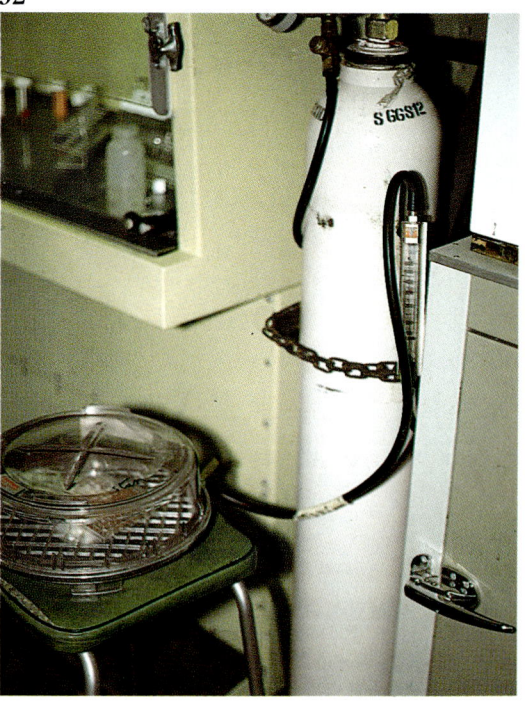

92 Testing for chloroquine sensitivity of *P. falciparum* The sensitivity of asexual intra-erythrocytic stages of *P. falciparum* to chloroquine may be measured by the response of the infection either *in vivo* or *in vitro*. The latter is readily performed in predosed microtitre plates which are incubated for up to 48 hours in a reduced oxygen tension. In this system, the drug sensitivity is judged by the level of inhibition of schizogony produced in different drug concentrations. This method may also be used with minor modifications for monitoring the response of other blood schizontocides (e.g. quinine).

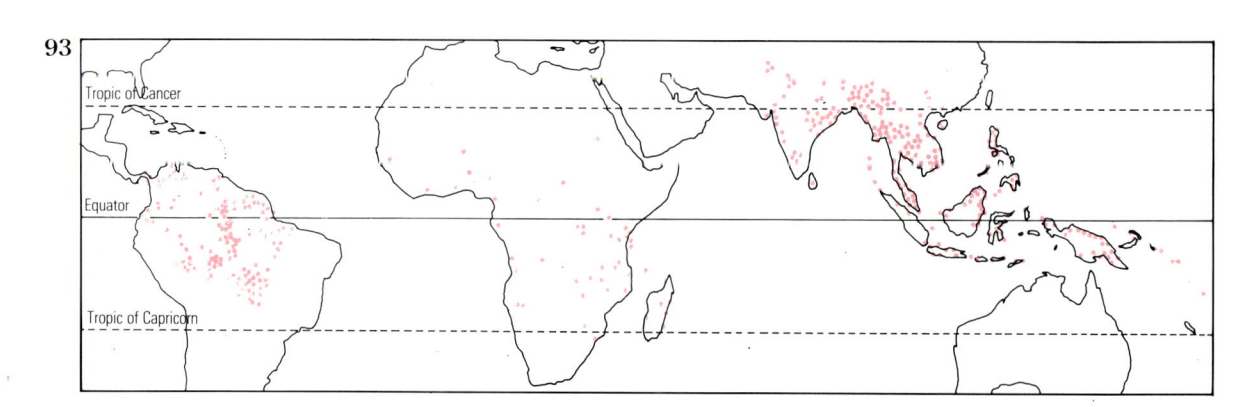

93 Distribution map of chloroquine resistance In the areas shown, falciparum malaria may not respond to prevention or treatment with chloroquine and alternative drugs in other chemical groups may have to be used. Since about 1960 this problem has increased seriously, both geographically and in the levels of resistance that are manifested to other drugs in addition to chloroquine. The situation is especially ominous in Africa where transmission is very intense.

P. vivax

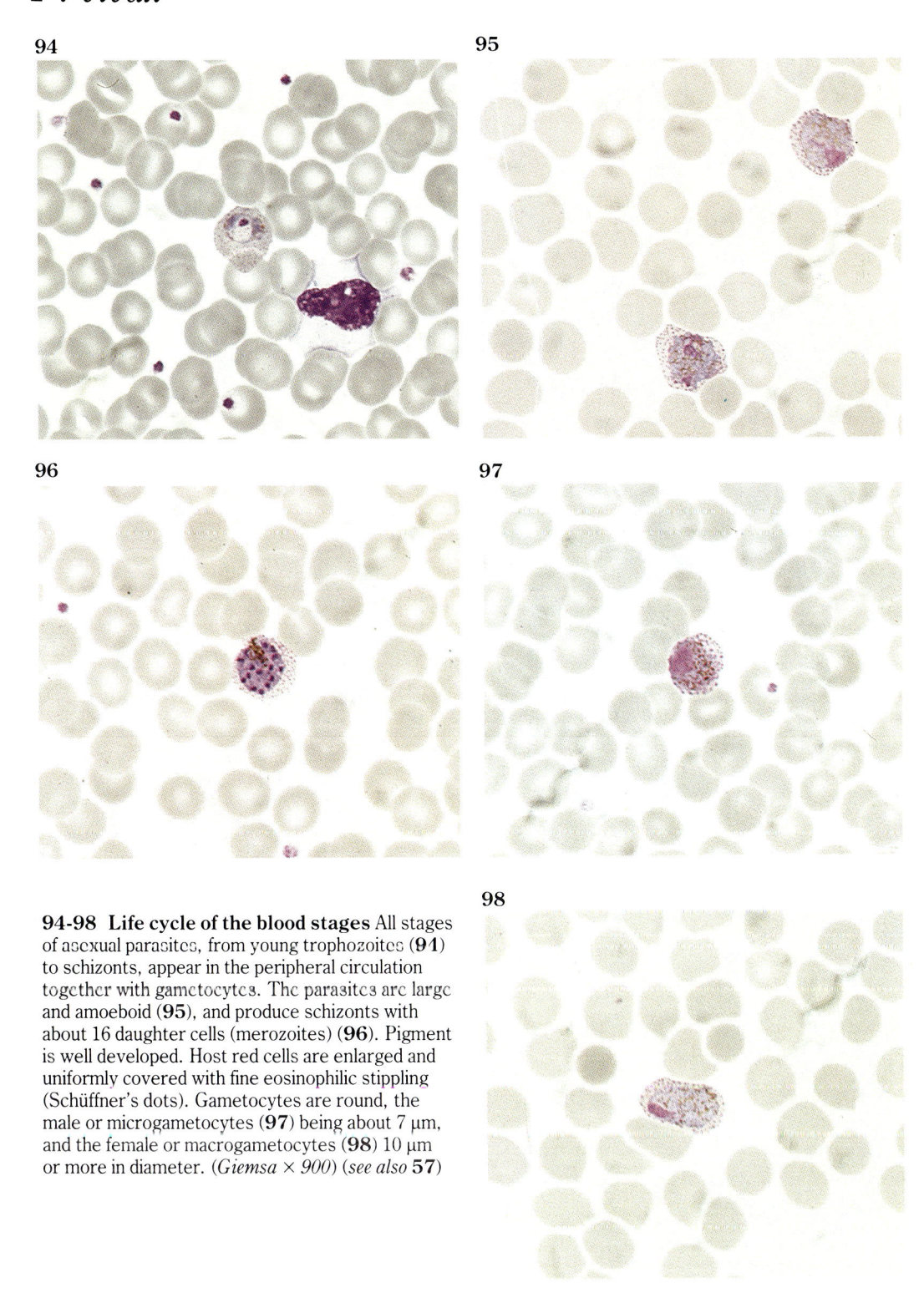

94

95

96

97

98

94-98 Life cycle of the blood stages All stages of asexual parasites, from young trophozoites (**94**) to schizonts, appear in the peripheral circulation together with gametocytes. The parasites are large and amoeboid (**95**), and produce schizonts with about 16 daughter cells (merozoites) (**96**). Pigment is well developed. Host red cells are enlarged and uniformly covered with fine eosinophilic stippling (Schüffner's dots). Gametocytes are round, the male or microgametocytes (**97**) being about 7 μm, and the female or macrogametocytes (**98**) 10 μm or more in diameter. (*Giemsa* × *900*) (*see also* **57**)

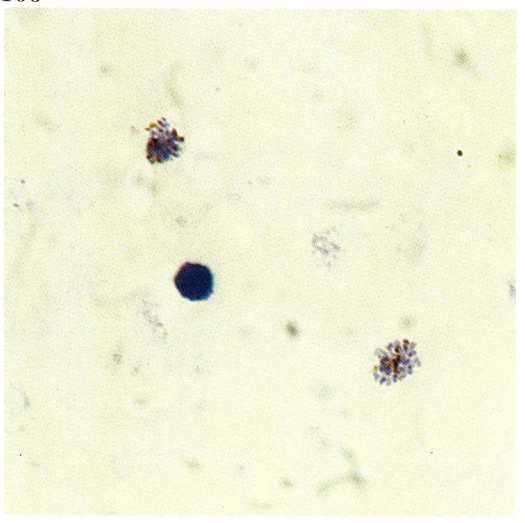

99-101 Thick blood film All stages may be present. Parasitaemia is often less heavy than in falciparum malaria. The parasites seen here are all in a single thick film. Amoeboid trophozoites (**99**) are seen in the thicker part and two schizonts (**100**) in a thinner part. Three polymorphs, a lymphocyte and (centre) a macrogametocyte are seen in **101**. Sometimes the Schüffner's dots can be seen in 'ghost cells' in the thinner parts of the film where the host cell has been haemolysed, as in this example. (*Field × 900*)

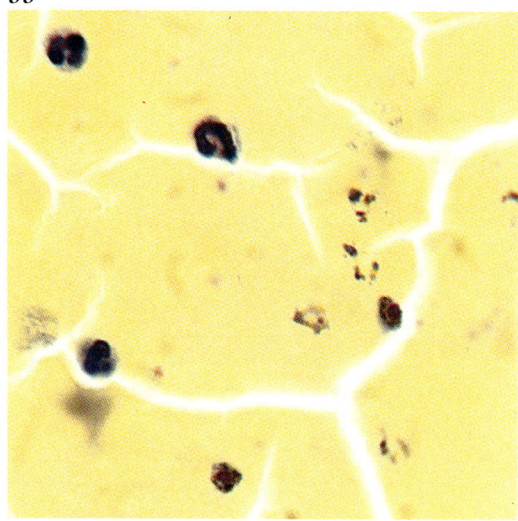

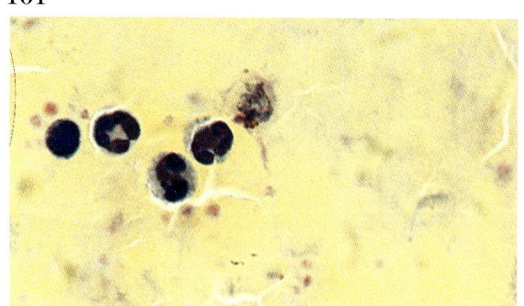

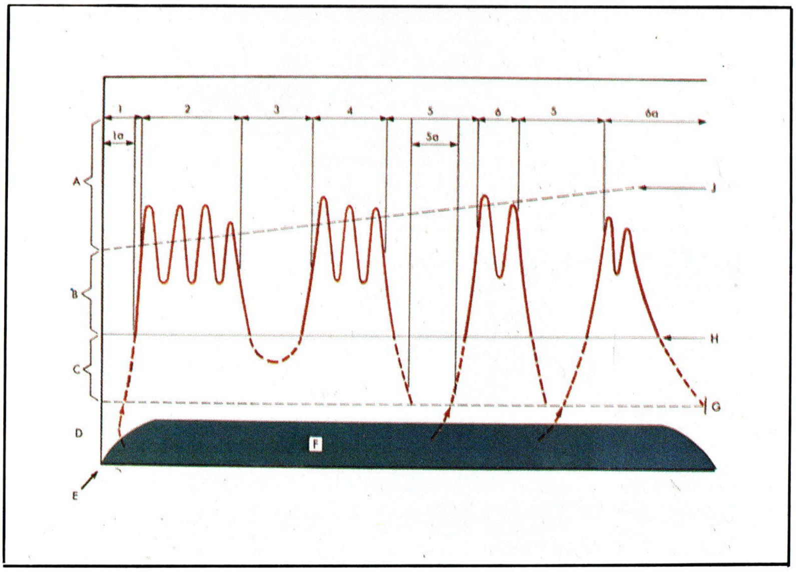

102 Diagram of relapse patterns in vivax malaria Relapses in vivax malaria are due to emergence of new blood forms from maturing secondary liver schizonts that develop at intervals of several months from hypnozoites. In tropical areas the first relapses may arise within three to four months of a primary attack but, in subtropical areas, usually only after nine months or more. A - Clinical symptoms; B - Overt parasitaemia; C - Subpatent parasitaemia; D - Primary tissue stages and hypnozoites in the liver; E - Sporozoite infection; F - Exo-erythrocytic schizogony arising from hypnozoites; G - Radical or spontaneous cure; H - Microscopic threshold; J - Clinical (pyrogenic) threshold rising with the increased immunity; 1 - Incubation period; 1a - Pre-patent period; 2 - Primary attack composed of paroxysms; 3 - Latent period (clinical latency); 4 - Recrudescence (short-term relapse); 5 - Latent period; 5a - Parasitic latency; 6 - Clinical recurrence (long-term relapse) followed by parasitic recurrence; 6a - Asymptomatic parasitic relapse.

P. ovale

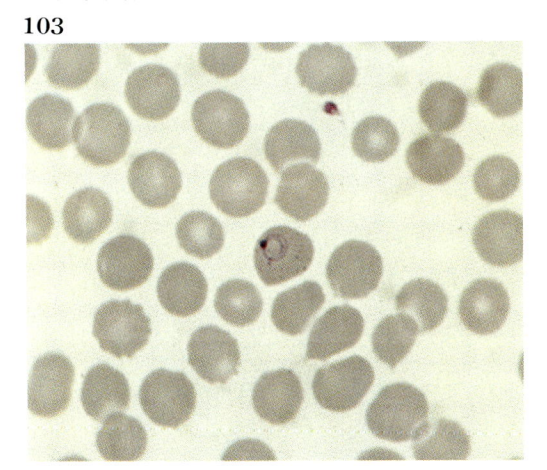

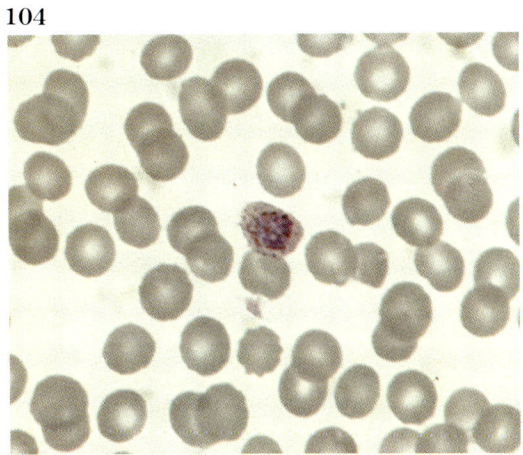

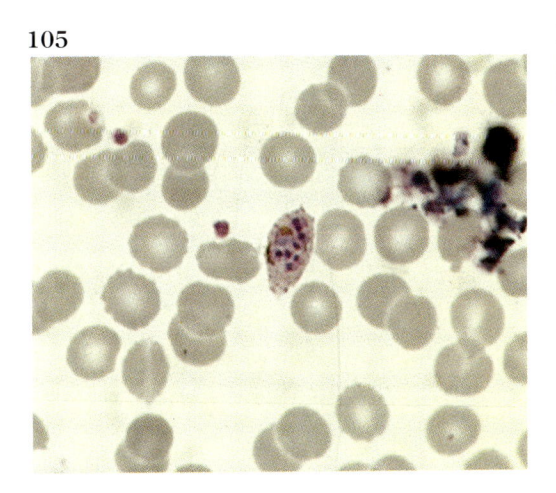

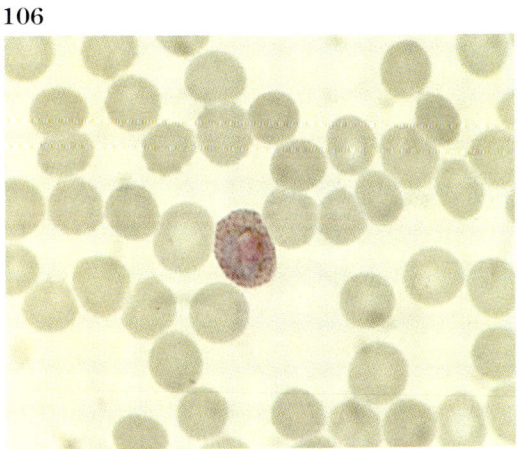

103-107 Life cycle of the blood stages Ring forms (**103**) have a prominent nucleus. The older parasites (**104**) differ from *P. vivax* in being more compact, and producing about eight merozoites at schizogony (**105**). Like *P. vivax*, the host red cells contain Schüffner's dots (sometimes called 'James' stippling') and tend to be ovoid and fimbriated. Micro- and macrogametocytes (**106 & 107**) are smaller than those of *P. vivax*. Relapses occur as in *P. vivax* but the disease tends to be more chronic. (*Leishman* × *900*)

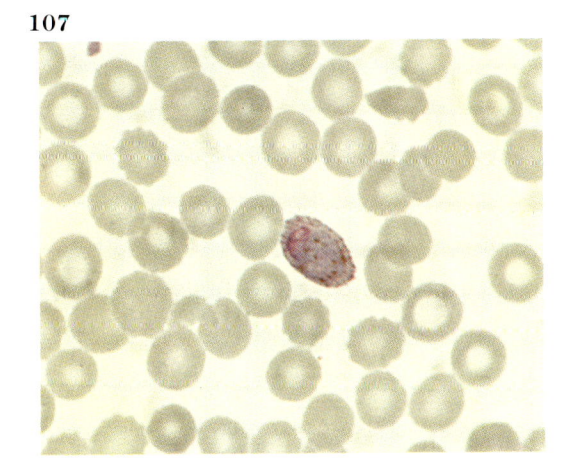

P. malariae

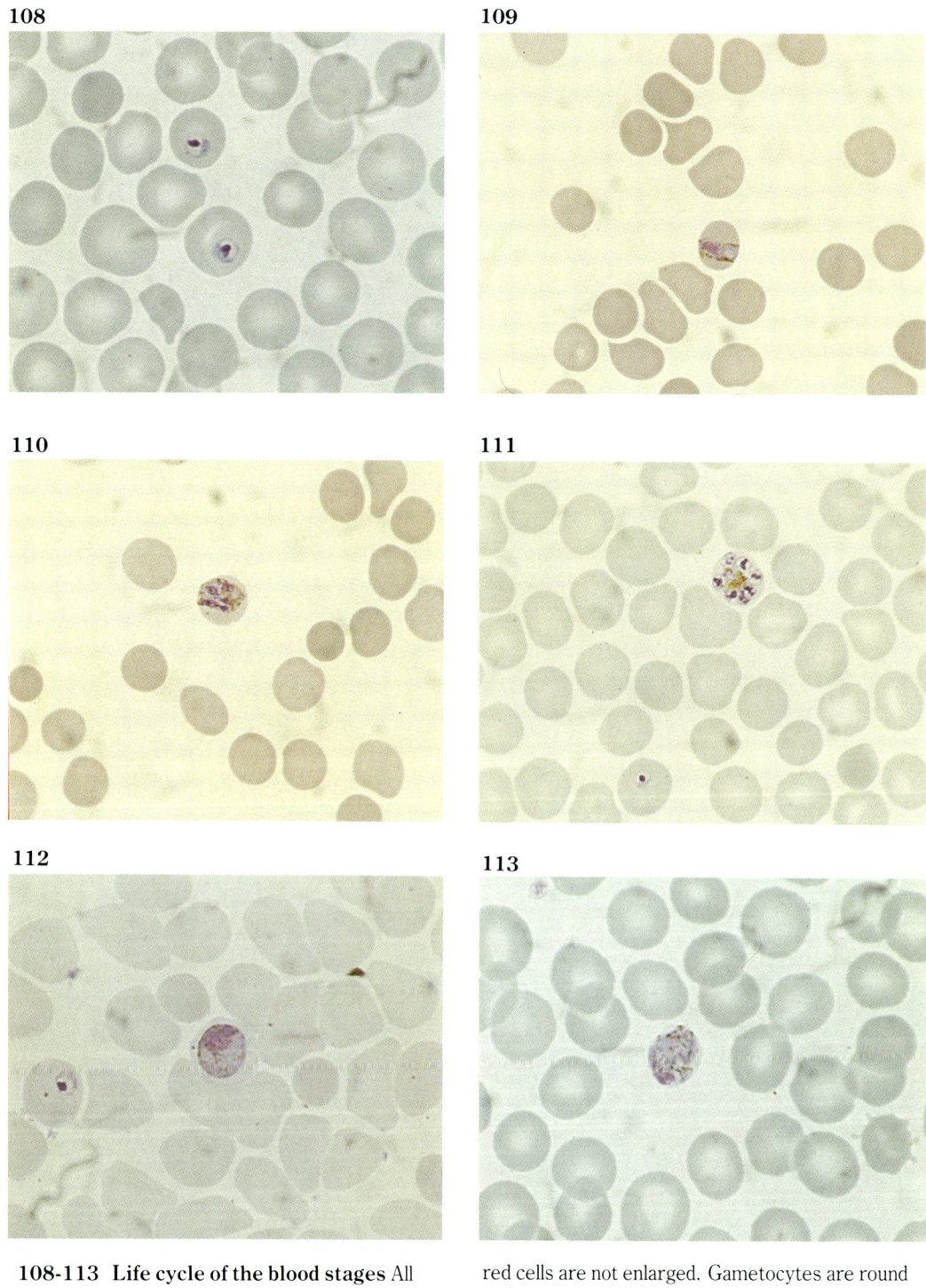

108-113 Life cycle of the blood stages All stages may appear in the peripheral circulation from young trophozoites (**108**) to compact schizonts (**111**) with eight merozoites. 'Band forms' (**109 & 110**) are common. With special staining a very fine stippling (Ziemann's dots) is sometimes seen. Host red cells are not enlarged. Gametocytes are round and compact with distinct blackish pigment, the females (**113**) usually staining a bluer colour, and the males (**112**) somewhat mauvish.
(*Leishman × 900*)

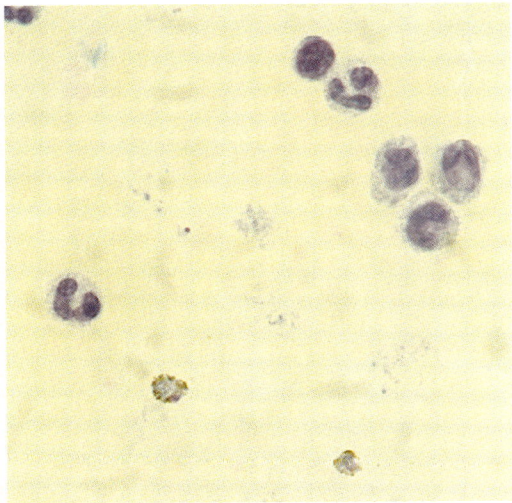

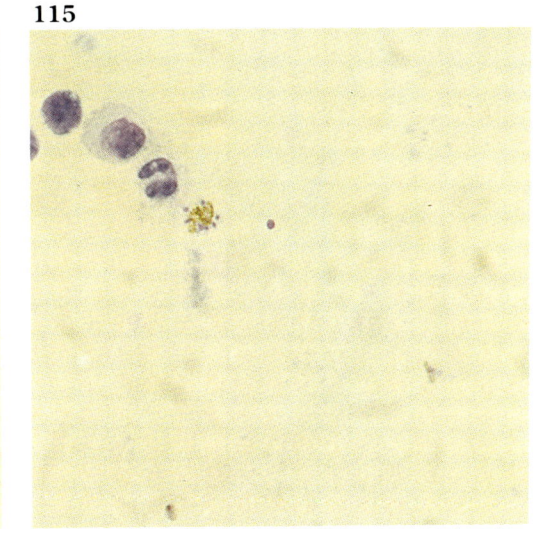

114-116 Thick blood films of *P. malariae* and *P. ovale* Younger parasites are easily recognised by their heavy pigment which may obscure the inner structure of older trophozoites and gametocytes (**114**). Schizonts containing about eight merozoites with a central mass of pigment (**115**) are characteristic. Differentiation of *P. ovale* from *P. malariae* is difficult in thick films in which the parasites are easily confused (cf. **116** with **114**). As in *P. vivax*, 'ghost cells' may be seen in thinner parts of the thick film but the contained *P. ovale* are more compact (cf. **116** with **101**). (Field × 900)

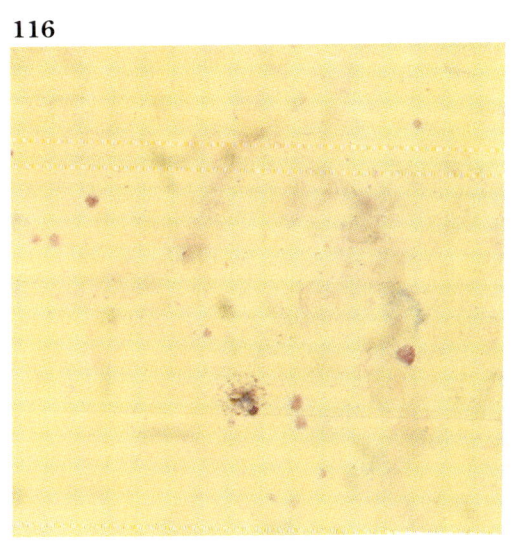

117 Ultrastructure of *P. malariae* trophozoite Very small but regular bosses occur on the surface of the host erythrocyte (possibly corresponding to the Ziemann's dots). (cf. 'knobs' on *P. falciparum*-infected red cells **67**). (× 11 000)

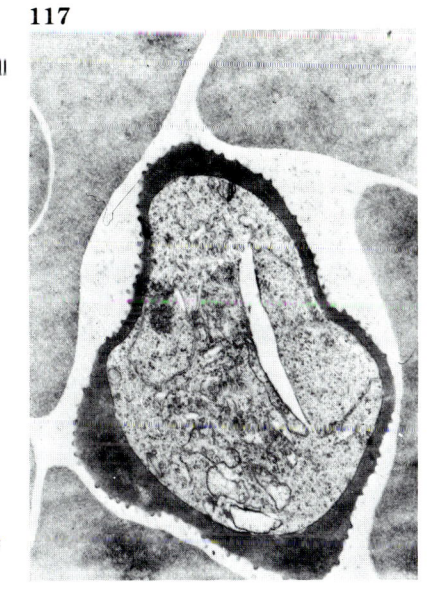

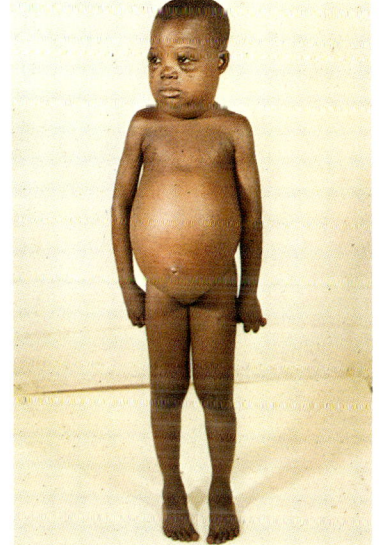

118 Nephrotic child with *P. malariae* infection A close association has been established between quartan malaria and the nephrotic syndrome in children. Note the gross oedema and ascites.

39

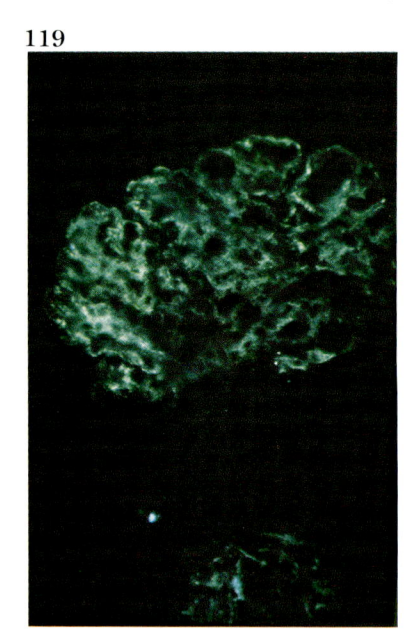

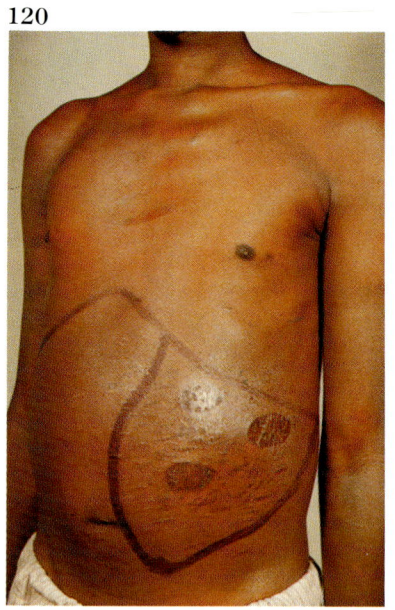

119 Immunofluorescence of immune complexes in kidney Immunofluorescent antibody techniques have demonstrated the deposition of immune complexes on the basement membrane of the glomeruli in 'quartan malarial nephrosis'. (× *350*)

120 'Tropical splenomegaly syndrome' (TSS) Gross enlargement of the spleen is a characteristic feature of the tropical splenomegaly syndrome (hyperreactive malarial splenomegaly, 'big spleen disease'). The syndrome is thought to be due to an abnormal immunological response to malaria infection. High IgM levels are invariably found. Note scars due to application of indigenous medicines.

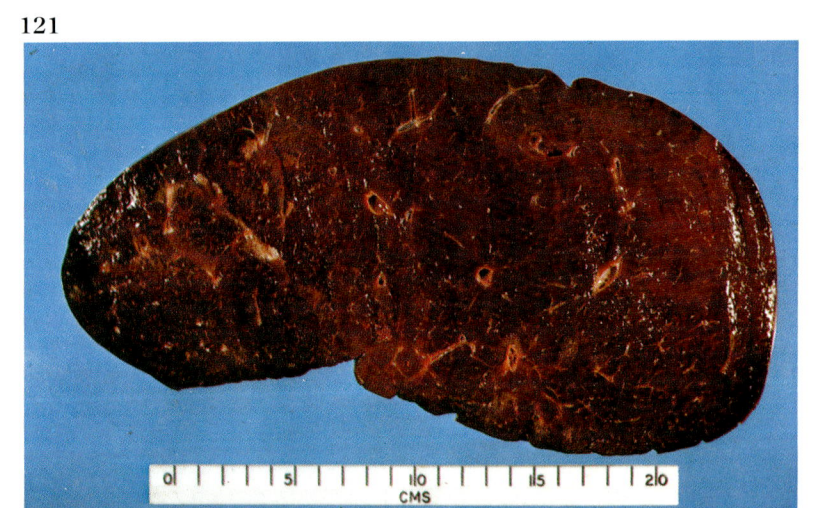

121 Massive spleen in TSS Regression of the enlarged spleen occurs when long-term antimalarial therapy is given.

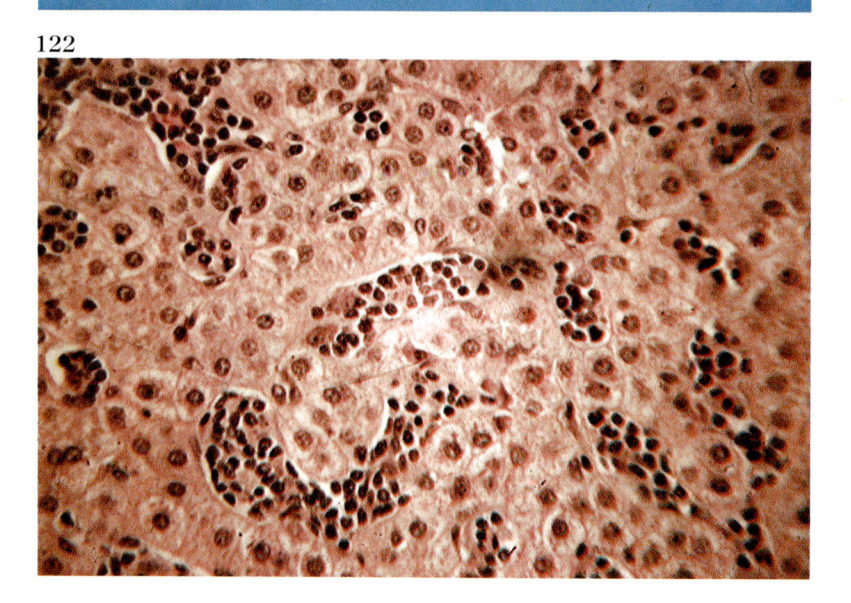

122 Section of liver in TSS Liver biopsy shows hepatic sinusoidal dilatation with marked infiltration of lymphocytes and hypertrophy of the Kupffer cells. (*H&E × 500*)

Babesiosis in Man

123 *Babesia divergens* in human blood Infection with species of *Babesia* from cattle or rodents is a rare occurrence in man. Parasites are transmitted by ticks. Infection in normal people may give rise to a self-limiting fever and parasitaemia (e.g. the rodent parasite *B. microti* on the eastern seaboard of the United States). Heavy red cell infection may develop, however, in splenectomised patients, leading to fatal haemolytic anaemia. This patient died from an infection acquired with the cattle parasite *B. divergens* in Scotland. (*Giemsa* × 900)

124a,b Unidentified *Babesia* species in human blood This unidentified *Babesia* was acquired in the South of France by a man who had been splenectomised some time previously and had evidence of a recent tick bite. His work brought him into frequent contact with dogs. This patient recovered with intensive antibabesial chemotherapy. (*Giemsa* × 900)

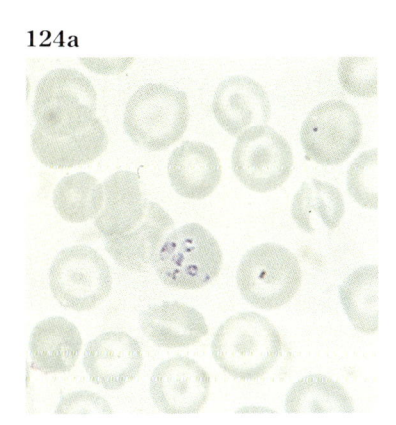

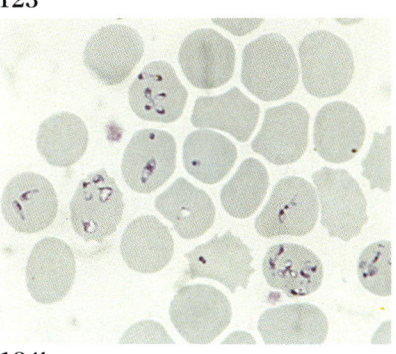

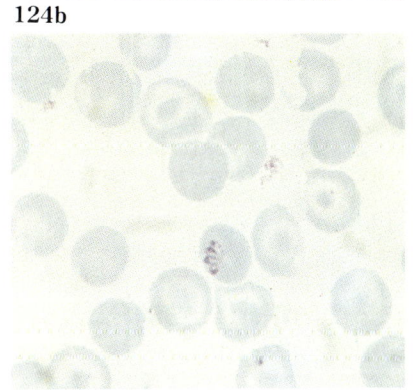

TRYPANOSOMIASIS (*See* Tables VI & VII)
African Trypanosomiasis

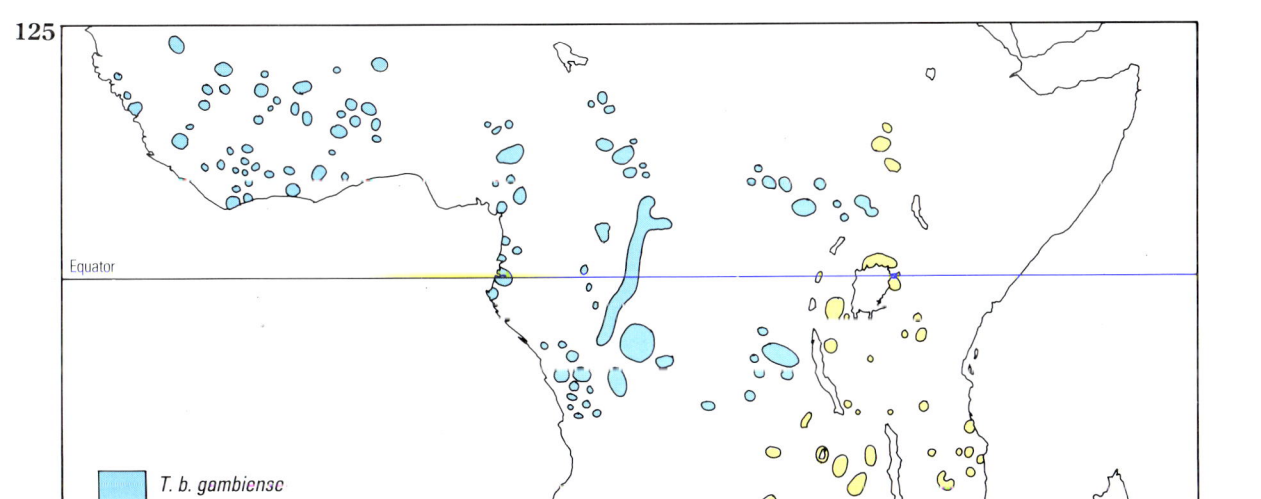

125 Distribution of infection in man African trypanosomiasis is confined to equatorial Africa with a patchy distribution depending upon detailed topographical conditions. It is caused by two subspecies of *Trypanosoma brucei*. *T. brucei* parasitises wild and domestic animals but does not infect man. The different subspecies can be distinguished with certainty only by biochemical techniques such as electrophoretic typing of their isoenzymes (*see* **172 & 535**). *T. b. gambiense* infection is widespread in West and Central Africa but *T. b. rhodesiense* is restricted to the East and East Central areas with some overlaps between the two.

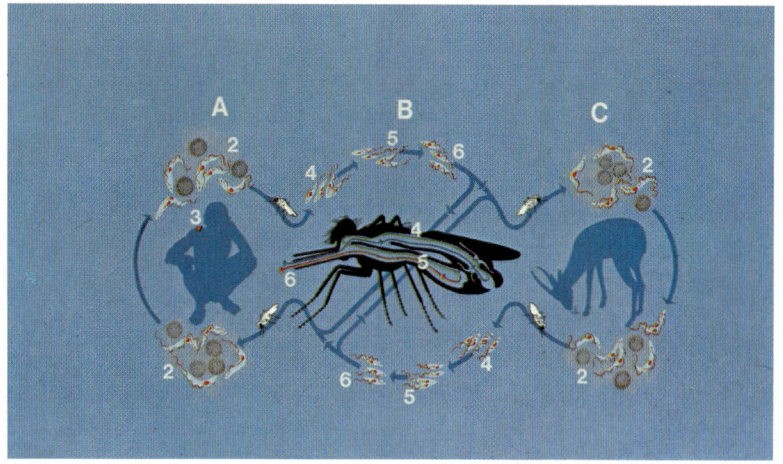

126 Life cycles of African trypanosomes A. Trypomastigote stages (2) of *T. b. gambiense* or *T. b. rhodesiense* are produced in the blood and tissue spaces of man when he is bitten by a tsetse fly. The parasites may be found in various glands (3) as well as in the blood. B. Trypomastigotes ingested by the tsetse fly transform into epimastigotes (4) which divide (5) during a complicated migration in the fly, eventually forming metacyclic trypomastigotes (6). These can infect another man or reservoir animals (C) in which the blood and tissues are invaded as in man (2). (*See also* **127-131, 134, 139**.)

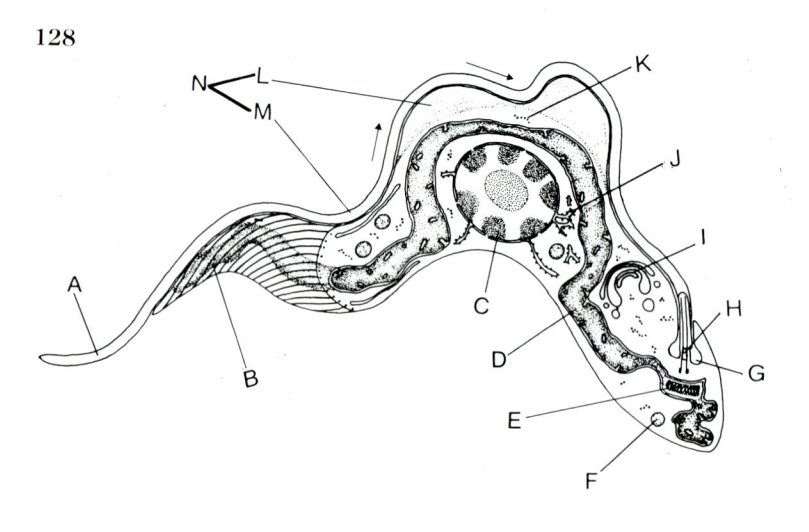

127 *T. b. rhodesiense* in human blood *T. b. gambiense*, *T. b. rhodesiense* (and *T. b. brucei* of animals) are virtually indistinguishable in blood films. Note the small kinetoplast and free flagellum. Both subspecies from man will infect guinea pigs but only *T. b. rhodesiense* is infective to rats, in which the parasites are polymorphic, i.e. long, thin, intermediate and short stumpy forms of trypomastigotes may coincide. (*Giemsa × 900*)

128 Diagram of ultrastructure of *T. b. gambiense* A - free flagellum; B - microtubules of pellicle; C - nucleus; D - mitochondrion; E - kinetoplast; F - cytoplasmic granule; G - reservoir; H - basal body of flagellum; I - Golgi apparatus; J - endoplasmic reticulum; K - ribosomes; L - fold of pellicle; M - attached flagellum; N - undulating membrane. (× 30 000)

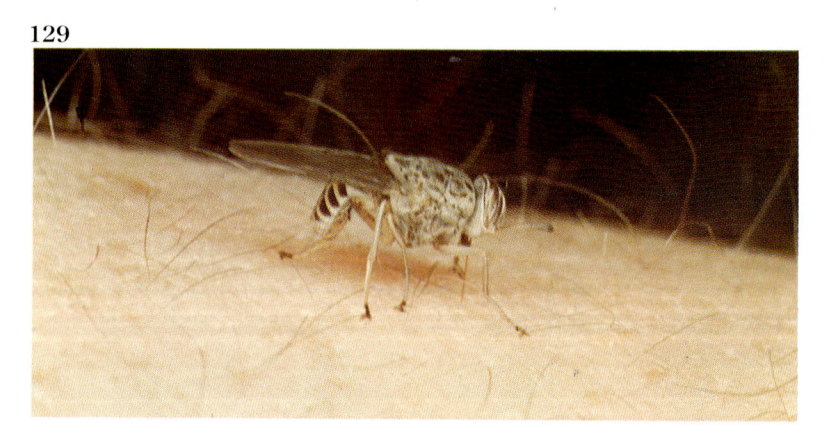

129 Tsetse fly feeding The common vectors of *T. b. gambiense* are *Glossina palpalis* and *G. tachinoides* in West Africa. *T. b. rhodesiense* is associated with *G. morsitans*, *G. swynnertoni* and *G. pallidipes*. Other, secondary vectors have more localised distributions. (× 4)

130 Trypanosomes in section of tsetse fly After ingestion by the tsetse fly, the trypomastigotes pass to the midgut. After asexual reproduction the parasites migrate forward between the peritrophic membrane and gut wall to re-enter the pharynx and proboscis. They migrate back into the salivary glands when they transform first into epimastigotes (*see* **155**), then to the infective stage (metacyclic trypomastigotes) (**131**). The section shows trypomastigotes massed at the entrance to the midgut ready to enter the proventriculus. (× 90) (*See also* **126**.)

131 Metacyclic trypanosomes in salivary 'probe' The infective stages are passed into the bite together with the saliva when the fly next feeds. They may be observed in saliva expressed from the proboscis of the fly onto a microscope slide. (× 900)

132 Larva, pre-pupa and pupa of *Glossina morsitans* A single larva develops inside the female tsetse fly and is deposited when mature in dry soil. Here it pupates and metamorphoses to the adult. (× 4)

133 Ecology of gambiense infection Gambiense trypanosomiasis is transmitted by riverine species of *Glossina* requiring optimum shade and humidity. Shady trees near lakes, rivers and pools of water are ideal habitats. The figure shows a typical site for transmission by *G. palpalis* in the hinterland of Liberia. Man-fly contact is intimate when villagers congregate around pools for collecting water or washing. Domestic pigs may serve as reservoirs. *G. tachinoides* is second in importance to *G. palpalis* as a vector of sleeping sickness. Rhodesiense trypanosomiasis can occur in scrub savannah country because the *Glossina* vectors are less dependent on moisture. Moreover, in such terrain wild animals and domestic cattle provide alternative feeding opportunities for the fly.

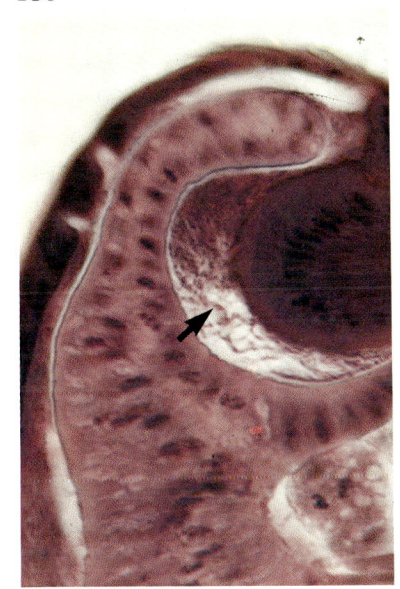

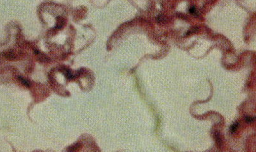

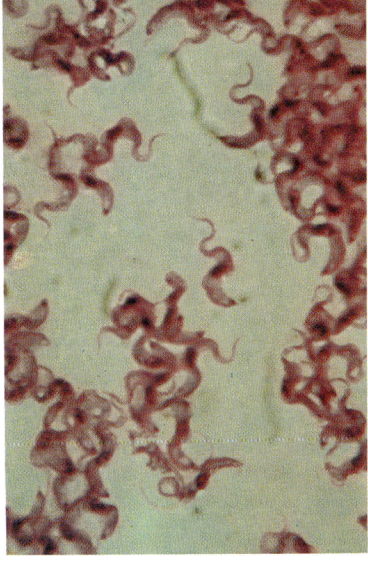

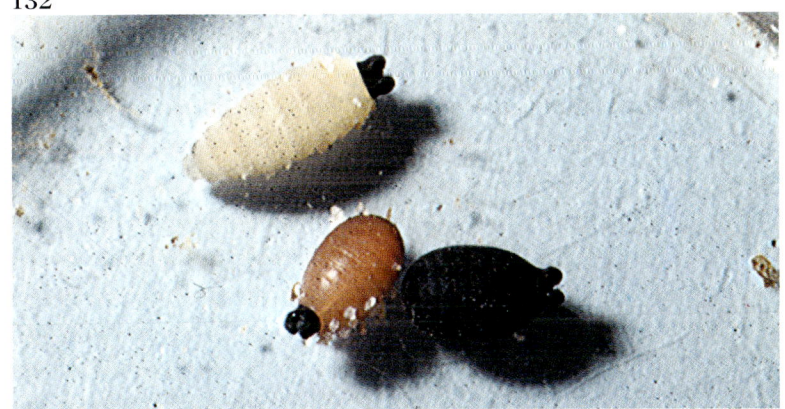

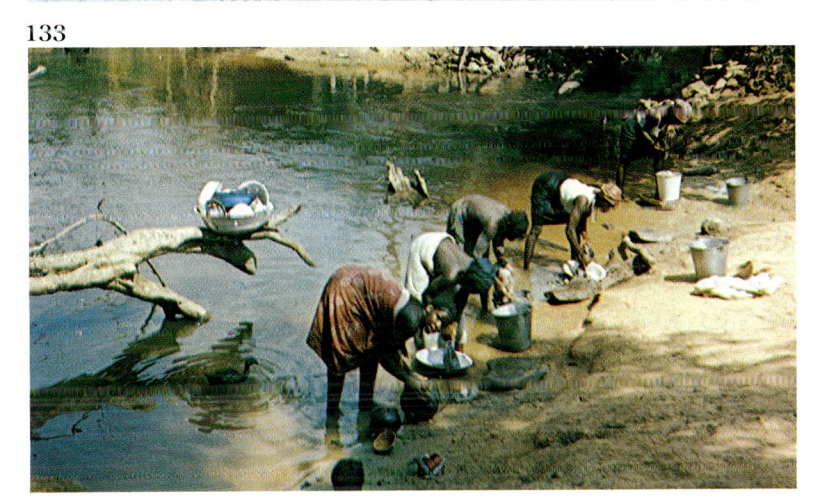

Trypanosomiasis due to other species is a serious disease of domestic animals, causing great economic loss and depriving human populations of much needed protein. *T. b. brucei*, *T. vivax* and *T. congolense* are the commonest parasites involved. Pigs may also be decimated by other species such as *T. suis* or *T. simiae*.

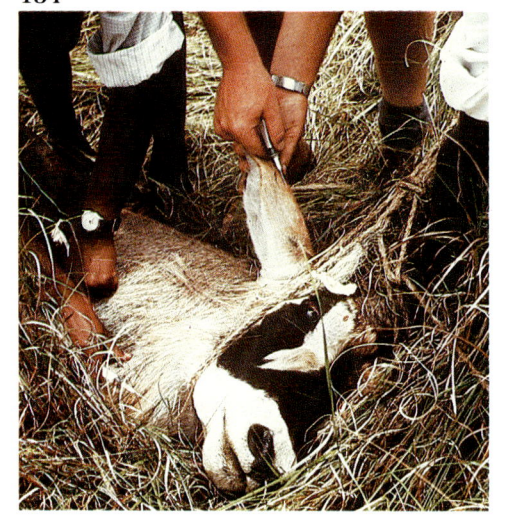

134 Blood sample being taken from antelope The reservoir of *T. b. rhodesiense* was long suspected to be wild animals. The first species found infected with this trypanosome was the bushbuck (*Tragelaphus scriptus*), but other species of game animals have since been found to harbour these parasites. This antelope was immobilised with an anaesthetic dart for a blood sample to be collected.

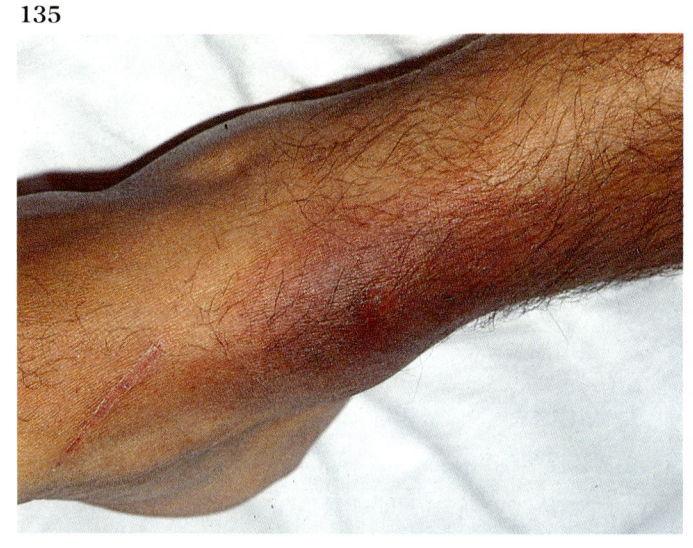

135 Trypanosomal chancre The bite reaction, the earliest clinical lesion, is known as a 'trypanosomal chancre'. It resembles a boil but is usually painless. Fluid aspirated from the nodule contains actively dividing trypanosomes.

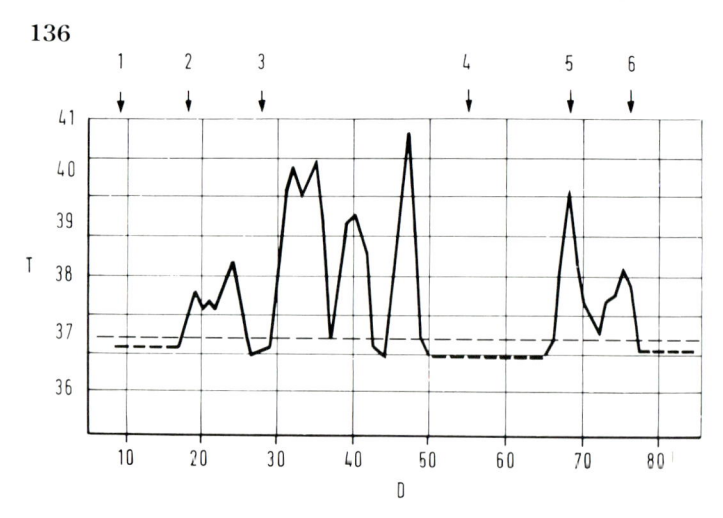

136 Temperature chart in a patient with trypanosomiasis Irregularly occurring episodes of pyrexia are often associated with the rash. Trypanosomes appear in the blood one to three weeks after infection. They may be scanty in gambiense but are commonly numerous in rhodesiense infection which is usually a more fulminating disease. 1 - headache; 2 - trypanosomal chancre; 3 - oedema of left eyelid; 4, 5, 6 - rash.

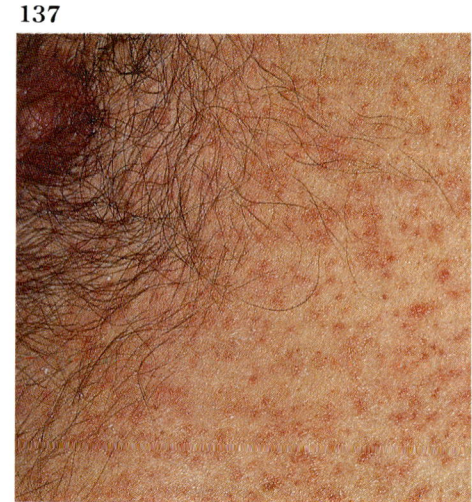

137 Trypanosomal rash In fair-skinned individuals each peak of fever may be accompanied by a remarkable skin eruption in the form of annular patches of erythema. In other cases the rash may be more generalised as seen here on the sixth day of an infection with *T. b. rhodesiense*.

138 Cervical lymphadenopathy
Enlargement of lymphatic glands, especially in the posterior triangle of the neck ('Winterbottom's sign') is an important clinical feature of *T. b. gambiense* infection which calls for diagnostic gland puncture.

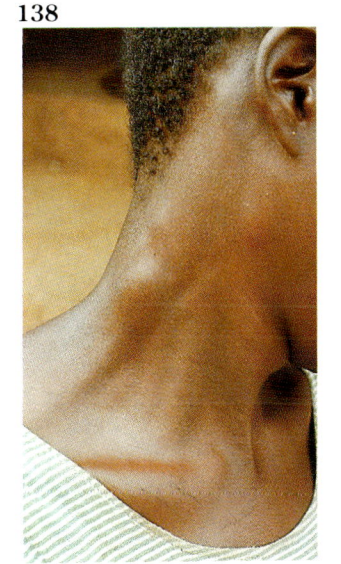

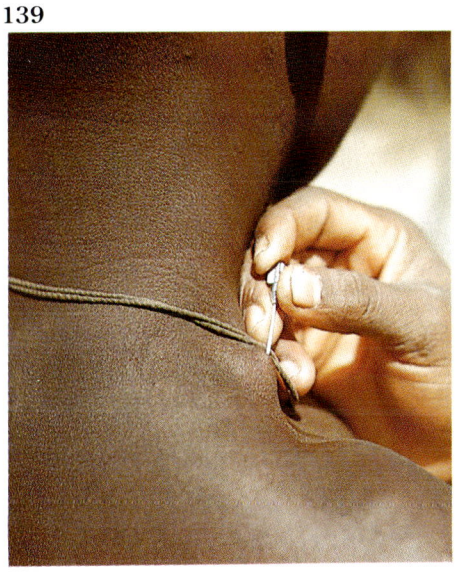

139 Gland puncture Examination of glandular aspirate is a valuable and simple means of providing an early diagnosis, especially in Gambian trypanosomiasis.

140 Trypanosomes in gland fluid
The trypanosomes are easily identified as actively motile organisms in the wet preparation of aspirated gland juice. Their identity can be confirmed by staining. (*Giemsa* × 1 250)

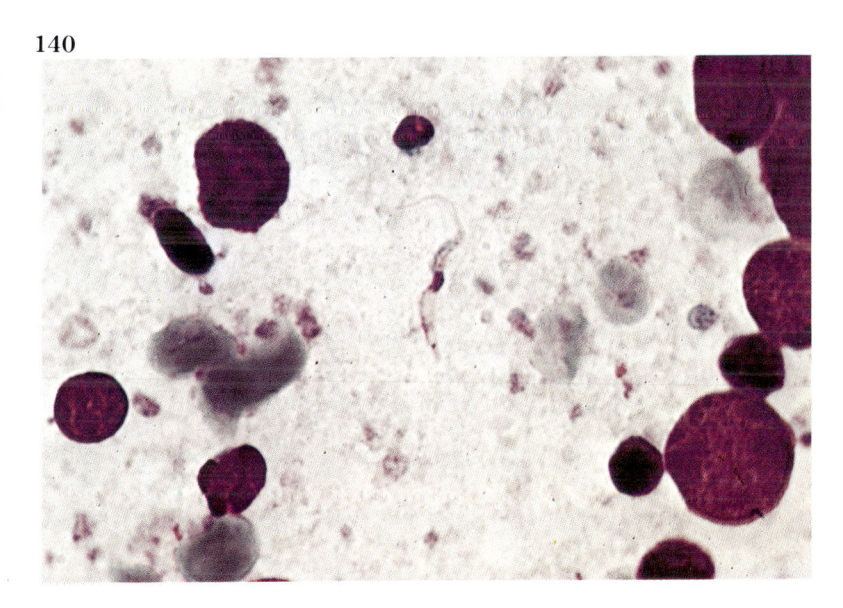

141 Sleeping sickness In the absence of treatment, the patient with gambiense infection becomes progressively more wasted and comatose, finally showing the classical picture of sleeping sickness as the CNS becomes involved. Although infection with *T. b. rhodesiense* often leads to death from toxic manifestations before CNS changes are evident, this man who was infected in Juba, southern Sudan, displayed early cerebral manifestations.

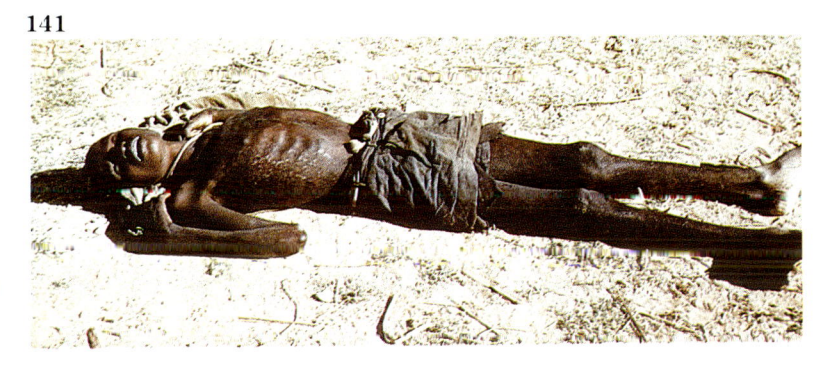

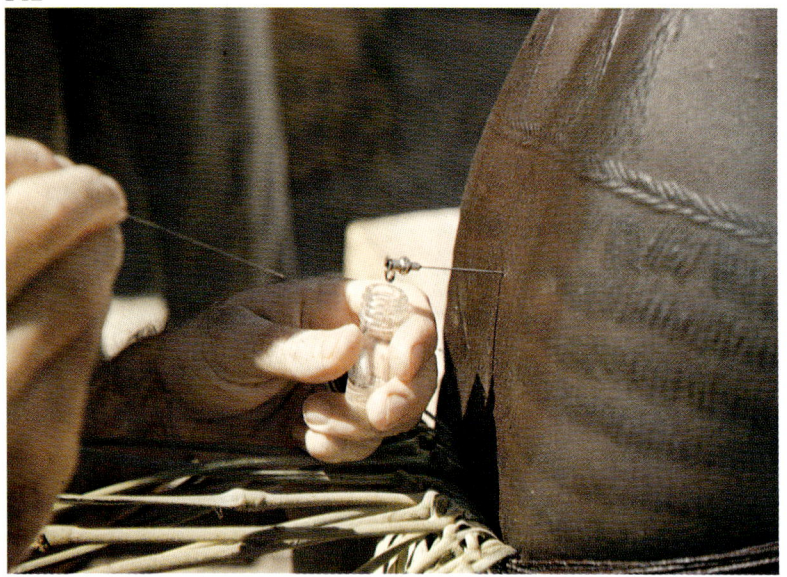

142 Lumbar puncture This procedure should be carried out to determine whether the CNS has been invaded. In such instances, the CSF will reveal a lymphocytic pleocytosis, an increased protein content and trypanosomes may be found in stained films of the centrifuge deposit. In *T. b. rhodesiense* infection, invasion of the CNS may occur within four to eight months, whereas several years usually elapse before meningoencephalitis develops in gambiense disease.

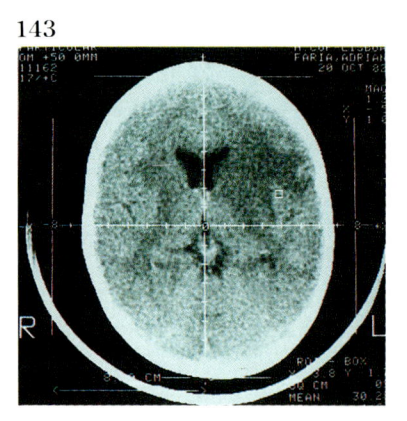

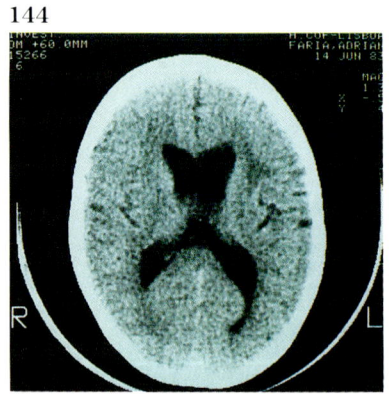

143 & 144 Cerebral changes in *T. b. rhodesiense* infection Computerised tomography shows evidence of cerebral involvement prior to treatment (**143**) and atrophic changes with hydrocephalus nine months after clinical cure (**144**) in this young child.

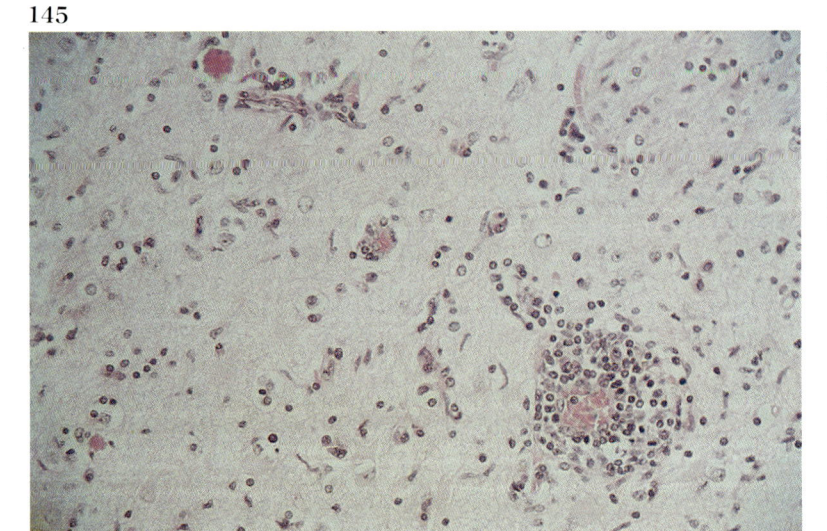

145 Microscopic changes in brain The leptomeninges are congested, there may be oedema and small haemorrhages are commonly present. The basic pathological change is a meningoencephalitis in which perivascular cuffing with round cells is often pronounced. (*H&E × 200*)

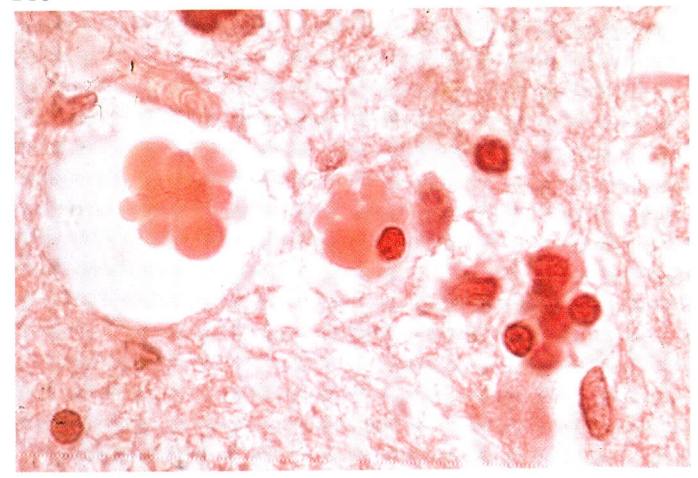

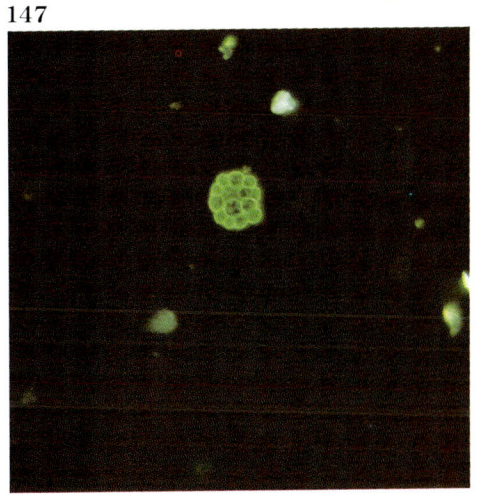

146 & 147 Morula cells in brain Scattered irregularly through the brain substance there occur large eosinophilic mononuclear cells (**146**) with eccentric nuclei known as morula cells of Mott. (*H&E × 2 000*) These are IgM-producing plasma cells as shown in this preparation (**147**) treated with anti-IgM antibody. (× *1 250*)

148 Card Agglutination Test for Trypanosomiasis (CATT) Antitrypanosomal IgM, which is raised both in the blood and the CSF in trypanosomiasis, can be detected by this simple test which is invaluable for rapid diagnosis, especially in field surveys. Other valuable serological aids are the CFT, quantitative IgM radial immunodiffusion assay and FAT. In the CATT test card shown here the presence of blue granular deposits in wells 4 and 8 are indicative of infection.

149 'Minocolumn' separation of trypanosomes The Sephadex 'minocolumn', which permits the detection of very small numbers of trypanosomes in specimens of blood or CSF, can be an invaluable diagnostic aid in individual patients and has even been employed in field surveys. Once eluted from the base of the column, even a single parasite is readily identified under the microscope.

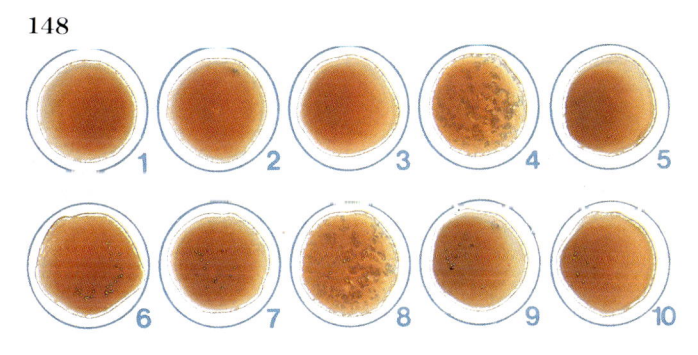

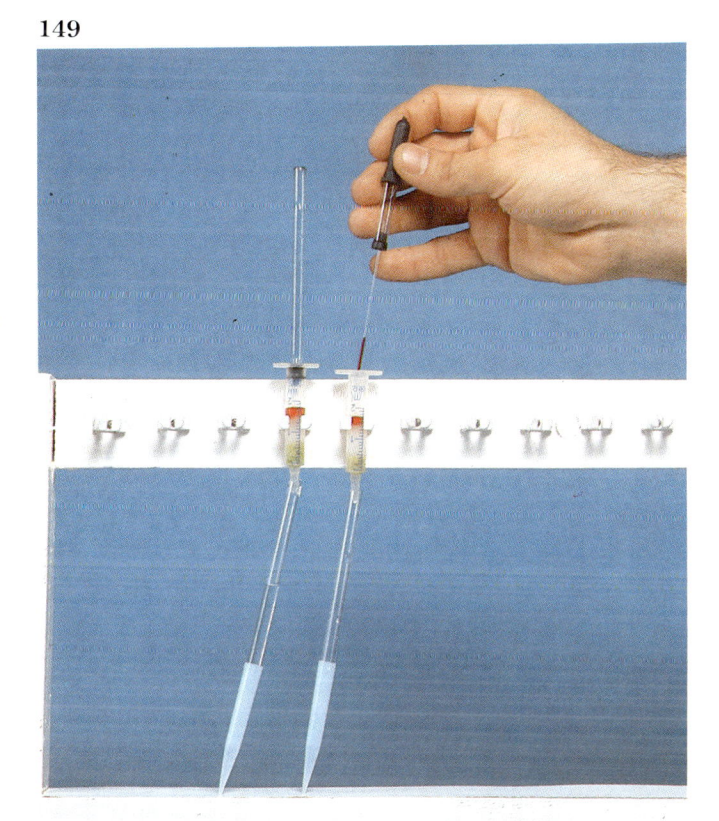

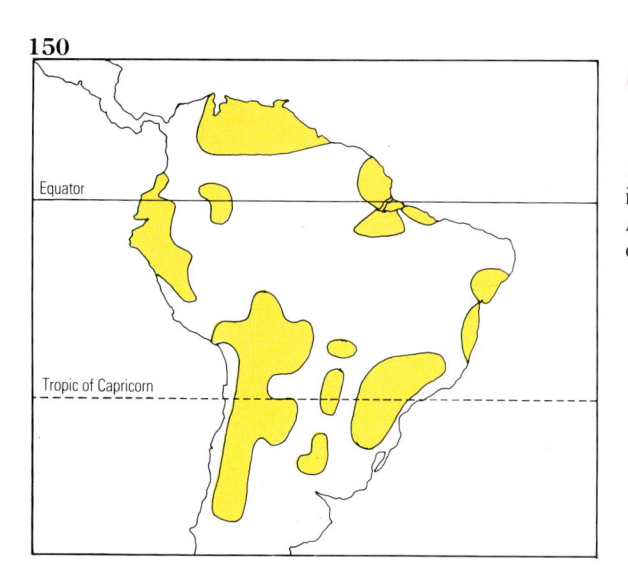

Chagas' Disease

150 Distribution of Chagas' disease Human infection is endemic in parts of Central and South America from the Andes to the Atlantic coast and as far south as the latitude of the River Plate.

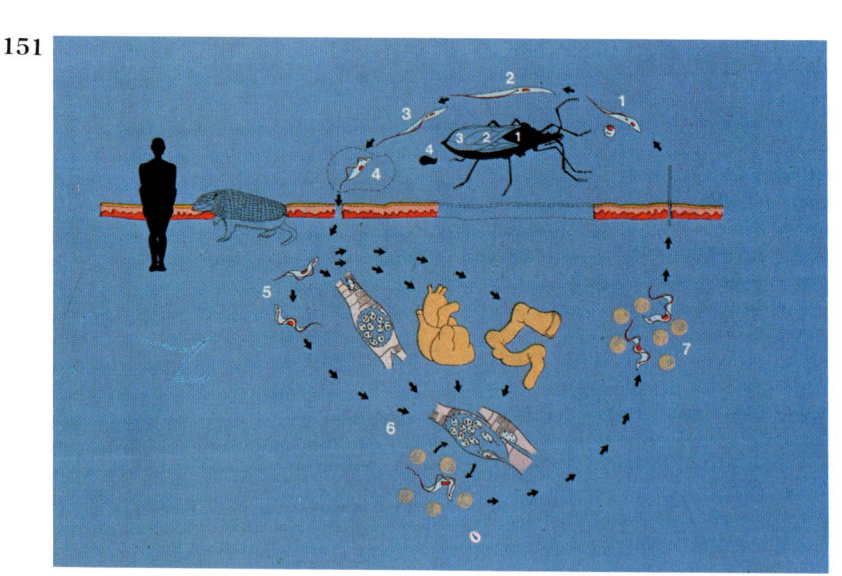

151 Life cycle in man and triatomid bugs Metacyclic trypanosomes (4) of *Trypanosomi cruzi* passed in the faeces of infected triatomid bugs (A) penetrate the skin or mucous membranes to reach the blood (5). They enter various muscular tissues, e.g. cardiac muscle (B), smooth muscle of the gut (C) or skeletal muscle (D). Here they transform to amastigotes which divide, producing pseudocysts. Subsequently, the daughter amastigotes transform back to trypomastigotes (6 & 7). These enter the blood from which they may reinvade muscular tissues, or be picked up by another triatomid bug when it feeds. In the bug the parasites transform to epimastigotes (1-3) which divide in the gut. Finally, some epimastigotes pass to the hindgut where they transform back to infective, metacyclic trypomastigotes (4) which are passed in the faeces as the bug next feeds.
(*See also* **152-155, 159**)

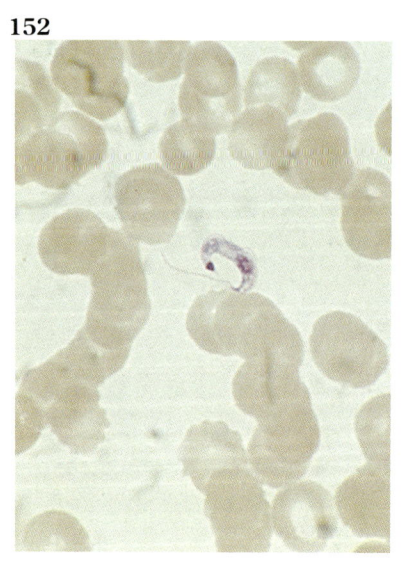

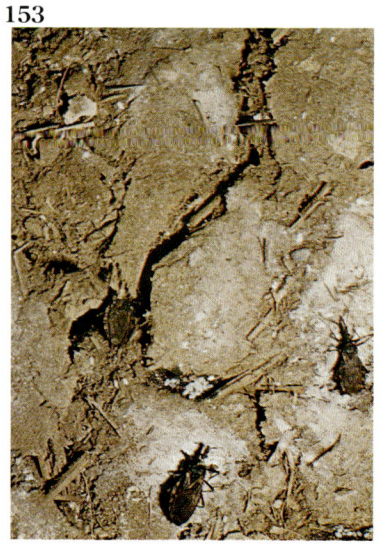

152 *T. cruzi* in human blood film The causative agent is *T. cruzi*. It occurs characteristically in blood films as short 'C' or 'S' shaped trypomastigotes with a prominent kinetoplast. It is otherwise monomorphic. (*Giemsa × 950*)

153 Ecology of vectors The favourite habitats of the reduviid bugs are cracks in the walls of mud huts in poor rural areas. Here the insects shelter and breed. Transmission occurs predominantly at night.

154 Typical vector biting
Reduviid bugs (also known as 'assassin' or 'kissing' bugs), particularly in the genera *Triatoma*, *Rhodnius* and *Panstrongylus*, transmit *T. cruzi* while feeding, not by inoculation but by faecal contamination. (× 3)

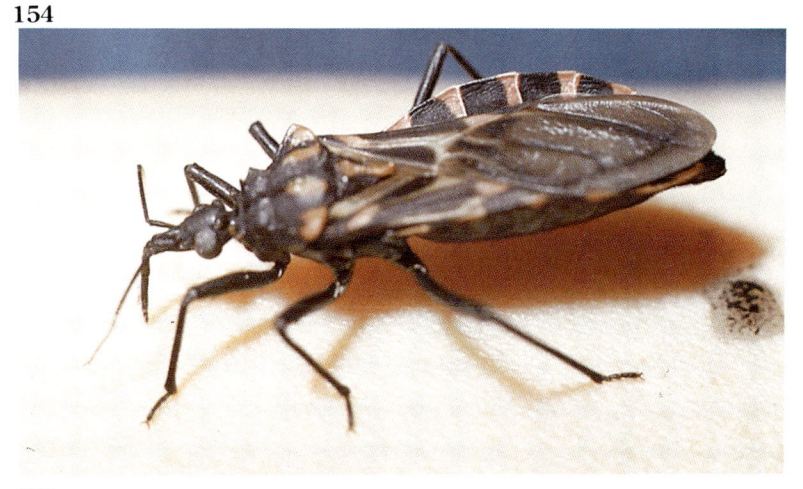

155 Metacyclic and epimastigote stages in faeces Infection is through contamination by metacyclic parasites (left) in bug faeces produced on the skin. These may invade the site of the bite or adjacent mucosa (e.g. the conjunctiva). (*Giemsa* × 1 500)

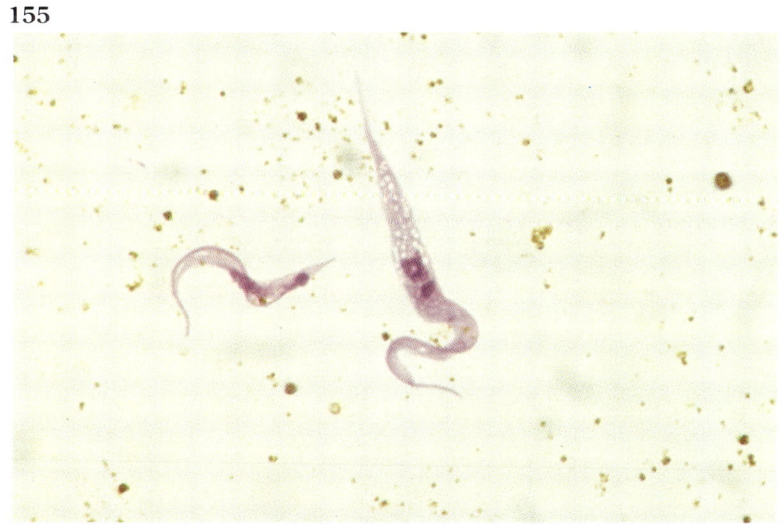

156 & 157 Reservoir hosts of *T. cruzi* Chagas' disease is a zoonosis. *T. cruzi* has an extensive mammalian reservoir both in wild hosts, especially armadillos (**156**) and opossums (**157**), as well as some domestic animals.

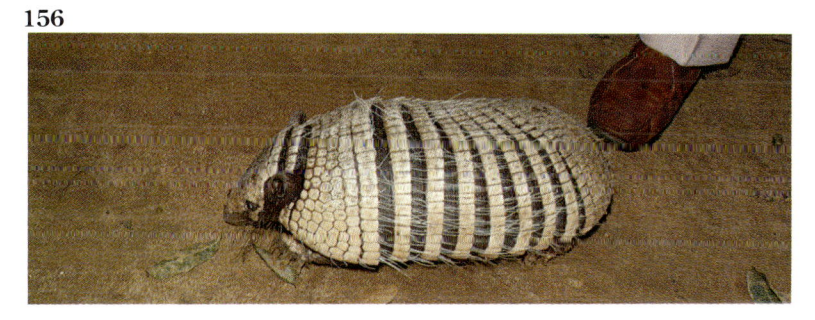

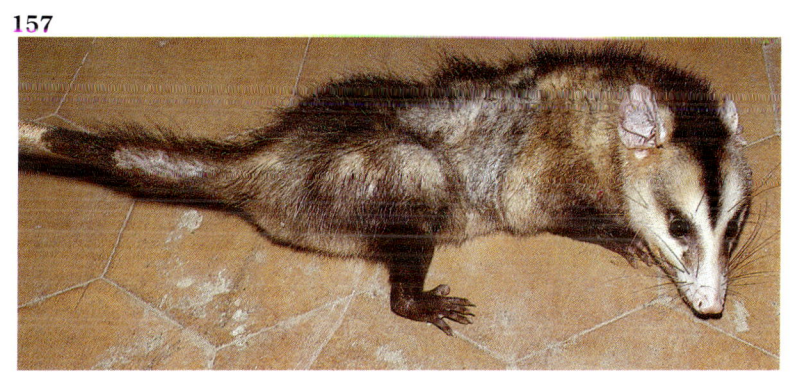

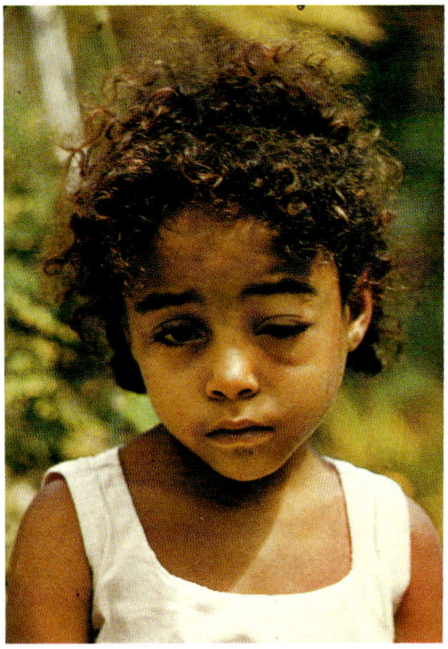

158 Romaña's sign The infection often begins with a local lesion, the chagoma. It causes marked local oedema which, should it occur in the region of the eye or within the conjunctival sac, is accompanied by swelling of the lids and chemosis. These unilateral periorbital changes constitute Romaña's sign.

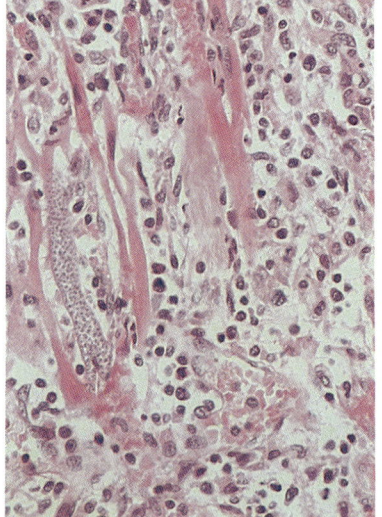

159 Amastigotes in heart muscle After a stage of initial parasitaemia associated with fever (often unrecognised), trypomastigotes pass to the cardiac muscle and smooth muscle lining the intestinal tract. Here they transform to the amastigote stage (Leishman-Donovan bodies) in which they multiply to form pseudocysts. In the heart this is associated with severe myocarditis, especially in the early stages of the infection. The severity of the acute myocarditis seems to seal the eventual fate of the sufferer from chronic cardiac changes. (*Giemsa × 200*).

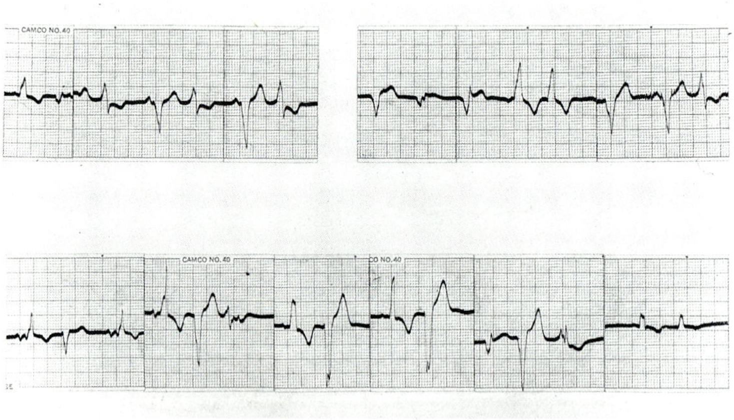

160 ECG showing heart block Dysrhythmias of various types and degrees are a characteristic feature of Chagas' disease. Complete heart block with Stokes-Adams attacks can occur and may result in sudden death.

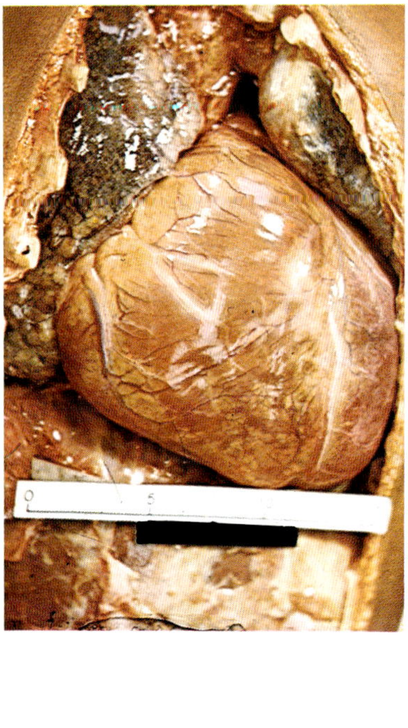

161 Cardiomegaly The heart shows gross enlargement and dilatation. The dilatation of the right atrium and both ventricles is marked in this specimen. The pathogenesis seems to be associated with a loss of autonomic control due to destruction of the ganglionic plexuses. Auto-antibodies are probably involved in this process (*see 163*).

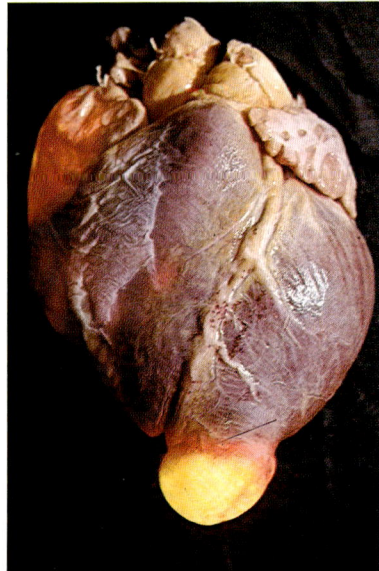

162 Apical aneurysm of heart Mural thrombi may be present at the apex of the left ventricle, with marked thinning of both ventricular walls. Apical aneurysmal formation is commonly seen.

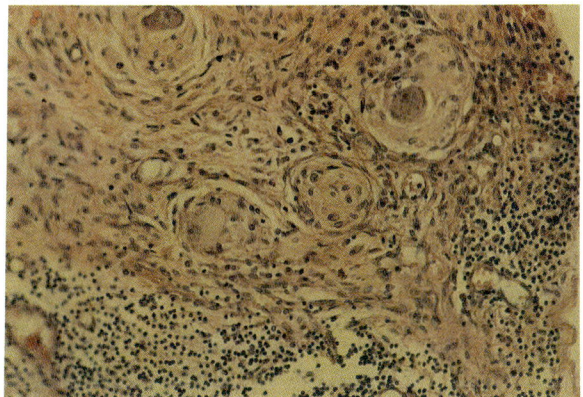

163 Sympathetic ganglion in wall of atrium
Degenerative changes in neuronal cells from a ganglion in the heart of a patient with Chagas' disease who died of sudden cardiac failure. Mononuclear cellular infiltration is conspicuous, especially round the capsule of the ganglion. (H&E × 150)

164 X-ray of mega-oesophagus Muscular degeneration and denervation of segments of the alimentary tract through destruction of the cells of Auerbach's plexus cause mega-oesophagus, megastomach, and megacolon, etc. which can be detected radiologically.

165 Post-mortem of patient with megacolon Gross megacolon is shown here in a woman who died of chronic Chagas' disease.

166 Xenodiagnosis Absolute confirmation of active infection is obtained by demonstrating that the patient can infect the vector (xenodiagnosis). Laboratory-bred, clean reduviid bugs are fed on patients suspected of having trypanosomiasis. Two weeks later the hindgut is dissected out and is examined for metacyclic trypanosomes.

167 ELISA test An ELISA test employing antigen from epimastigotes of *T. cruzi* cultivated *in vitro* is widely used, and is one of the most sensitive means of diagnosis. It can indicate past or present infection and does not necessarily imply the presence of parasites. Five positive reactions are shown in this microtitre plate in which an immunoperoxidase procedure was followed. The Machado-Guerreiro test is no longer in general use.

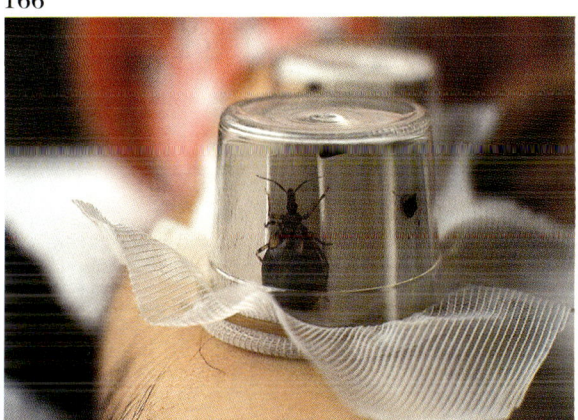

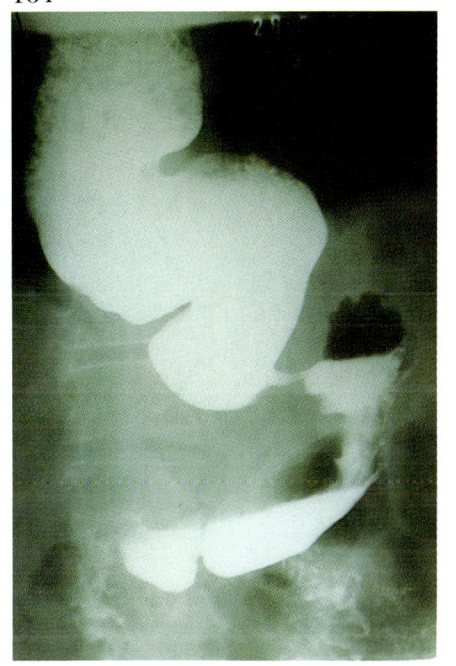

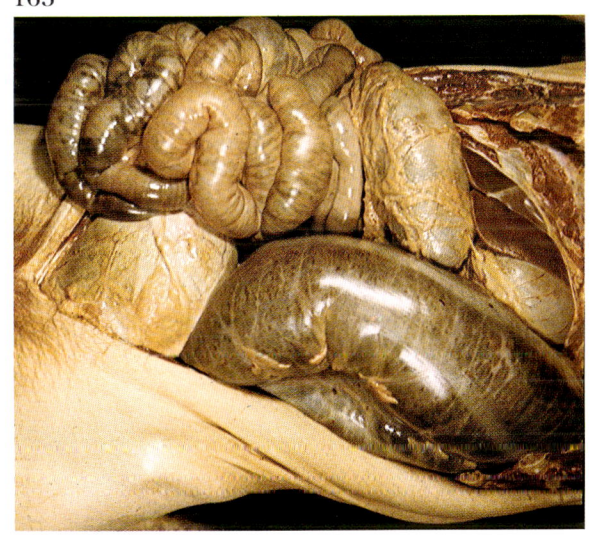

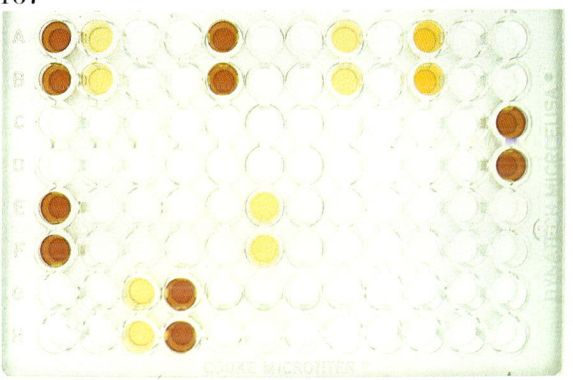

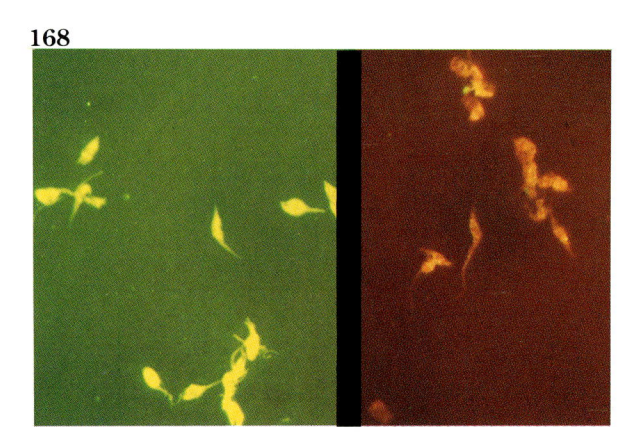

168 Immunofluorescence of *T. cruzi* Fluorescent antibody tests may also be employed using whole cultured epimastigotes as the antigen. (× *600*) (*Right*: negative control)

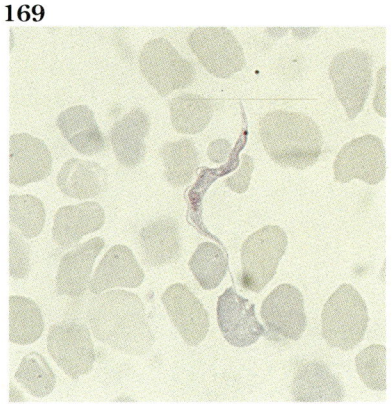

169 *Trypanosoma rangeli*
T. rangeli is a long, slender trypanosome also transmitted by reduviid bugs from wild animals to man. It is readily distinguished by its shape from *T. cruzi* in blood films and appears to be non-pathogenic to man.
(*Giemsa × 950*)

LEISHMANIASIS (*See* Table VIII)

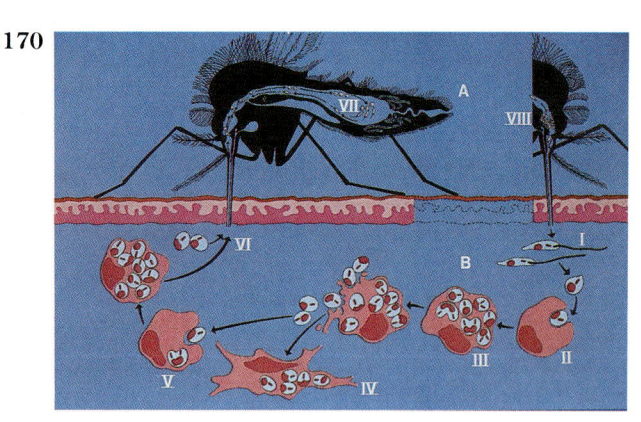

170 Life cycle of *Leishmania* Promastigotes (I) enter the skin of a vertebrate host (B) when the sandfly (A) bites, and transform into amastigotes which are phagocytosed by macrophages (II). In the macrophages the amastigotes divide (III), finally rupturing the host cell. They then enter either macrophages of the reticuloendothelial organs (IV) or of the skin (V) where they continue to divide. Some parasites circulate in mononuclear macrophages of the blood, and are picked up in these, or with skin macrophages (VI) when another sandfly bites. In the fly (A) they transform into promastigotes in the midgut, then migrate forward or backward (depending upon the species of *Leishmania*) to attach to the gut wall and multiply as promastigotes. Finally, they migrate forward to the pharynx and proboscis (VIII) from which they enter the skin of a new vertebrate host when the fly takes another meal. (*See also* **171, 173, 178, 193, 194, 207 & 221**.)

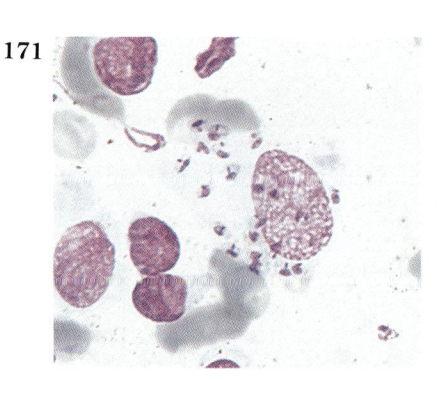

171 Amastigotes of *L. infantum* in a macrophage from dog skin
The amastigotes of different species are very similar on light microscopy, apart from their sizes, and can be distinguished even by experts only to a limited degree. (*Giemsa × 950*).

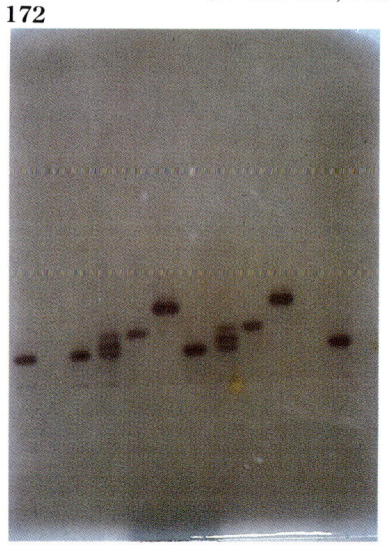

172 Isoenzyme electrophoresis, a tool for biochemical taxonomy
A widely used method for identifying species of *Leishmania* (also of considerable value for other parasites, e.g. trypanosomes, amoebae, schistosomes and their molluscan hosts) is the characterisation of isoenzymes by electrophoresis on starch gel or other bases. This figure of duplicate specimens of five *Leishmania* isolates illustrates banding of glucose phosphate isomerase in four distinct patterns, each of which indicates a different species. Two of the pairs are identical.

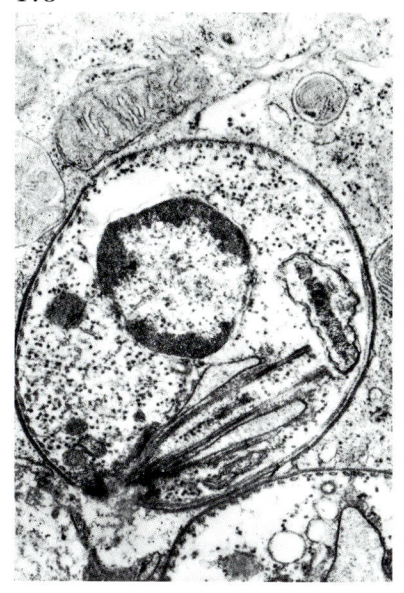

173 Ultrastructure of amastigotes Leishmanial amastigotes are seen within a parasitophorous vacuole in the host cell. The short flagellum (or mastigote) does not extend beyond the outer cell membrane in this stage. ($\times$ 30 000).

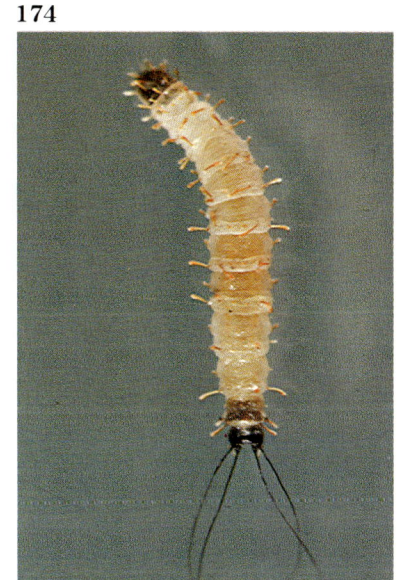

174 Sandfly larva *Leishmania* are transmitted by sandflies of the genus *Phlebotomus* in the Old World and Far East, and *Lutzomyia* in the New World. The photograph shows the larva of *P. perfiliewi* which is a vector of leishmaniasis in Southern Europe. In dry areas the larvae occupy cracks and crevices which provide a humid, cool microclimate. Forest species possibly prefer leaf mould on the forest floor. ($\times$ 10)

175 Pupa of *Lutzomyia longipalpis* *Lu. longipalpis* transmits visceral leishmaniasis in Brazil. ($\times$ 10)

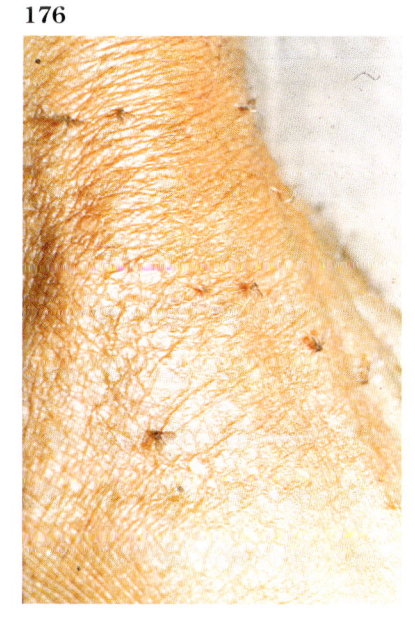

176 Adult female *Lu. longipalpis* biting This figure gives an impression of the small size of these flies. (*natural size*)

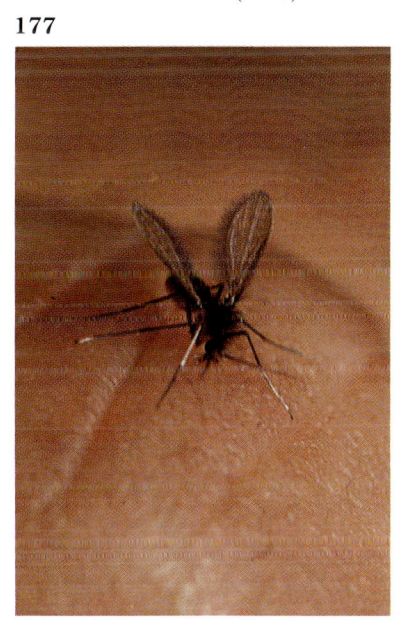

177 Close up view of *Lu. longipalpis* ($\times$ 10)

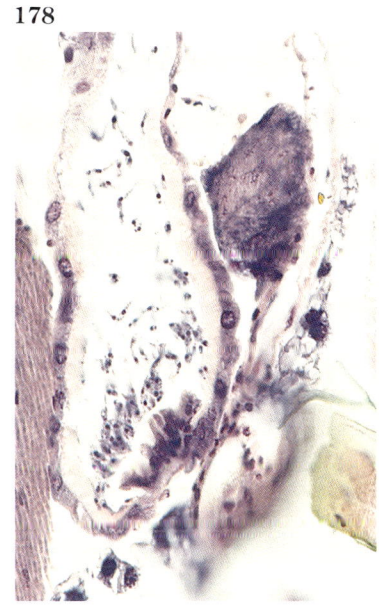

178 Promastigotes in vector midgut In the midgut of the poikilothermic vector, amastigotes transform to promastigotes which then divide asexually. (*Giemsa* $\times$ 1 150)

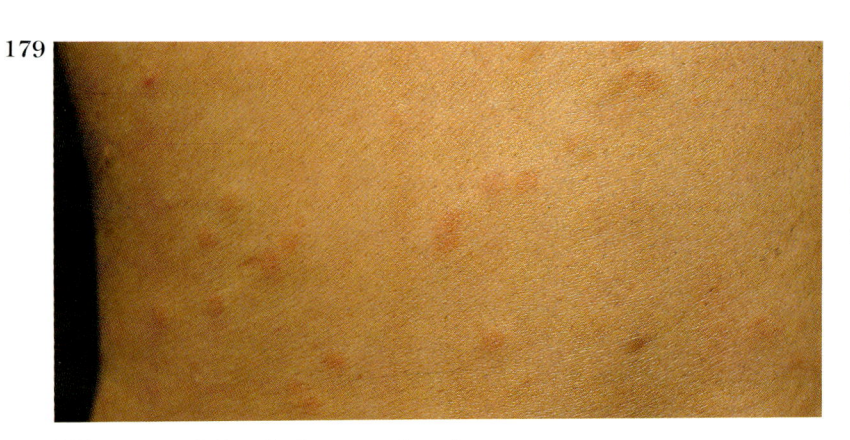

179 Reaction to sandfly bites A persistent macule appears at the site of each bite, even from an uninfected fly. This may be the starting point of the lesion in simple cutaneous leishmaniasis. Multiple primary lesions occur when the sandfly probes repeatedly in the course of feeding.

Visceral Leishmaniasis
(Kala-azar, Dum-Dum Fever, Black Sickness)

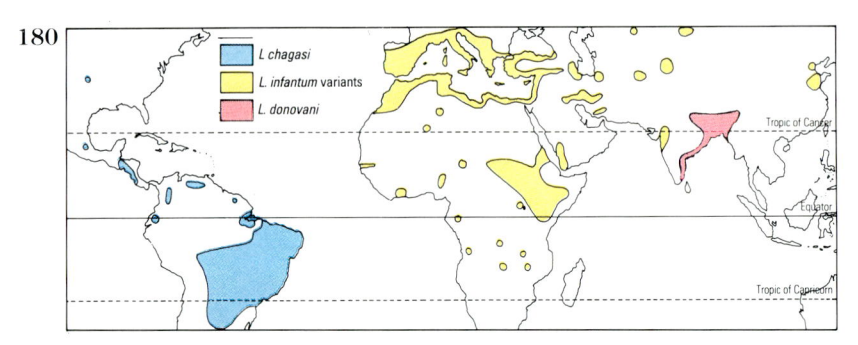

180 Distribution Visceral leishmaniasis caused by parasites of the *L. donovani-L. infantum* complex occurs in the Mediterranean littorals, the Middle East and adjacent parts of the USSR, the Sudan, East Africa, the Indian subcontinent and China, and South America ('*L. chagasi*') (see **Table VIII**). An arid warm environment provides ideal ecological conditions for the breeding of many species of sandflies. Zoonotic kala-azar due to *L. infantum* and *L. chagasi* is commonly associated with dry, rocky, hill country where cases are typically scattered. In India, *L. donovani* is essentially an anthroponosis. This type of kala-azar may occur in severe epidemic fashion as can kala-azar in the Sudan.

181 Ecology of kala-azar in India In parts of India (e.g. North Bihar) new epidemics of kala-azar have occurred in recent years. The close association between man and his domestic animals in this Bihari village favours the growth of populations of the local vector of *L. donovani*, *Phlebotomus argentipes*.

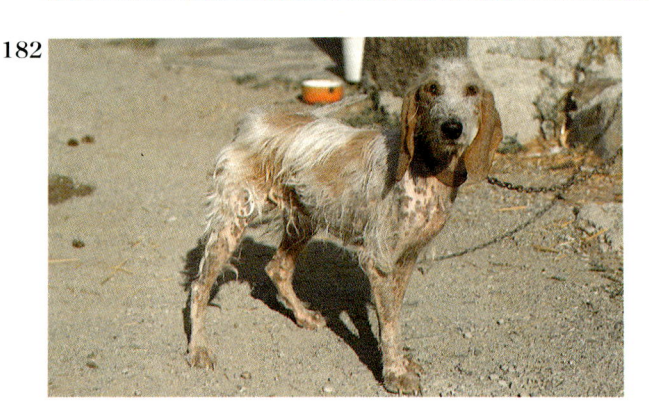

182 Reservoirs of zoonotic *L. infantum* The massive loss of hair, overgrowth of nails and generally poor condition of this dog in the Cevennes area of France are typical of chronic *L. infantum* infection. Several varieties of this parasite occurring in the Old World are distinguishable by isoenzyme typing. They can give rise to different clinical syndromes in man (e.g. cutaneous or mucocutaneous lesions, rather than kala-azar). In addition to dogs, wild carnivores and various species of rodents may serve as reservoirs for the different varieties (zymodemes) (see **Table VIII**).

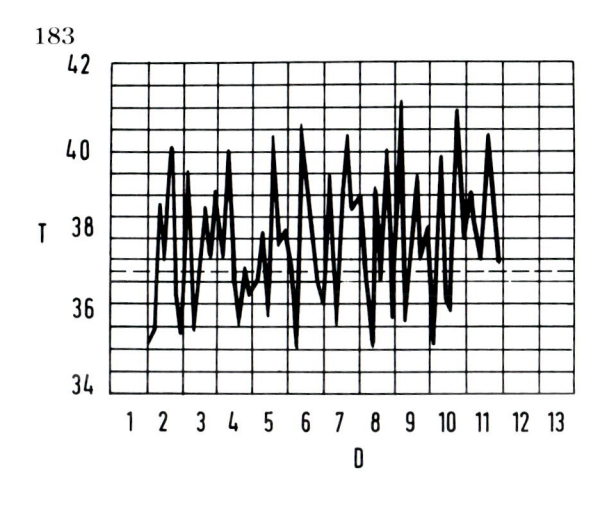

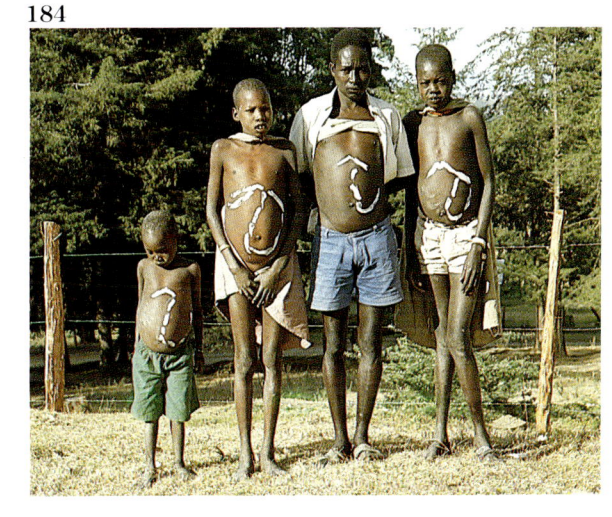

183 Temperature chart in kala-azar The temperature chart shows a double peak every 24 hours. Despite the high temperature, the patient often looks remarkably well and has a good appetite. A leucopenia with a relative lymphocytosis is often present. Kala-azar should be suspected if this picture is seen in an HIV-positive patient. (*See also* **828**.)

184 Clinical picture of kala-azar in Kenya Increasing enlargement of the spleen and liver is a characteristic feature while, in dark-complexioned subjects, deepening skin pigmentation is seen—hence the synonym of kala-azar, the 'black sickness'. A generalised lymphadenopathy is common in African kala-azar

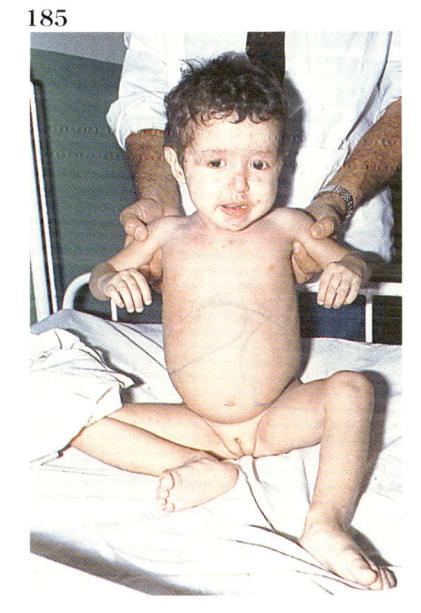

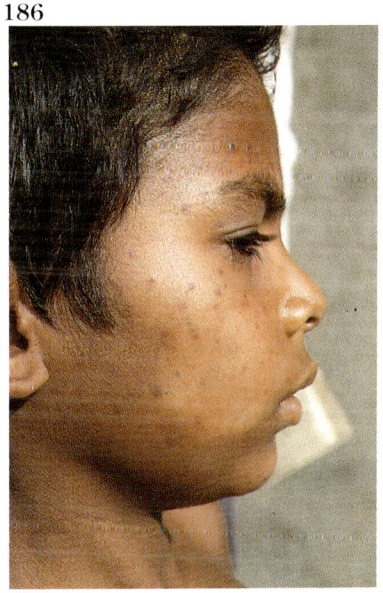

185 Infantile kala-azar Children present with chronic, irregular fever, anaemia, leucopenia and thrombocytopenia, a moderately enlarged, non-tender liver, and a greatly enlarged firm spleen. If left untreated, the infection is often fatal, commonly from secondary infections. This infant was infected in the northeast of Brazil.

186 Purpura in kala-azar The condition may present as a petechial rash if the thrombocytopenia is severe, as in this Indian boy. Petechial haemorrhages of the retina also occur not infrequently.

187 Post kala-azar dermal leishmaniasis (PKDL) This syndrome is a sequel to visceral leishmaniasis that may arise several years following successful treatment of the primary *L. donovani* infection, as in this Indian woman. Dermal lesions vary greatly in appearance and may contain amastigotes in large numbers. Some patients with hypopigmented macules may serve as reservoirs for fresh epidemics if conditions occur that favour sandfly breeding and transmission.

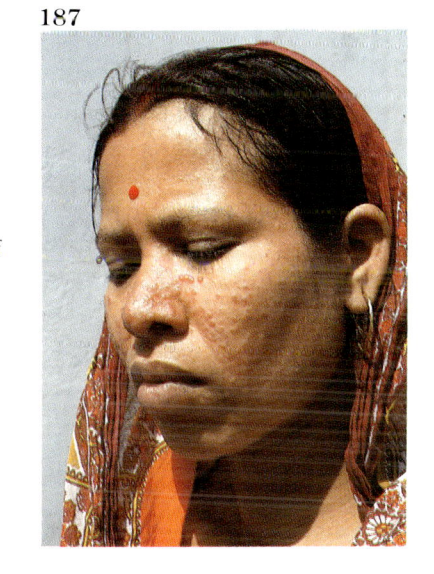

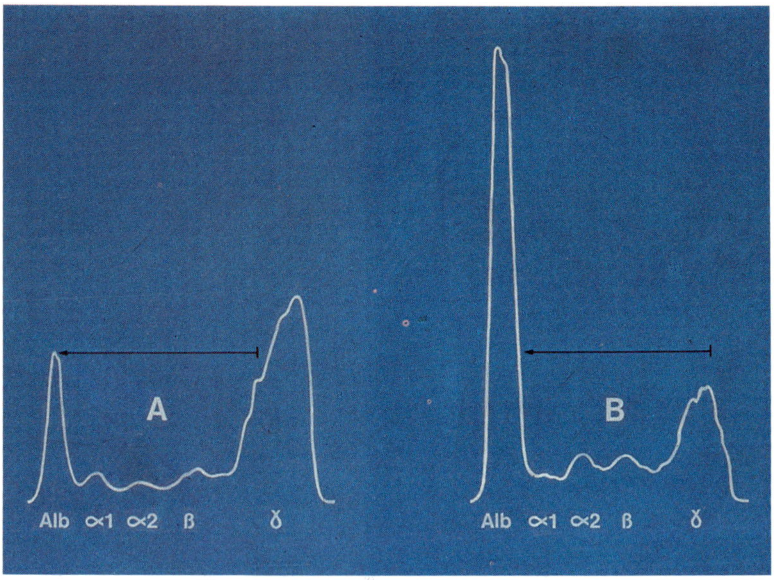

188 PKDL in a Chinese patient
The patient was completely cured by chemotherapy. This response differentiates the condition from the anergic, 'diffusa' type of leishmaniasis (*see* **220**).

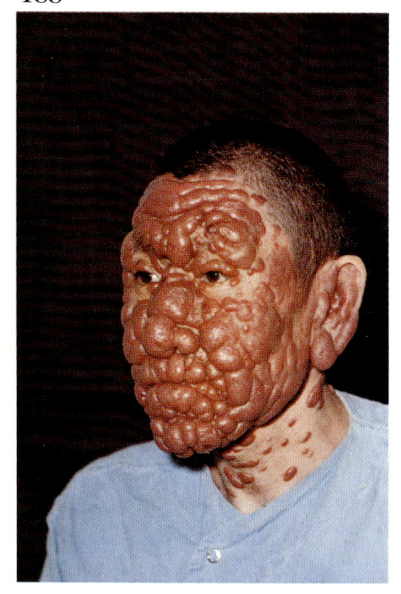

189 Serum proteins before and after treatment of kala-azar Large quantities of IgG are produced by patients with kala-azar and the A/G ratio is reversed. This may be demonstrated by electrophoresis.

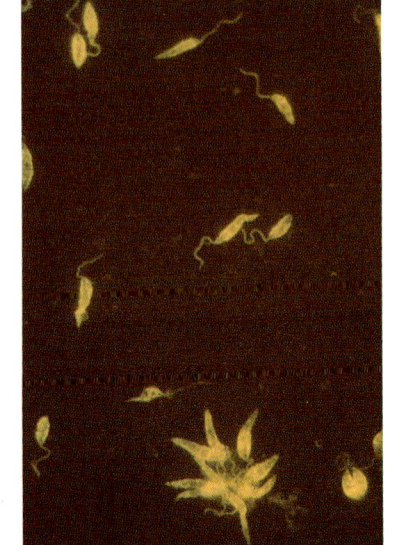

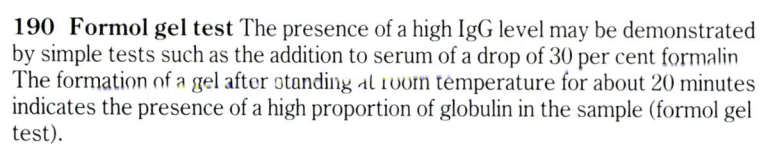

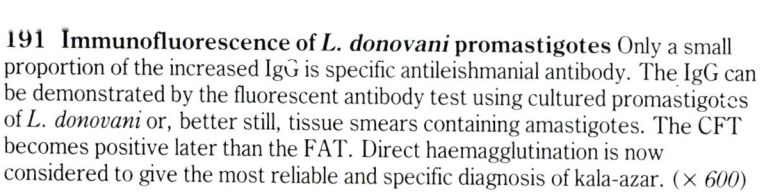

190 Formol gel test The presence of a high IgG level may be demonstrated by simple tests such as the addition to serum of a drop of 30 per cent formalin The formation of a gel after standing at room temperature for about 20 minutes indicates the presence of a high proportion of globulin in the sample (formol gel test).

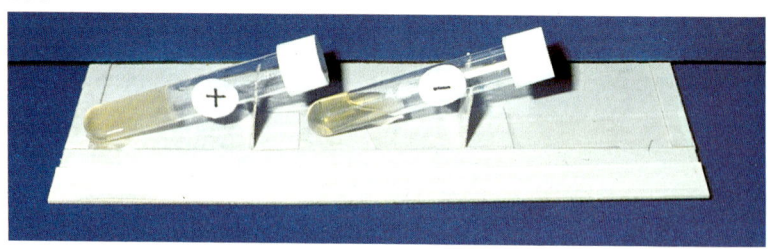

191 Immunofluorescence of *L. donovani* promastigotes Only a small proportion of the increased IgG is specific antileishmanial antibody. The IgG can be demonstrated by the fluorescent antibody test using cultured promastigotes of *L. donovani* or, better still, tissue smears containing amastigotes. The CFT becomes positive later than the FAT. Direct haemagglutination is now considered to give the most reliable and specific diagnosis of kala-azar. (× *600*)

192 Iliac crest puncture of bone marrow The principal means of diagnosis of kala-azar is the detection of amastigotes in bone marrow, spleen or blood. The organisms are recognised in dried smears of material stained with a Romanowsky stain by their characteristic morphology.

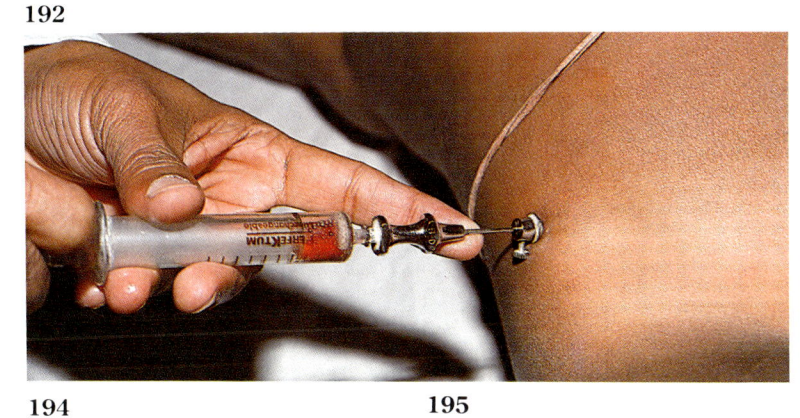

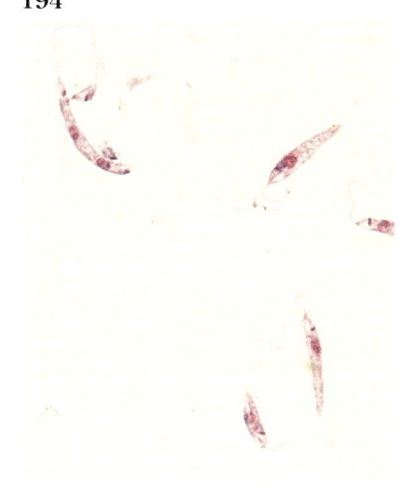

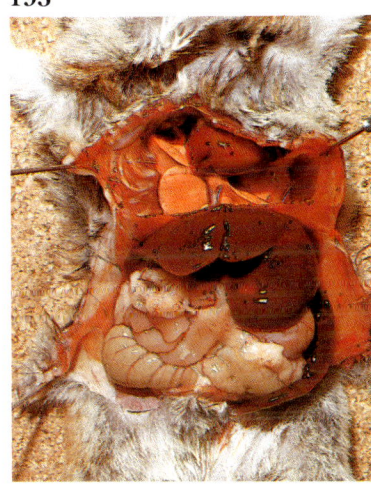

193 *L. infantum* in macrophage from bone marrow While typically found in macrophages as shown here, isolated extracellular amastigotes from disrupted host cells are commonly seen in such preparations. (*Giemsa* × *950*)

194 Promastigotes in NNN culture After inoculation of aspirated material into appropriate media such as blood agar (NNN medium, i.e. Novy-Nicolle-MacNeal) and incubation at 28°C for one to four weeks, promastigotes may appear in the fluid overlay. *L. donovani* is more readily isolated in culture than *L. infantum*, which sometimes grows better in Schneider's insect tissue culture medium than in NNN. (*Giemsa* × *950*)

195 Diagnosis by animal inoculation The parasites may be isolated by intrasplenic inoculation into hamsters. After four to six weeks, characteristic visceral lesions are seen macroscopically and amastigotes are found in large numbers in smears of the liver and spleen. This picture taken at autopsy shows a greatly enlarged spleen and liver.

Old World Cutaneous Leishmaniasis

196 Distribution Cutaneous leishmaniasis in the Old World is caused by *L. major*, *L. tropica*, *L. aethiopica* and certain zymodemes of the *L. infantum* complex (*see* **Table VIII**). All except *L. tropica* are essentially zoonoses that occur in scattered foci throughout the tropical and subtropical belts. Depending upon the locality, cutaneous leishmaniasis is known as Oriental sore, Aleppo button, Bouton de Biskra, Baghdad boil, Delhi sore, etc.

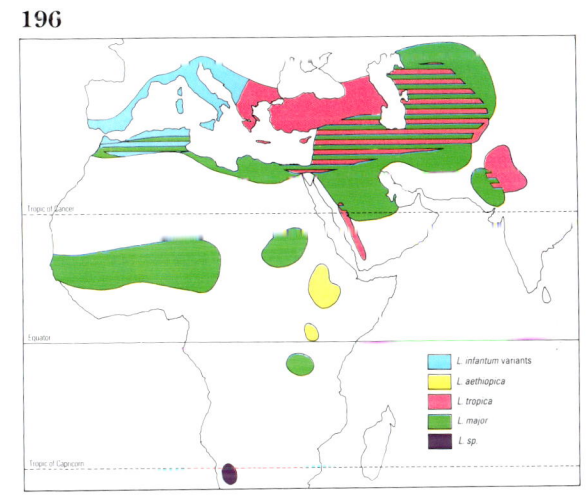

57

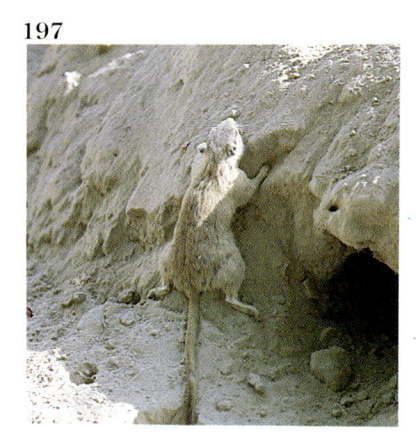

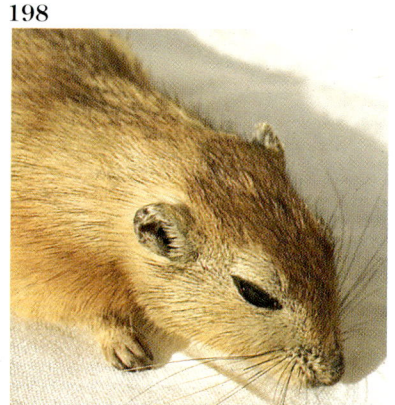

197 Animal reservoirs of *L. major* Various rodent species, such as this 'great gerbil', *Rhombomys opimus*, of eastern Iran and neighbouring parts of the USSR and the 'fat-tailed sand rat', *Psammomys obesus* (see **198**) in Libya, Israel and Saudi Arabia, are important reservoirs of *L. major*.

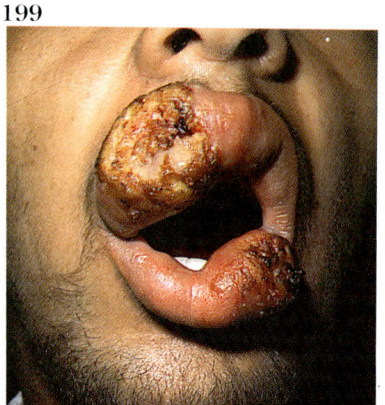

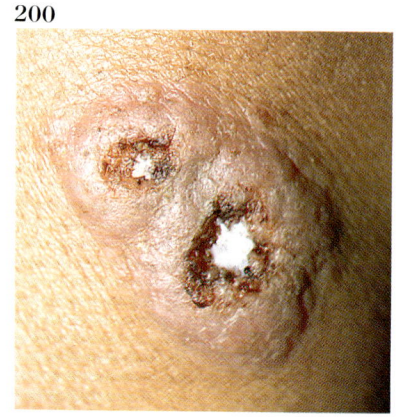

198 Ear lesion on *Psammomys obesus* These rodents and the sandflies that rest in their burrows are responsible for outbreaks of zoonotic cutaneous leishmaniasis (ZCL) in newly urbanised areas that intrude on their normal habitat, arid or even semi-desert terrain. The burrows provide ideal breeding and resting sites for for sandfly vectors such as *Phlebotomus papatasi* that transmit *L. major*, the species causing ZCL. Sandflies also rest during the day in cool deep crevices in the ground, between rocks, in caves, cellars, house walls, etc. Although the eroded ear seen here is typical of *L. major* in its natural host, many infected animals have no obvious skin lesions.

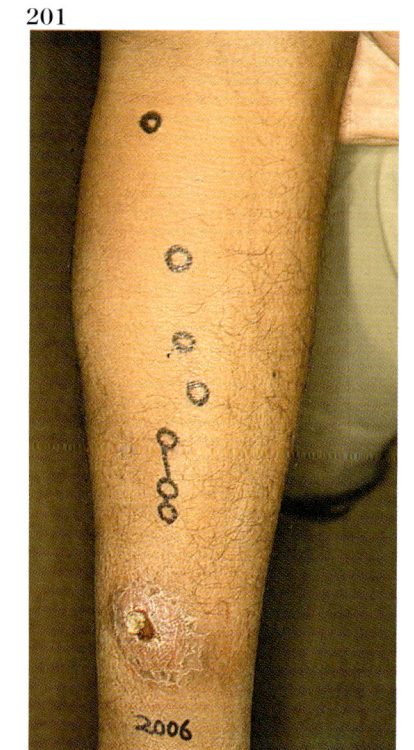

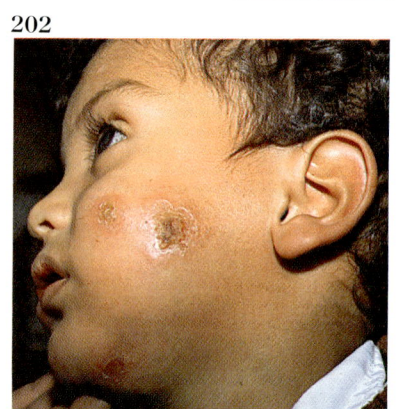

199 'Wet' lesion of mouth *L. major* occurs most commonly in rural areas, causing moist, ulcerative lesions which may be extensive and sometimes involve the epithelium of lips and nose.

200 Nodulo-ulcerative lesions of *L. major* These are the commonest types of lesion caused by *L. major*. The prominent 'rolled' edge of the lesions is the best area in which to demonstrate the parasites.

201 Lymphatic spread of *L. major* The ink marks indicate a line of subcutaneous nodules along the lymphatic passing proximally from the lesion on the lower part of this man's arm. The nodules usually resolve without complications when the primary lesion heals with or without specific therapy.

202 Simple 'dry' lesion of *L. tropica* This parasite often produces dry, usually self-healing lesions which, unlike the infection seen here, are usually single. This form was commonly seen in and around towns from North Africa and the Middle East to the USSR, Afghanistan and western states of India, especially in mountainous areas.

203 Leishmaniasis recidivans
Infection with *L. tropica* may become very chronic, a hyperallergic reaction leading to lupus-like lesions such as seen in this child in Israel.

204 Mucocutaneous leishmaniasis in Ethiopia In addition to simple cutaneous lesions due to infection with *L. aethiopica*, other forms are seen in the Ethiopian highlands where rock hyraxes are the reservoirs. It has not yet been ascertained whether the mucocutaneous condition seen here is due to this or another species of *Leishmania* (*see also* **220**).

205 Dry lesion on nose of woman in Southern France This lesion proved to be due to a zymodeme of the *L. infantum* complex.

206 Typical healed cutaneous lesion An atrophic, papery, slightly depressed scar results when healing occurs. This man was probably infected with *L. tropica* which healed spontaneously.

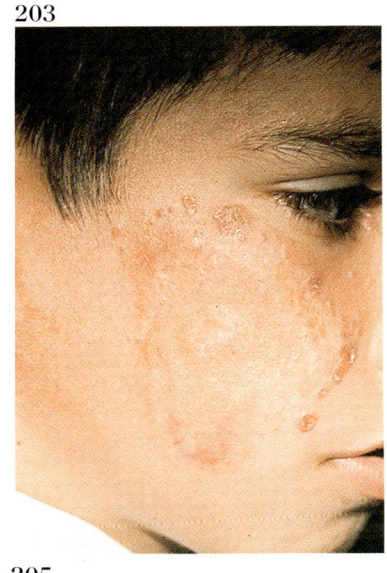

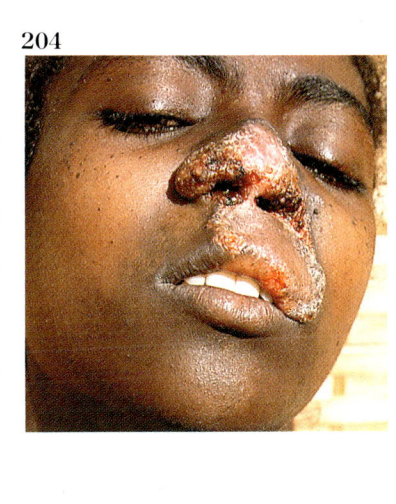

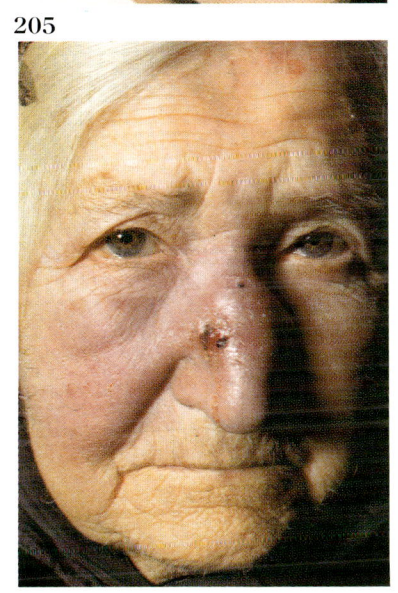

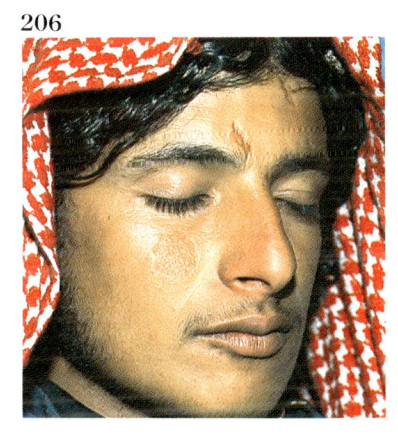

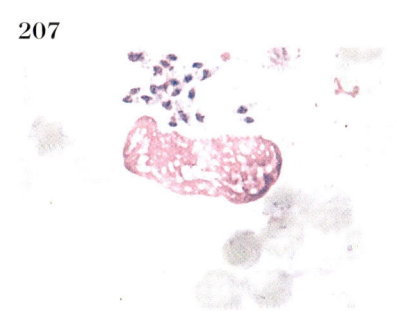

207 Amastigotes in macrophages from skin The diagnosis is confirmed by demonstrating amastigotes in smears made from the cutaneous lesions (*see comment,* **200**). Various simple techniques such as biopsy by dental broach or skin slit and scrape can be used. (*Giemsa × 950*)

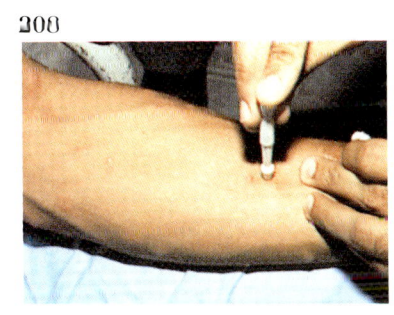

208 Punch biopsy A piece of tissue may be removed under local anaesthetic with a disposable skin punch for histology, culture and the direct demonstration of amastigotes.

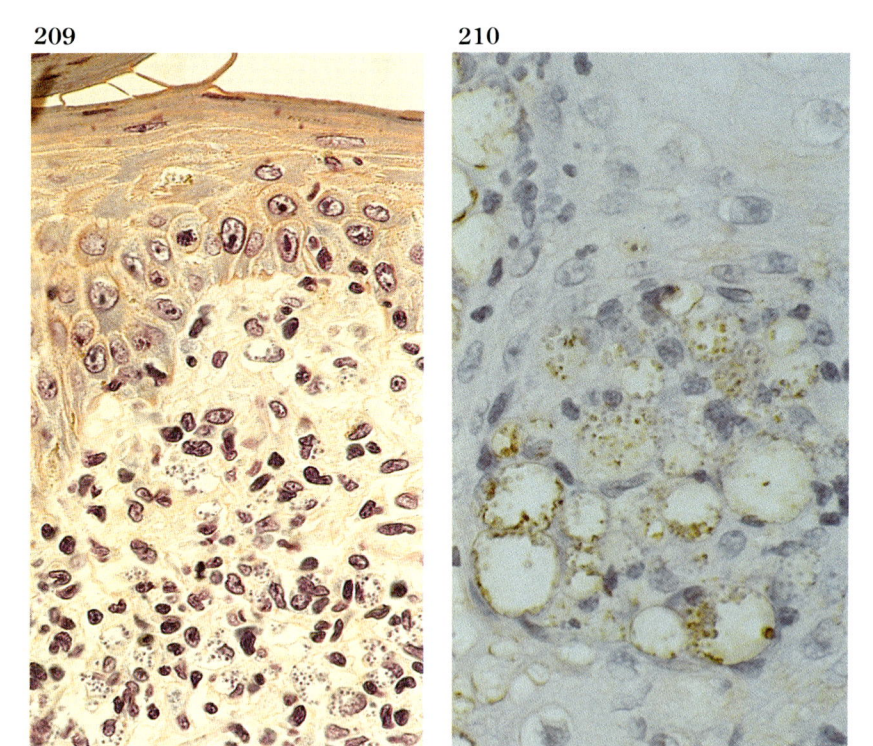

209 Parasitised macrophages in skin section Many parasitised macrophages can be seen in this section from an acute lesion caused by *L. major*. (H&E × 250)

210 Immunoperoxidase staining of *Leishmania* This procedure is very useful to demonstrate small numbers of amastigotes in tissue sections in which H&E staining is often unsatisfactory. The section shown here has many brown-staining amastigotes in parasitophorous vacuoles within mauve-staining macrophages. (× 320)

211 Montenegro test The diagnosis may be assisted by the injection of an intradermal antigen prepared from cultured promastigotes of *L. major* or other species. This produces a typical cell-mediated response (Montenegro test) in most cases of active cutaneous disease within one to two months of its onset and the test usually remains positive for life. It is negative in the active stages of kala-azar, but may become faintly positive during the course of treatment, especially in East African patients. The reaction shown in the upper (antigen) site is maximum after 48 hours. The lower site is the control.

New World Cutaneous Leishmaniasis

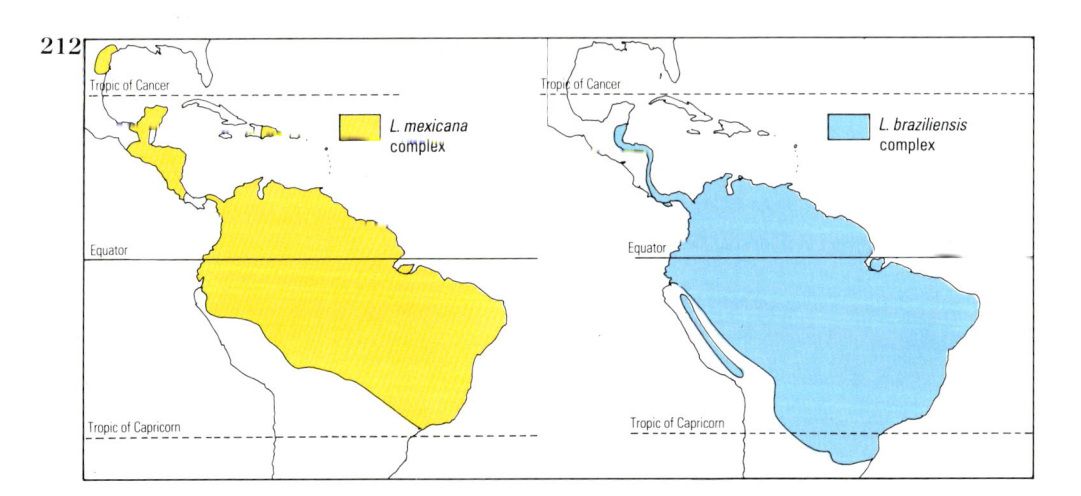

212 Distribution (including Espundia) New World cutaneous and mucocutaneous leishmaniasis ('Espundia') occur focally from Texas (USA) and Mexico southwards throughout Central America and South America as far south as São Paulo state of Brazil. The disease is limited by the Andean chain to the West except in Peru where a special form of cutaneous disease, 'Uta', is found on the western slopes of the Andes. (*See* **Table VIII**.)

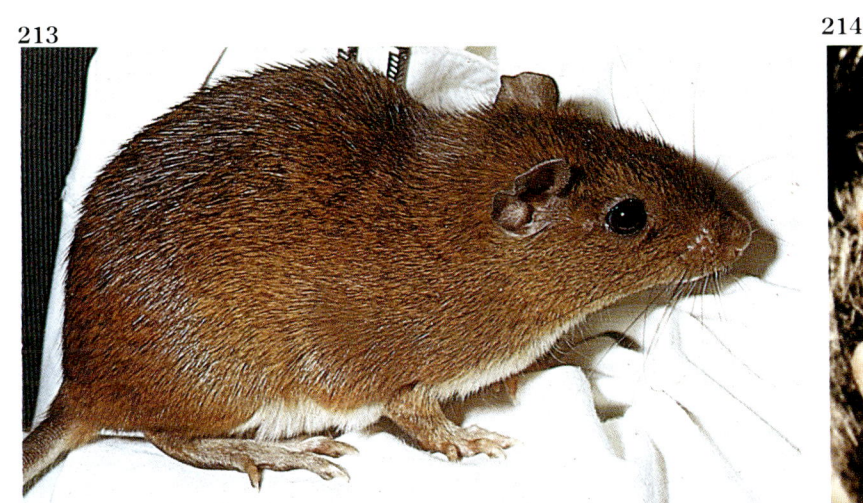

213 Rodent reservoir of *L. amazonensis* in the Brazilian rain forest
Most cutaneous leishmaniases in the New World are zoonoses associated with rodents of the rain forest. *L. amazonensis* has been isolated from this species, *Proechimys guyanensis*, in the Amazon basin of Brazil.

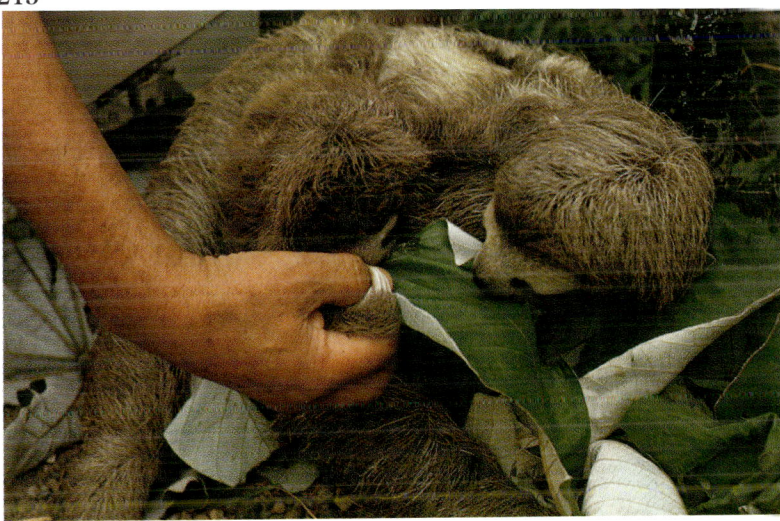

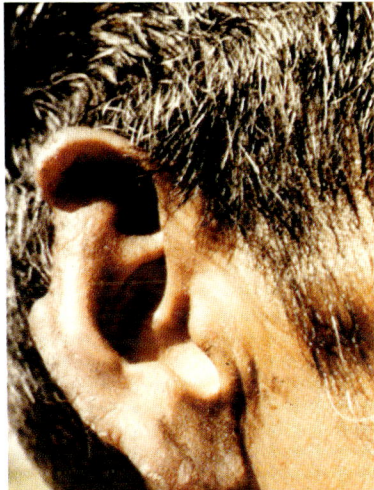

214 Chiclero's ulcer Forest workers collecting gum from wild chicle trees commonly sleep near the forest floor and are bitten on exposed parts of the head by vectors that normally maintain transmission of *L. mexicana* among the forest rodents. Ulcers leading to erosion of the auricular cartilage are known as 'chiclero's ulcers'.

215 Arboreal animals as reservoirs In other areas, e.g. Panama, Brazil, and the Guyanas, a wide variety of arboreal animals serve as reservoirs for *L. panamensis* and *L. guyanensis*. The hosts include species of monkeys, marmosets, ant-eaters and such bizarre animals as the three-toed sloth shown here in Panama.

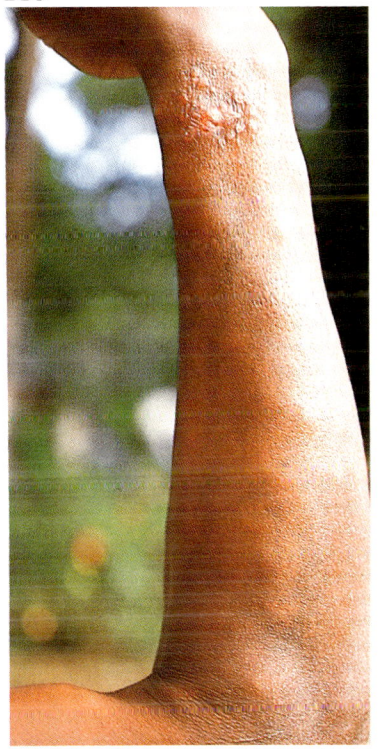

216 'Sporotrichoid' dissemination As noted for *L. major* (**201**), lymphatic spread may occur also with New World species. This patient was infected with *L. guyanensis*, the agent of 'Pian bois'. In such infections the lymphatic nodules may ulcerate, resulting in chains of 'sporotrichoid' lesions.

Mucocutaneous Leishmaniasis

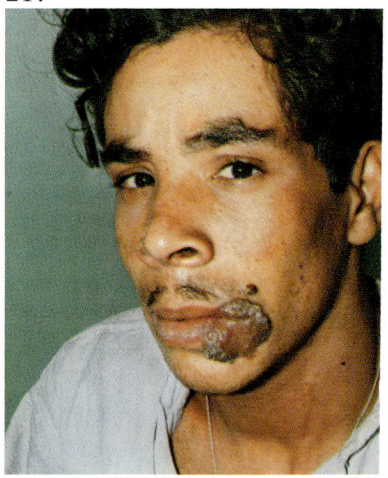

217 Early lesion of Espundia The lesions of mucocutaneous leishmaniasis due to infection with *L. braziliensis* may first become evident as ulcers involving the mucocutaneous junctions of the mouth and nose.

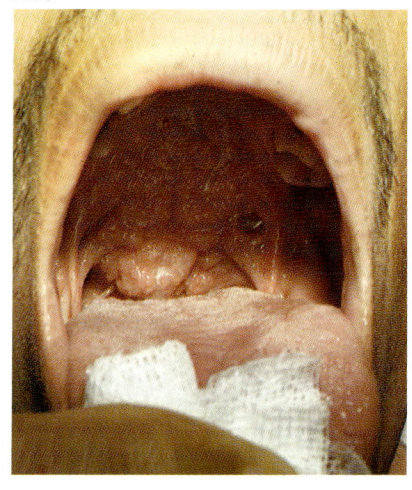

218 Pharyngeal involvement Ulceration often extends to the pharynx and soft palate, and the first symptoms may be related to tissue destruction in this area. This man had the scar of a large ulcer which had apparently healed on his leg some 30 years before.

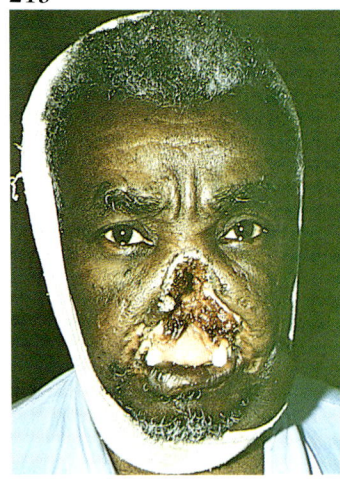

219 Destructive Espundia Gross destruction of the nose, including the septum and palate, may follow inadequate treatment of *L. braziliensis* infection. Many patients with this disease respond very poorly, if at all, to any form of chemotherapy and reparative plastic surgery is called for. The tissue destruction is probably due to cytotoxic immune complexes formed in this hyperallergic response.

Diffuse Cutaneous Leishmaniasis (DCL)

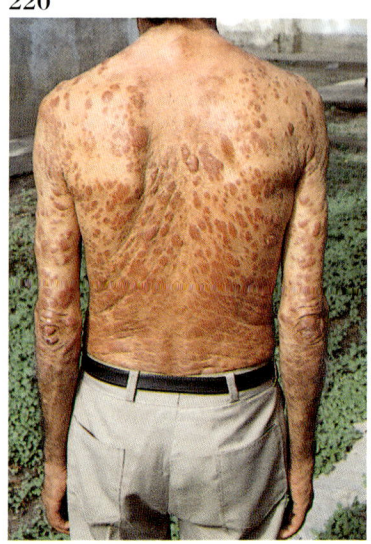

220 DCL in the New World In rare individuals, a highly specific failure of cell-mediated immunity may result in the development of chronic disseminated disease, 'Leishmaniasis diffusa', resembling lepromatous leprosy, following infection with parasites of the *L. mexicana* complex. In such cases chemotherapy, at best, produces only a temporary remission and complete cure to date is unknown. This Brazilian patient first developed lesions due to *L. amazonensis* more than 20 years before this picture was made. A similar syndrome occurs in Ethiopia and western Kenya in patients infected with *L. aethiopica*. DCL never affects the mucosae and is thus readily distinguished from Espundia or PKDL (cf. **187 & 188**).

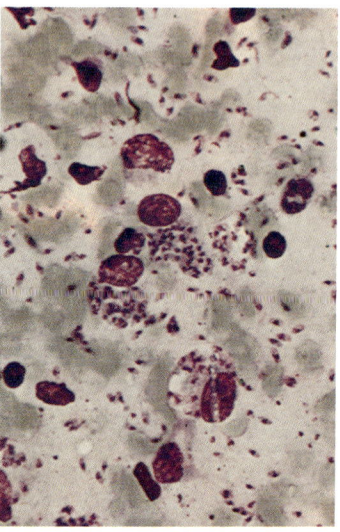

221 Skin smear in DCL This smear from a skin biopsy from an Ethiopian patient with DCL shows large numbers of amastigotes. Parasites are rarely so numerous in biopsies from patients with other forms of cutaneous leishmaniasis. (*Giemsa × 500*)

NEMATODES—THE FILARIASES (See Tables IX & X)

Wuchereria bancrofti, Brugia malayi and *Brugia timori*

222 Distribution *W. bancrofti* is widely distributed throughout the tropics. Although normally nocturnal, a subperiodic diurnal form occurs in the eastern Pacific.
B. malayi has only been recognised in Asia. The periodic form occurs in India, SE Asia and Japan. The subperiodic form occurs only in Malaysia, Borneo and the Philippines.
B. timori is localised to islands of the Lesser Sunda group of Indonesia and Timor.

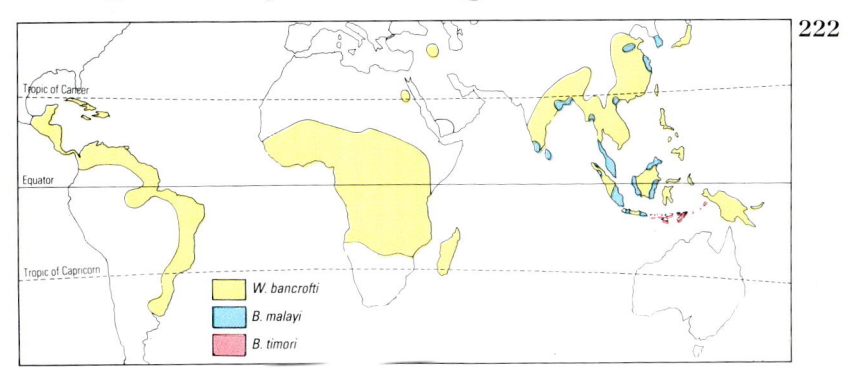

223 Newly-hatched female *Culex quinquefasciatus*. (See also **232**.) (× 3)

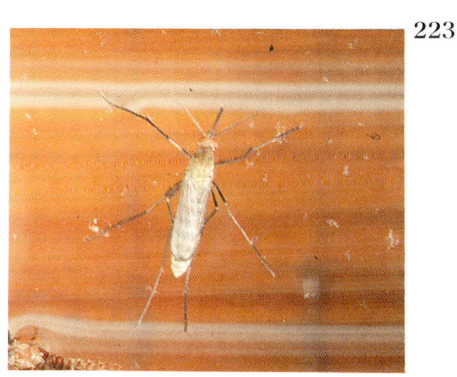

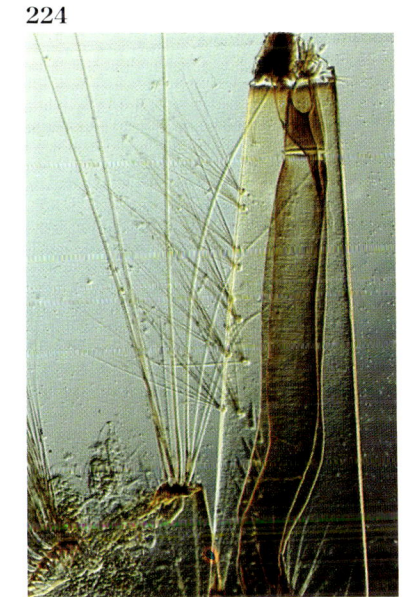

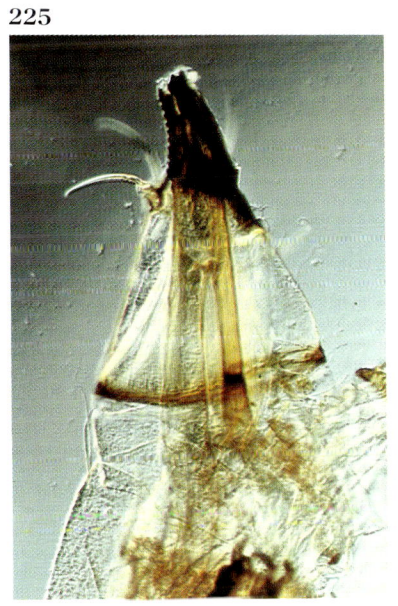

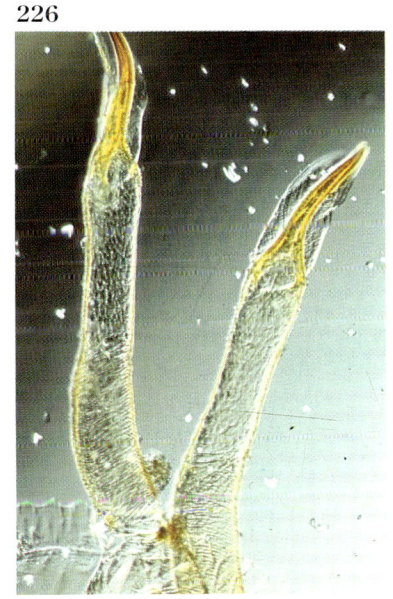

224-226 Aquatic stages of *Culex* and *Mansonia* Unlike *Anopheles* mosquitoes (*see* **6**) or those of *Culex* (**224**), *Mansonia* larvae (**225**) and pupae (**226**) are attached by their breathing tubes (siphons) to underwater roots, stems and leaves of aquatic plants. Note the saw-edged tips of the siphons used to penetrate the plants. Their ideal breeding habitats are open swamps with *Pistia*, water lilies and other aquatic plants. (× 60) (See also **2-13**.)

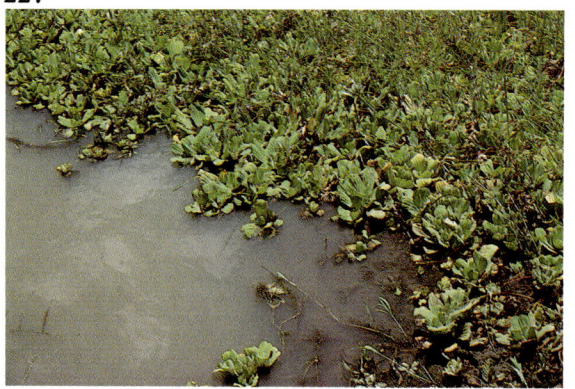

227 *Mansonia* breeding site *Pistia* growing at the edge of a swamp in western Kenya.

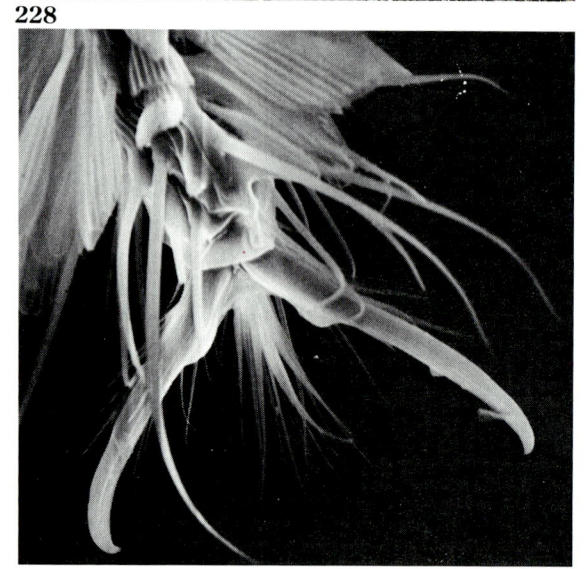

228 & 229 Tarsal claws of *Aedes* and *Culex* The tarsal claws of *Aedes* (**228**) have strong hooks and a simple pulvillus. ($\times$ *1 000*) *Culex* (**229**) has fleshy pulvilli and no hooks. ($\times$ *1 300*) (In these scanning electron micrographs the hooks are not seen in the *Aedes*. The contrast between the simple pulvillus of *Aedes* and the complex pulvillus of *Culex* is clearly demonstrated.)

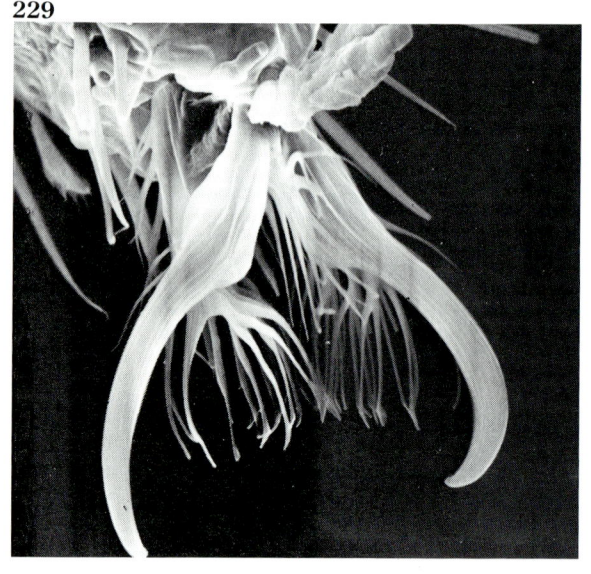

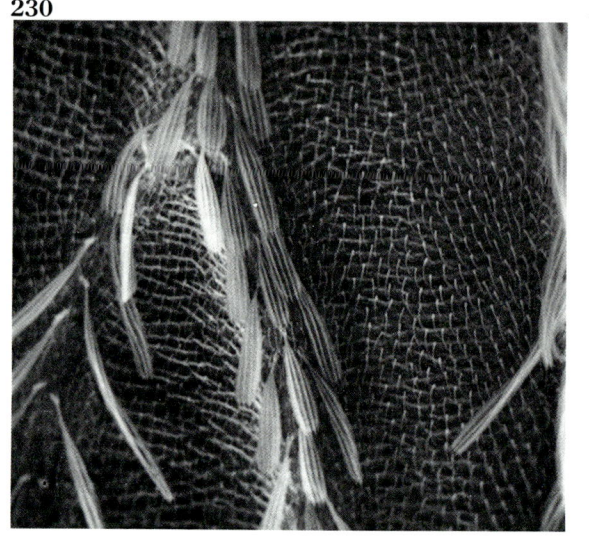

230 & 231 Wing scales of *Culex* and *Mansonia* The adults are distinguished from other culicines by the typical large wing scales. *Culex* (**230**); *Mansonia* (**231**). ($\times$ *370*)

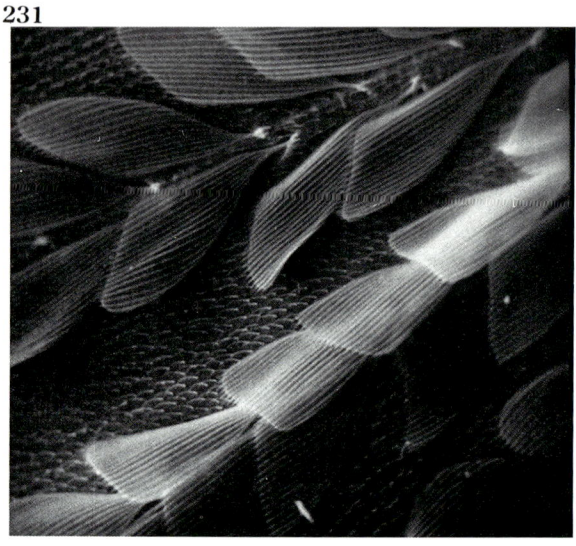

232 Peridomestic culicine breeding site near Delhi Septic pits and drains containing stagnant water are ideal breeding grounds for *Culex quinquefasciatus* which is a peridomestic vector of bancroftian filariasis.

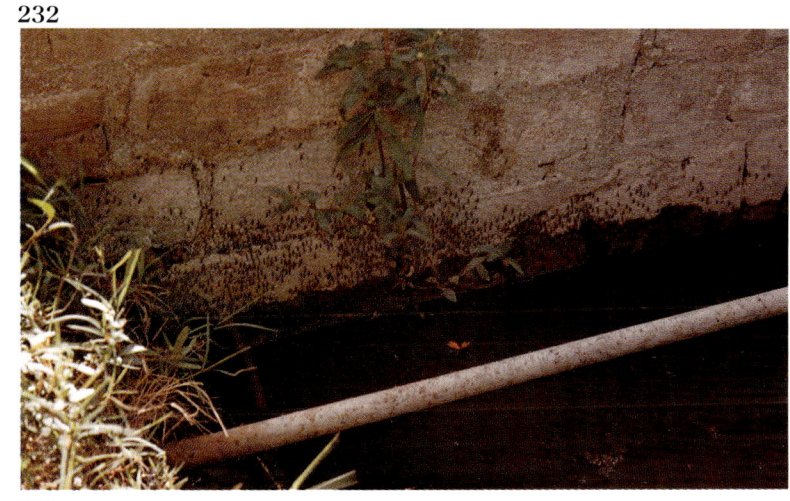

233 Life cycle of *Wuchereria bancrofti* and *Brugia malayi* Third-stage infective larvae (a) enter the mouthparts of the mosquito from which they penetrate the skin when the insect bites (b). They enter the lymphatics where the worms mature into thread-like adults (c) which can live for many years. Blockage of lymphatic vessels by the adult worms leads to elephantiasis (d) in some individuals. Larvae (e) are produced in the female worms and transform to microfilariae (f) which enter the peripheral circulation. From there they are picked up by mosquitoes with a blood meal (g). The microfilariae (h) penetrate the insect's gut wall to develop in the thoracic muscles (ij) in which they mature to the third-stage larvae. (See also **235-238, 245, 250-252**.)

234 Female *Aedes* (*Stegomyia*) *polynesiensis* Night biting *Culex quinquefasciatus* and various species of *Anopheles* are the main vectors of the nocturnal periodic form of *W. bancrofti*. Day biting *Aedes polynesiensis* transmits the subperiodic form of *W. bancrofti* in various Pacific islands. Species of *Mansonia* are the main vectors of *B. malayi*. Compare the hump-backed stance with that of *Anopheles* (**58**). (× 5)

235 Larvae in mosquito thorax Ingested microfilariae exsheath, migrate from the midgut, and penetrate the thoracic muscles where they mature to sausage-shaped first- and second-stage larvae. (× 140)

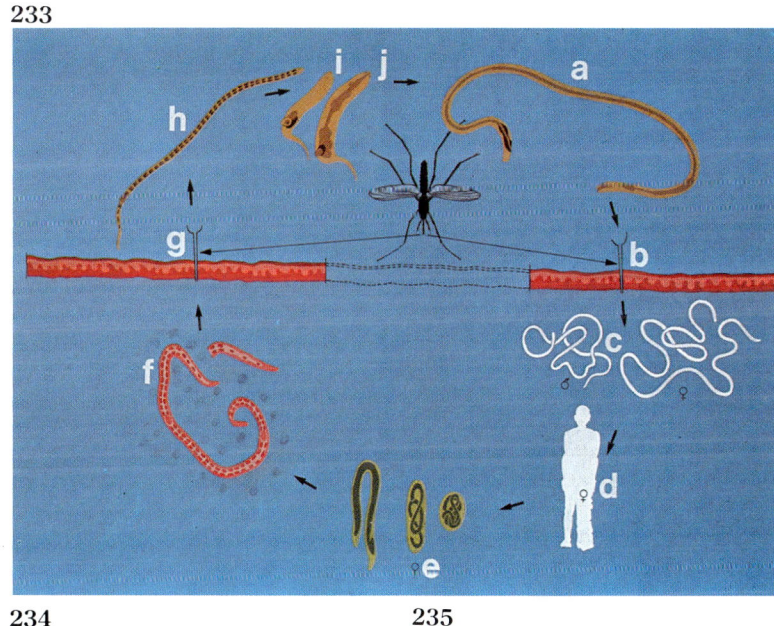

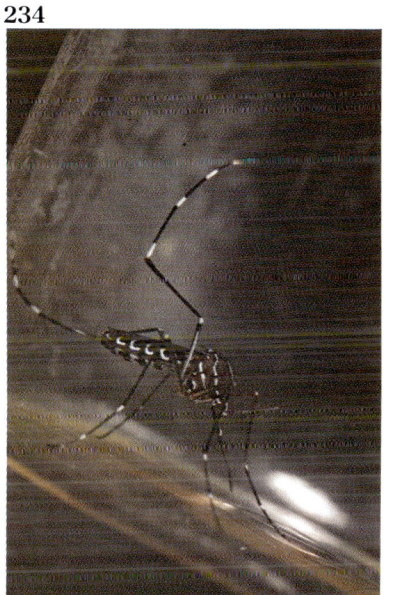

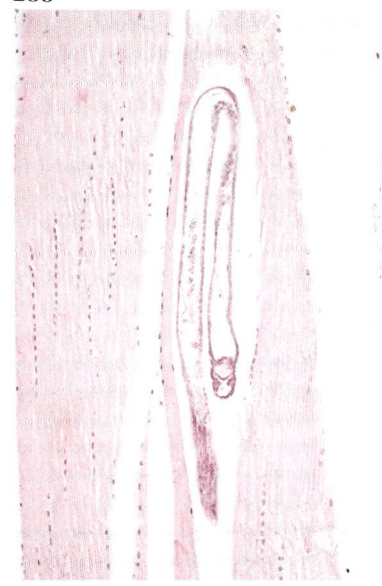

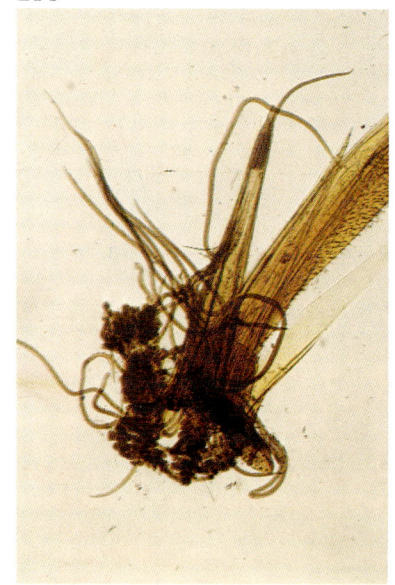

236 Infective larvae After about two weeks the larvae develop into third-stage, filariform larvae which enter the mosquito's proboscis. These infective larvae later penetrate the skin of a new host through the puncture wound made when the mosquito bites. ($\times 20$)

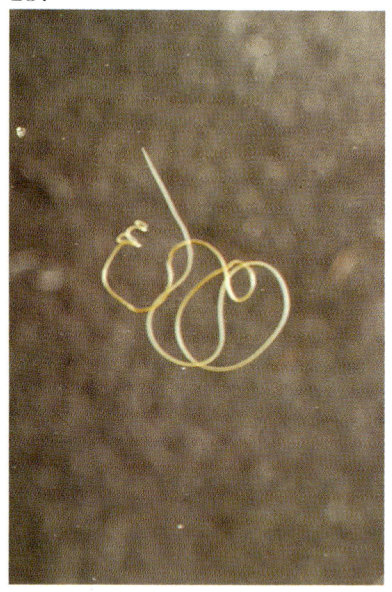

237 & 238 Male and female *W. bancrofti* adults On maturation the infective larvae copulate and the adult filariae become localised in lymph glands, e.g. in the groin. Adult male *W. bancrofti* (**237**) are about 4 cm long, females 8 to 10 cm (**238**). ($\times 8$)

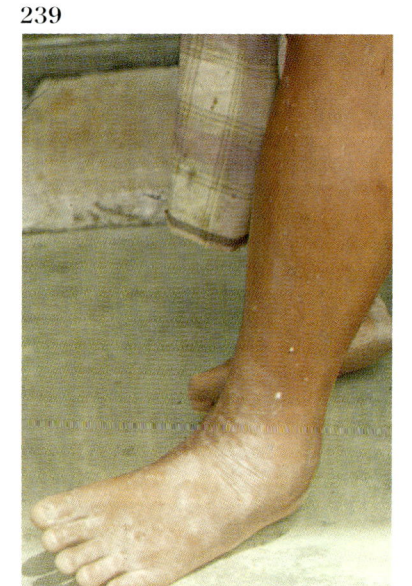

239 Lymphangitis Acute involvement of lymphatic vessels is common, especially in the extremities. In association with lymphangitis there is almost always some local lymphadenitis and fever.

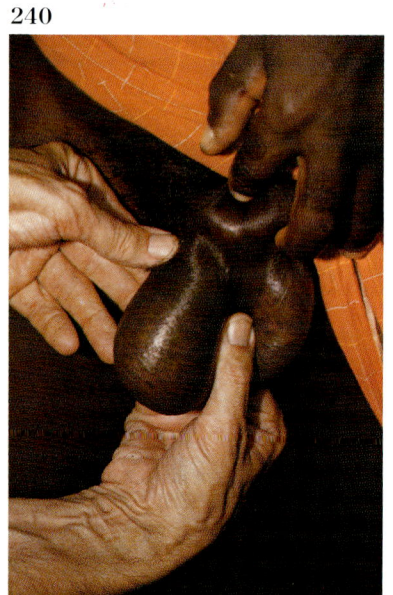

240 Hydrocele In the acute stages orchitis may occur. It is commonly associated with hydrocele and microfilariae may be found in the hydrocele fluid.

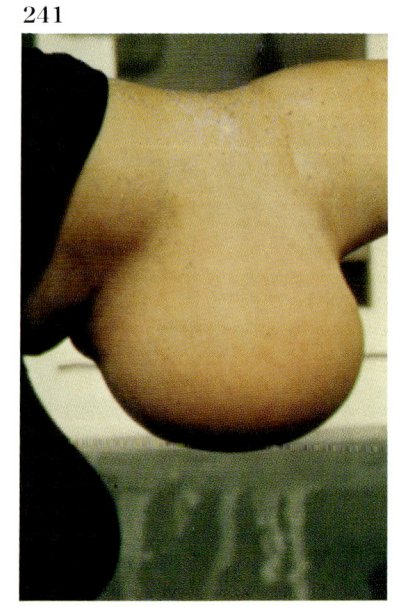

241 Elephantiasis of right epitrochlear gland in a Fijian A feature which is unusually frequent in the South Pacific and is also due to *W. bancrofti* is gross enlargement of the epitrochlear lymph node.

242 Elephantiasis of the leg and scrotum due to *W. bancrofti* in Tahiti Severe elephantiasis of the scrotum may produce gross and incapacitating deformity that requires radical surgery to remove the surplus tissue.

243 Early elephantiasis due to *B. malayi* In regions of high endemicity, lymphatic obstruction may occur, especially in the leg, progressing in chronic cases to the grotesque extreme called 'elephantiasis'. This may also arise in the arm, breast or scrotum. By this late stage microfilariae are rarely found in blood films.

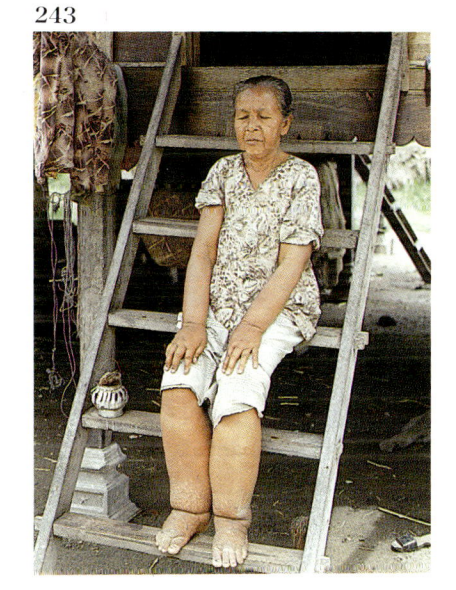

244 Massive elephantiasis due to *B. malayi* As in that caused by *W. bancrofti* (see **242**), the enlargement is commonly unilateral.

245 *W. bancrofti* in inguinal lymph gland Note the marked cellular reaction in this section, including multinucleated giant cells. (*H&E* × 20)

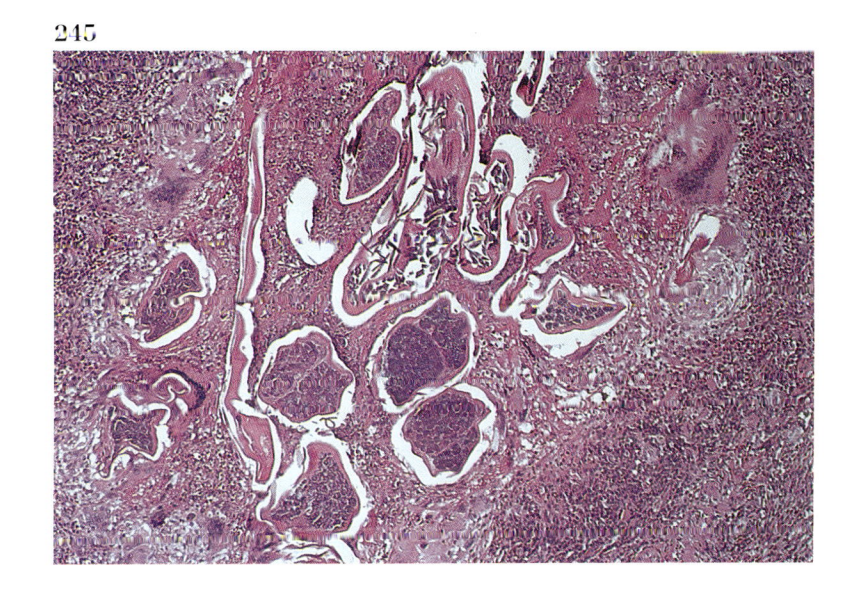

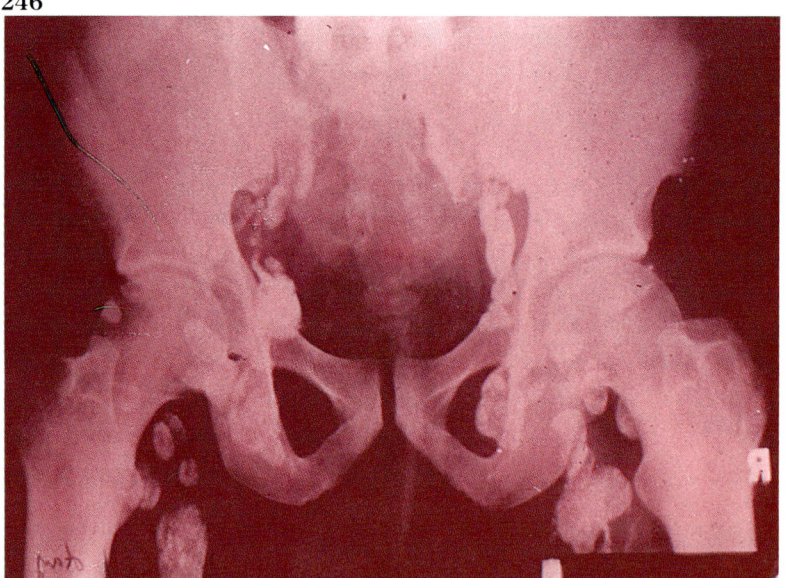

246 Calcified lymph nodes
Numerous calcified nodes are seen in this X-ray of a patient with chronic *W. bancrofti* infection.

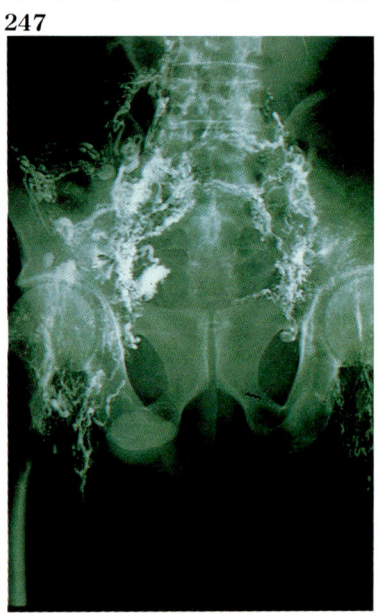

247 Lymphogram in patient with chyluria Obstruction of the cisterna chyli or its tributaries may occur, giving rise to chyluria.

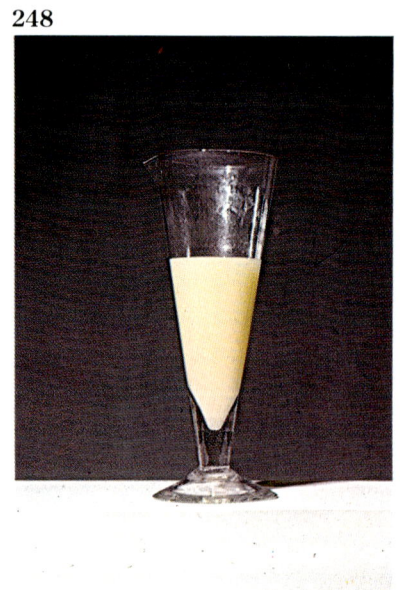

248 Urine containing lymph The dilated lymph vessels rupture and discharge chyle into the urinary tract, thus producing the milky appearance known as chyluria.

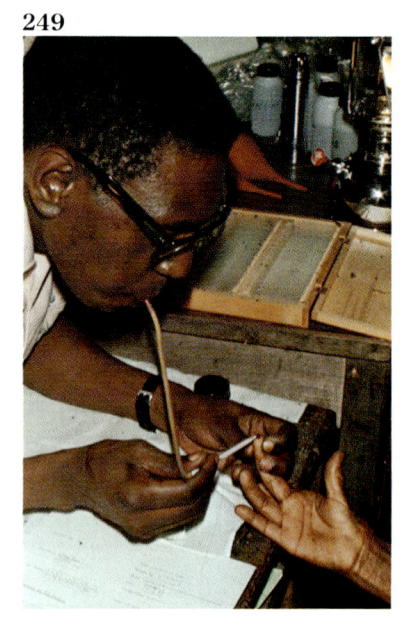

249 Microfilarial counts
Identification of microfilariae and parasite counts per unit quantity of blood are necessary for the epidemiological evaluation of filariasis (although not for individual diagnosis). Twenty cu mm pipettes are commonly used to make a thick blood film of specified size. This picture was taken during a night survey in an area endemic for *W. bancrofti*.

250-254 Microfilariae in blood films If microfilariae are present in the peripheral circulation they can usually be found by examining a fresh preparation of blood taken between 10 pm and midnight. The worms may be seen in a wet preparation but morphological differentiation is only possible after suitable staining with a Romanowsky stain (Leishman or Giemsa), or haematoxylin.
W. bancrofti (**250**); *B. malayi* (**251 & 252**); *L. loa* (**253 & 254**); (× 1 150) (*See* **Table X** and **299-301** for skin snip technique for other species.)

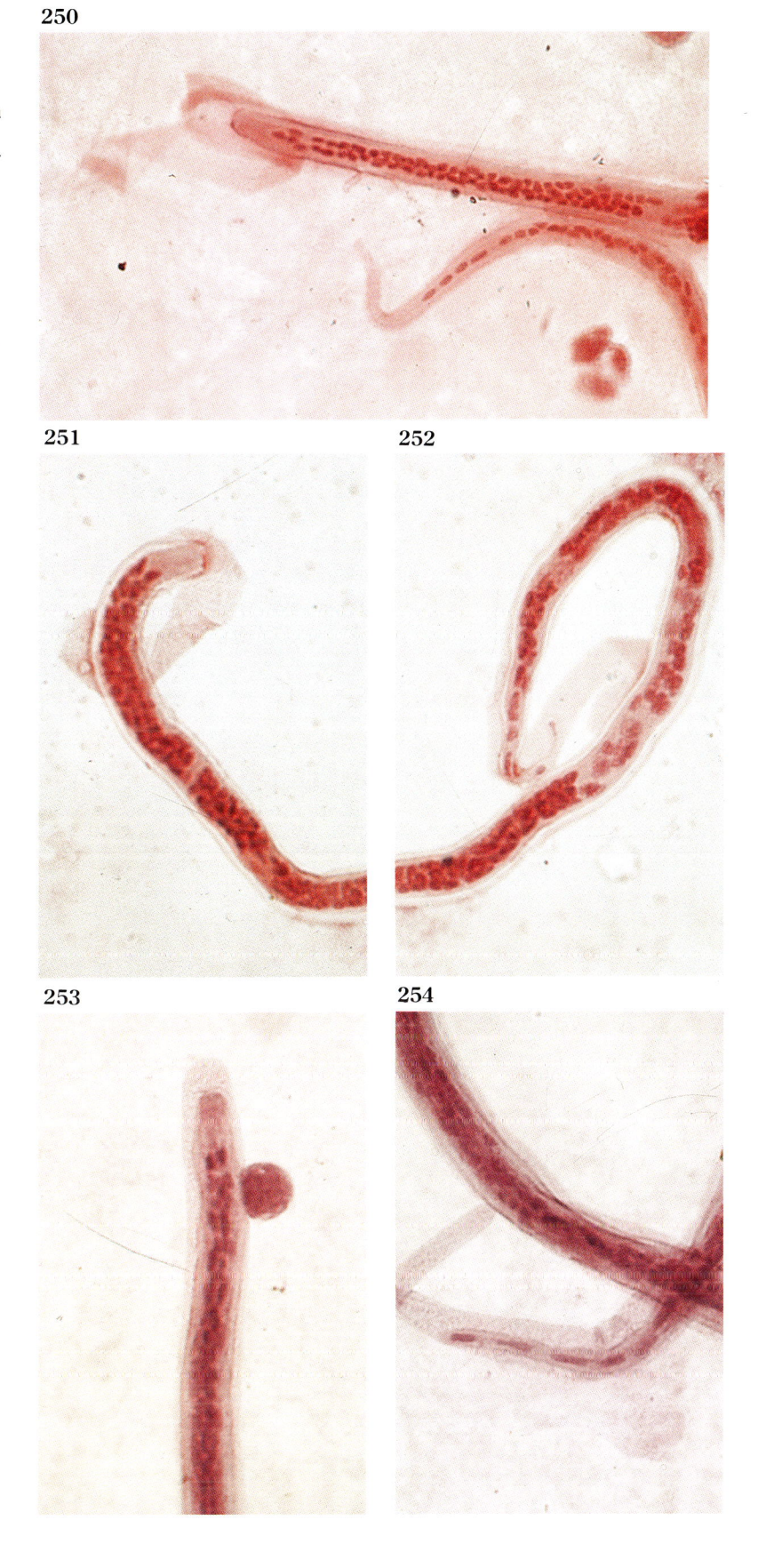

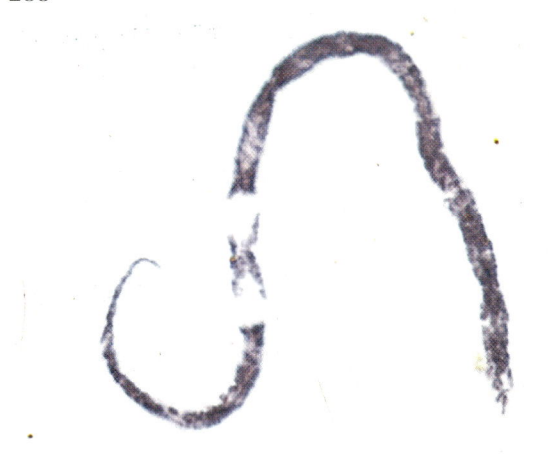

255 Microfilaria of *Mansonella ozzardi* (*Haematoxylin* × 1 150).

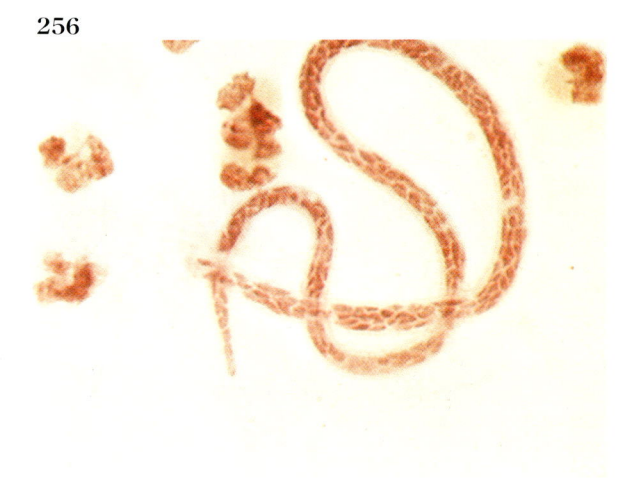

256 Microfilaria of *M. perstans* (*Giemsa* × 1 150).

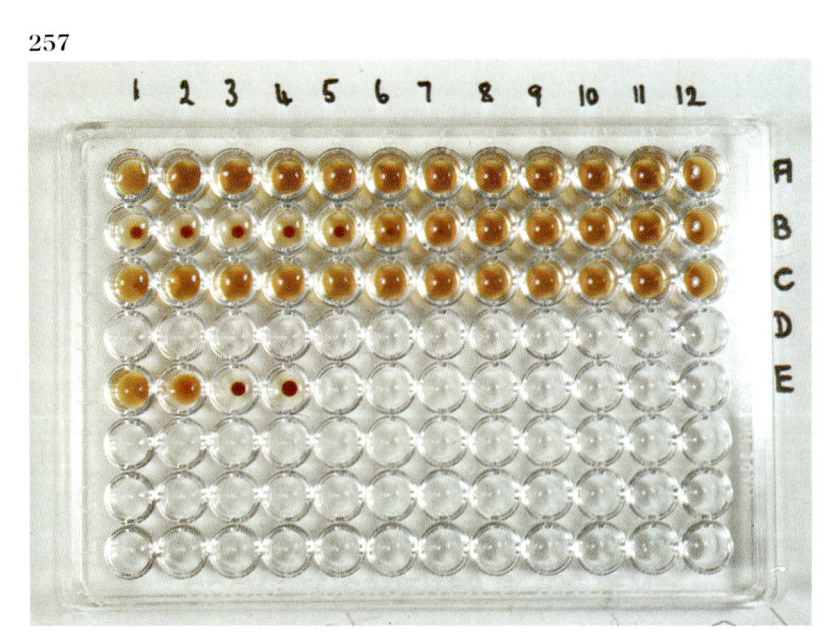

257 Serological diagnosis of filariasis The Complement Fixation Test using *Dirofilaria immitis* of the dog as antigen will confirm a diagnosis of filariasis, but it does not distinguish between the different species of filaria. (Row A is a negative control serum; row B shows a positive titre of 1/64; row C is a negative reaction from another patient; E is complement control.)

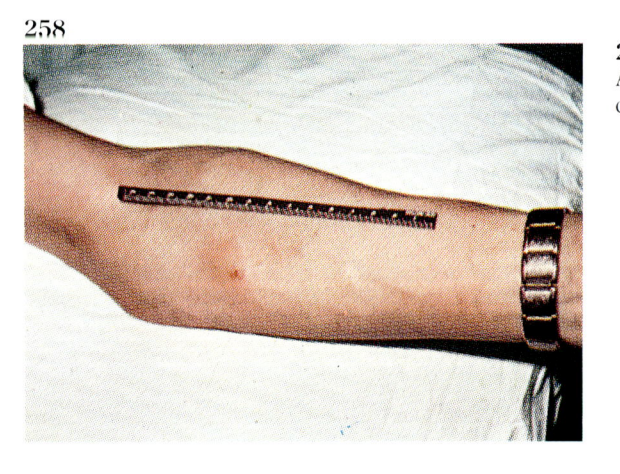

258 Positive skin test with *Dirofilaria* antigen A similar antigen may also be used to demonstrate delayed cutaneous hypersensitivity.

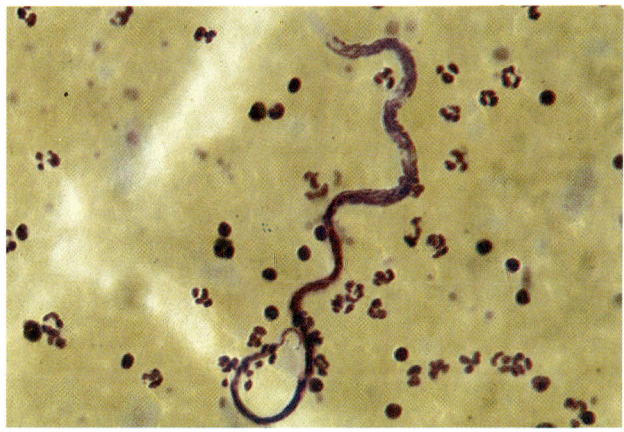

259 B. timori microfilariae The sheathed microfilaria of B. timori is easily distinguished from that of B. malayi and W. bancrofti by its large size, the lack of staining of the sheath of B. timori in Giemsa stain, and the distribution of the nuclei in the posterior end. B. timori, like B. malayi, has two distinct nuclei in the tail (cf. **250** & **252**). (× 375)

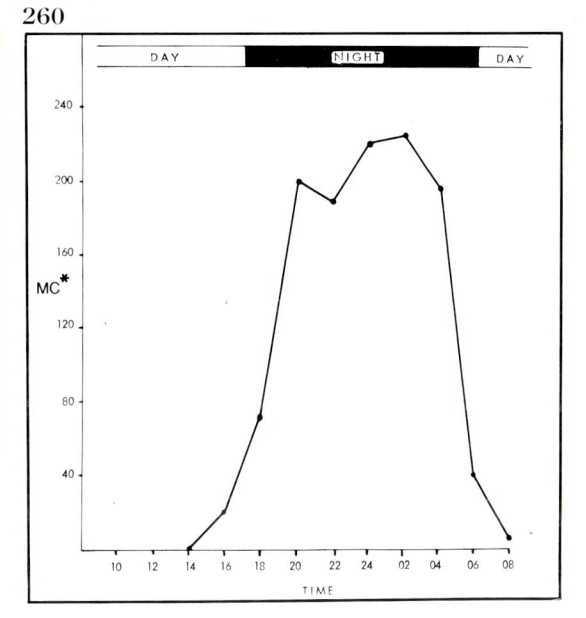

260 Circadian rhythm In B. timori, as in B. malayi or typical W. bancrofti infection, parasite counts reveal a marked nocturnal periodicity. (In the diurnal, subperiodic type of W. bancrofti, microfilariae are readily seen in blood taken during the day.) *Microfilaria as percentage of mean daily count (average of 10 patients).

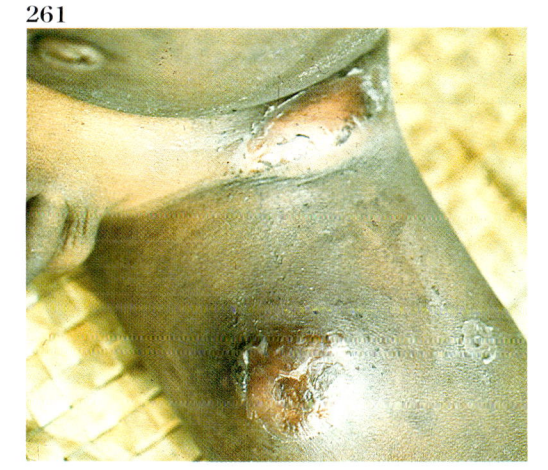

261 Abscesses in groin and thigh due to B. timori Both this species and W. bancrofti are found in some Indonesian islands (see **222**) where up to 25 per cent of village populations have been found infected with B. timori. The clinical disease resembles that caused by B. malayi except that abscess formation is fairly common in the early stages along the line of the great saphenous vein in the upper thigh (as seen here), while chronic lymphoedema is commoner rather than frank elephantiasis in later cases. This parasite is transmitted by Anopheles barbirostris.

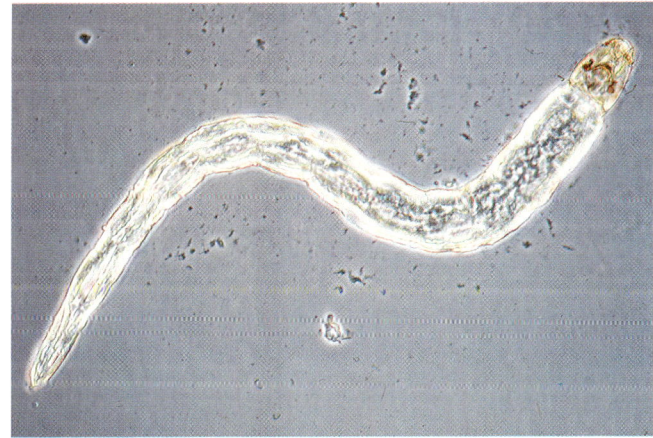

Mansonella perstans

262 Larvae of Culicoides M. perstans is found in tropical Africa and coastal regions of Central and South America. The vectors of M. perstans are small speckled wing flies of the genus Culicoides of which C. austeni and C. grahami appear to be the main vectors in West Africa. The aquatic stages are commonly found in tree holes, leaf axils and other small natural water containers. (× 120)

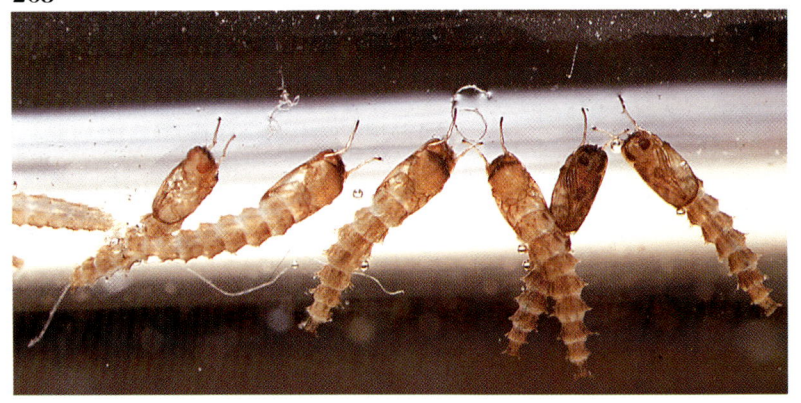

263 Pupae of *Culicoides* (× 12)

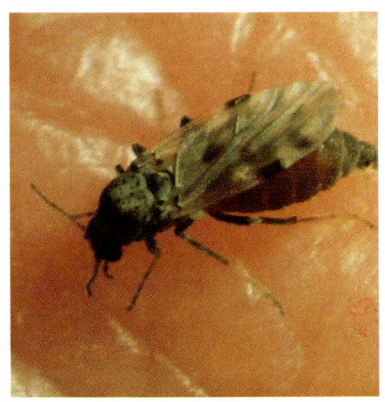

264 Adult *Culicoides* biting (× 25)

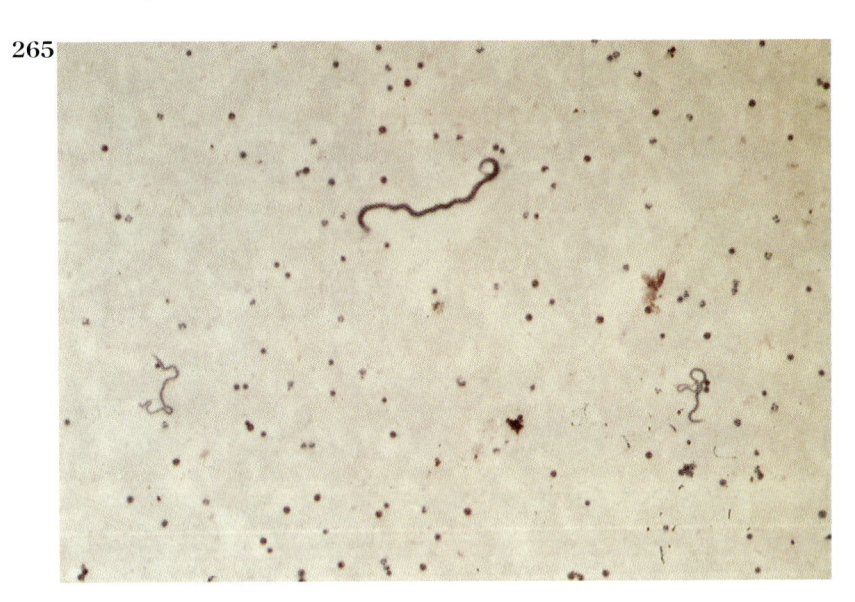

265 *M. perstans* and *Loa loa* in blood film The unsheathed microfilaria of *M. perstans* is readily distinguished from the sheathed microfilaria of *Loa loa* (or that of *W. bancrofti*) in blood films by its smaller size, even at a fairly low magnification. Multiple infections with several species of blood-dwelling microfilariae are common. *M. perstans* infection is usually asymptomatic and may last many years. Males measure about 45 mm in length, females about 70 to 80 mm. (*Giemsa* × 125)

Loaiasis

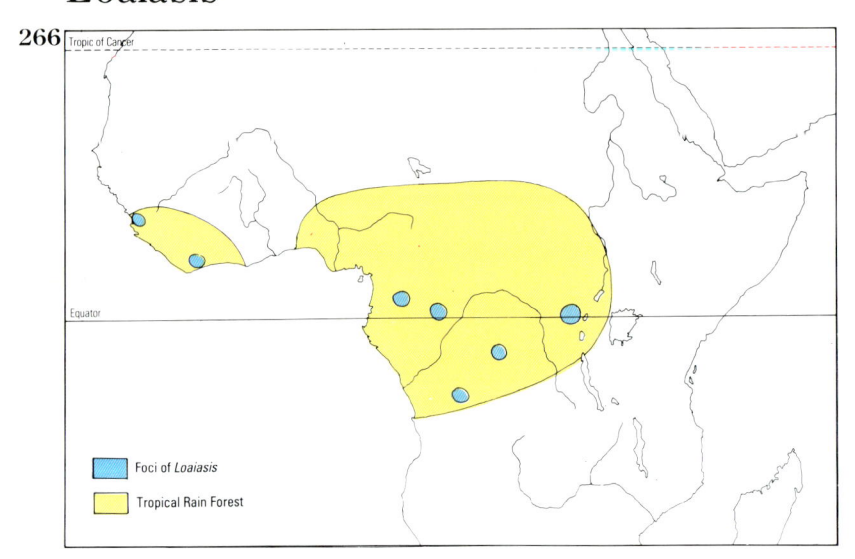

266 Distribution of loaiasis Loaiasis is confined to Africa, extending from the Gulf of Guinea in the West to the Great Lakes in the East. Infection with an almost identical parasite is common in these areas in certain monkeys such as the mandrill.

267 Life cycle of *Loa loa* When the *Chrysops* fly bites, the infective third-stage larvae (a) enter the vertebrate host (b) where they mature into adults (c) within about one year. The adults live for 4 to 12 years. The females (about 7 cm long) migrate through the subcutaneous tissues and may cross the front of the eye under the conjunctiva (d). Microfilariae (f) develop from larvae (e) in the female and circulate in the blood with which they are picked up by another fly (g). In the gut of the fly the microfilariae (h) exsheath and enter the fat bodies in which they mature first to 'sausage-like' forms (ij), then infective third-stage larvae (a). The larvae infect a new host when the *Chrysops* takes another blood meal.

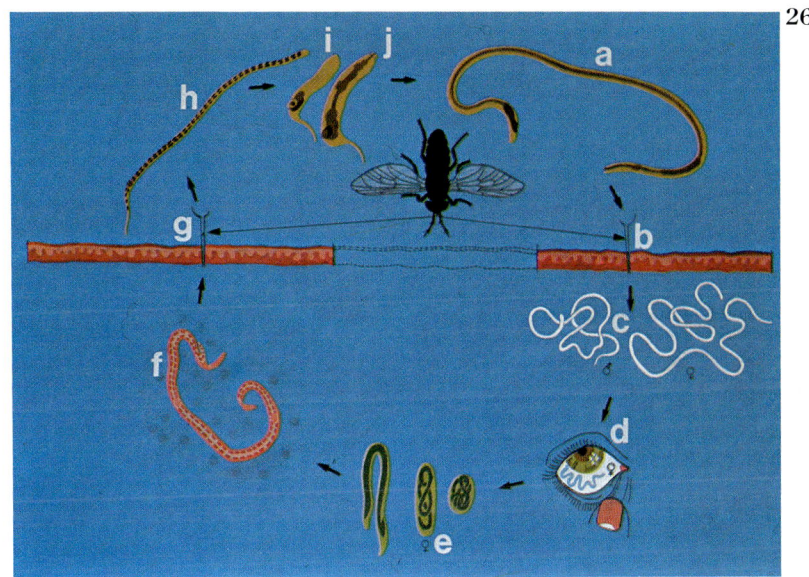

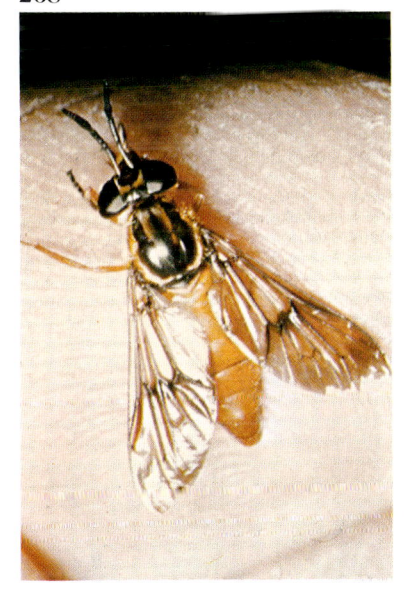

268 Female *Chrysops dimidiata* biting Tabanid flies of the genus *Chrysops*, particularly *C. dimidiata* and *C. silacea*, transmit loaiasis. The flies live in the canopy of primary rain forests. (× 4)

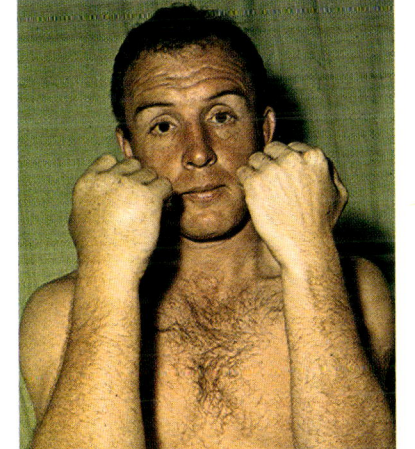

269 Calabar swelling in right hand and arm Recurrent large swellings lasting about three days are characteristic and indicate the tracks of the migrating adults in the connective tissue. They are most frequently seen in the hand, wrists and forearm. A marked eosinophilia (60 to 90 per cent) accompanies this phase of the infection.

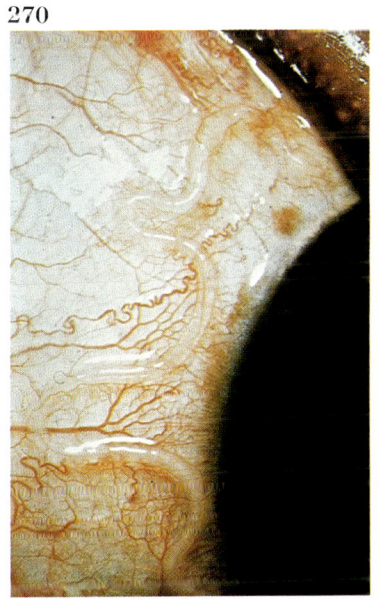

270 Adult *Loa loa* in the eye The movement of the adult worm under the conjunctiva gives rise to considerable irritation and congestion.

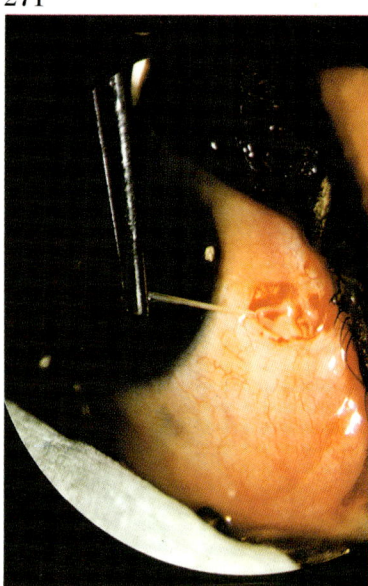

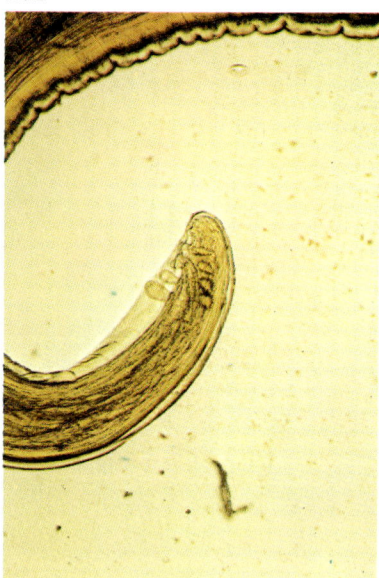

271 Extraction of worm The adult worm can be extracted with fine forceps after anaesthetising the conjunctiva.

272 Tail of male *Loa loa* (× 90)

Onchocerciasis

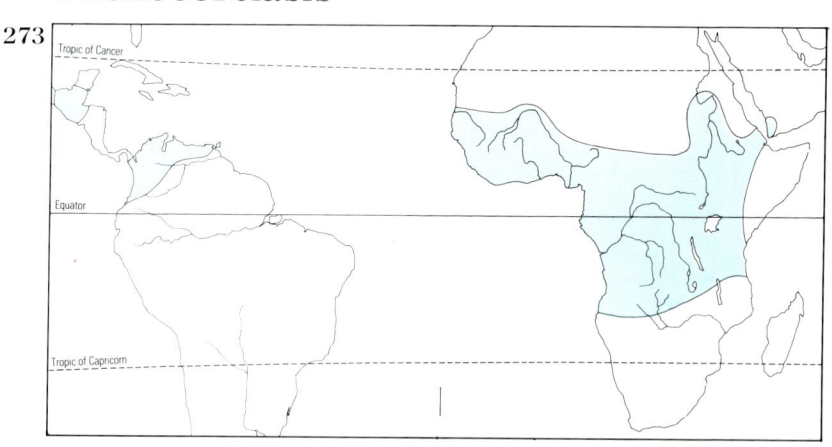

273 Distribution of onchocerciasis *Onchocerca volvulus* is a tissue-dwelling nematode, the microfilariae of which are found predominantly in the skin and eye. Onchocerciasis has a focal distribution in Africa and South America. It is endemic in West Africa, equatorial and East Africa and in the Sudan. A small focus is known also in Yemen. It occurs in Central America and in parts of Venezuela and Colombia.

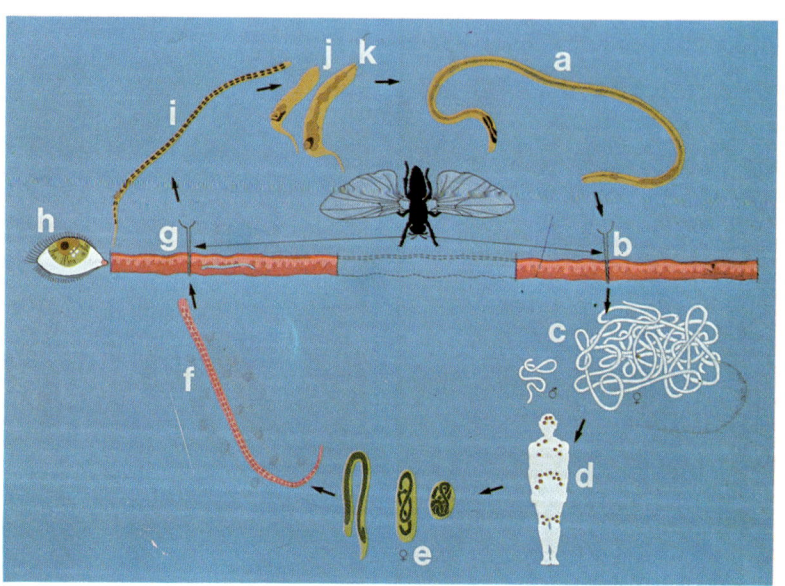

274 Life cycle of *Onchocerca volvulus* The infective, third-stage larvae (a) enter the skin following the bite of the blackfly vector, *Simulium* (b). The larvae migrate to the subcutaneous tissues where they mature into thread-like adult males and females (c) in about one year, enclosed in fibrous nodules (d). Larvae (e) developing in the females form unsheathed microfilariae (f) which live in the skin (g) and eye (h). When microfilariae are picked up from the skin by another *Simulium* (i) they develop through several stages (jk) in the thoracic muscles to become infective, third-stage larvae (a) in about 6 to 12 days. (*See also* **277, 283-285, 301-303**.)

275 & 276 Aquatic stages of the vectors The filarial worm is transmitted by *Simulium* or 'Buffalo flies'. Species of the *S. damnosum* complex are the vectors in West Africa, *S. naevei* in East Africa, and *S. ochraceum* and *S. metallicum* in Central and South America. The larvae (**275**) and the pupae (**276**) are attached to submerged objects in fast running water from which they extract oxygen through head filaments. ($\times 6$) (*See also* **279, 280**.)

277 Adult *Simulium damnosum* ($\times 10$)

278 Typical locality of *Simulium* in West Africa Fast-moving, highly oxygenated water in streams, rivers, waterfalls, etc. provides the essential ecological environment. The figure shows a branch of the Upper Volta river. In some hyperendemic villages in West Africa a third of all adults may be blinded by onchocerciasis Widescale vector control of onchocerciasis using temephos (Abate) has reduced transmission considerably in seven West African countries. As a further control measure for the future, it has been shown that treatment with a single oral dose of ivermectin reduces and maintains microfilaria counts at low levels for up to one year.

279 Eggs of *Simulium* The black eggs are seen attached to a narrow leaf just below the surface of rapidly flowing water.

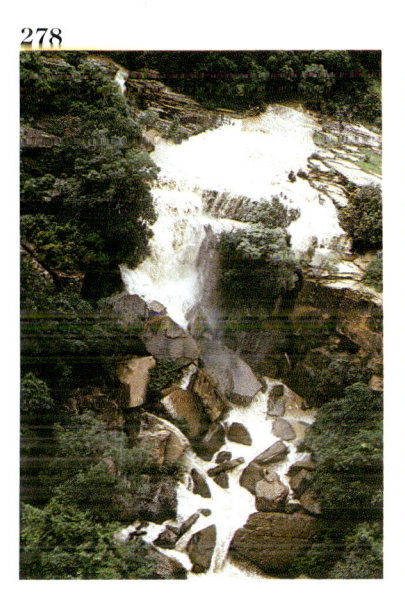

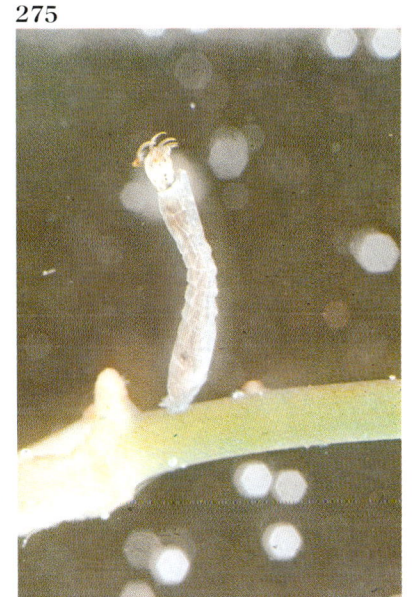

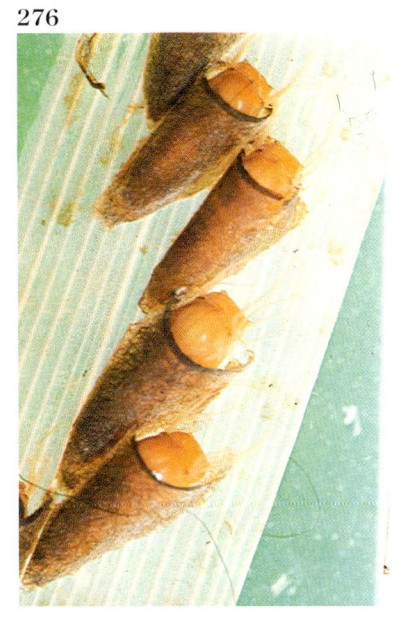

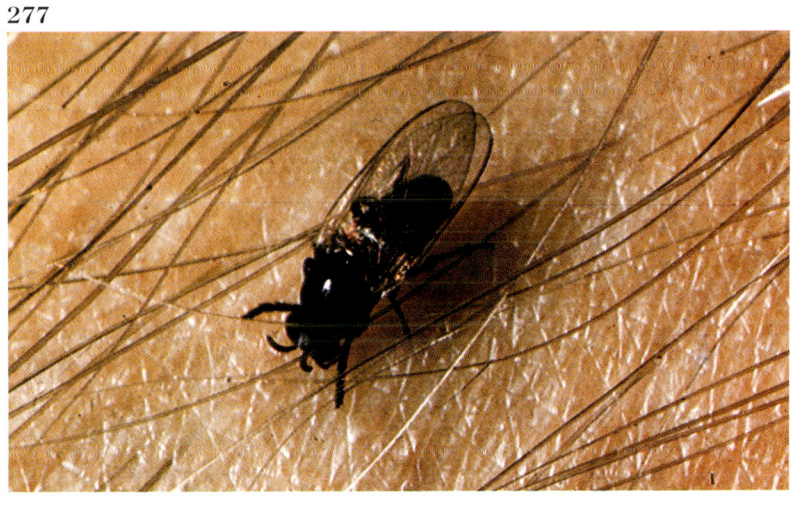

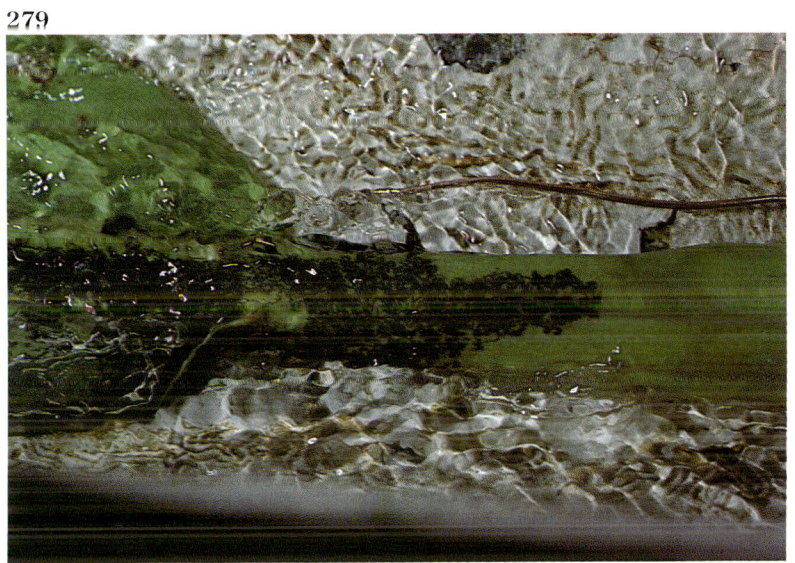

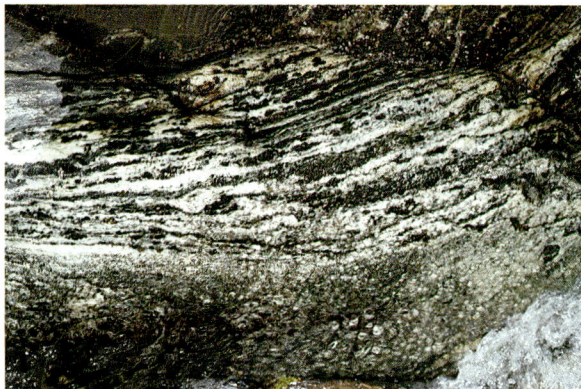

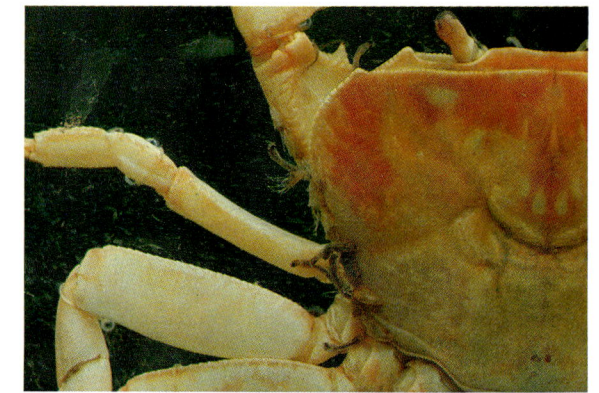

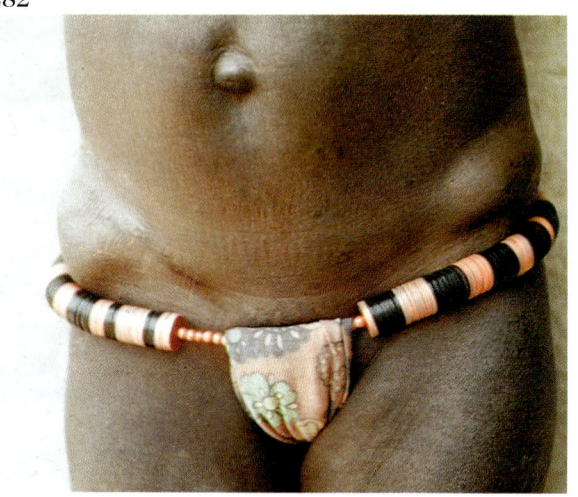

280 *Simulium* larvae and pupae attached to rocks Rapidly moving river in the dry season showing stone boulders in the bed of the stream which, by causing eddies in the water, provide enough oxygenation to permit the *Simulium* to survive while the river level is low.

281 *Simulium* larvae on a crab In East Africa larvae and pupae of the *S. naevei* complex are attached to fresh-water crabs.

282 *Onchocerca* nodules on iliac crests The adult filariae become encapsulated in fibrous material which forms nodules in the subcutaneous tissues. They are found predominantly in the lower part of the body in Africa, while in South and Central America they are more commonly found on the head and upper trunk.

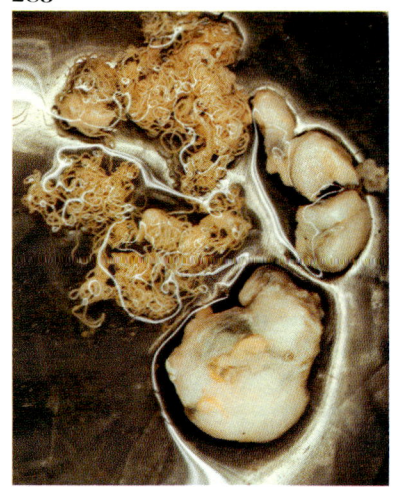

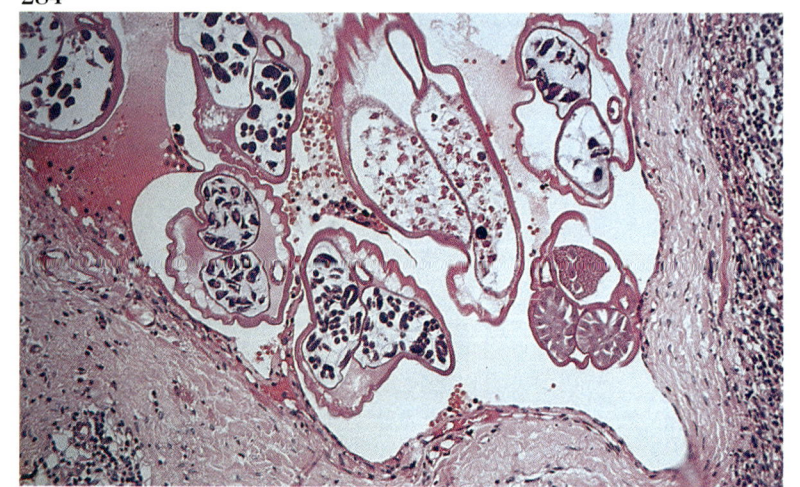

283 Macroscopic section of nodule In this gross section of a nodule the adult worms are seen entwined. (× 2)

284 Transverse section of nodule A microscope section through an onchocercal nodule, showing adult worms and microfilariae. (× 40)

285 Microfilariae in skin biopsy The microfilariae migrate to the skin and the eye. (H&E × 350)

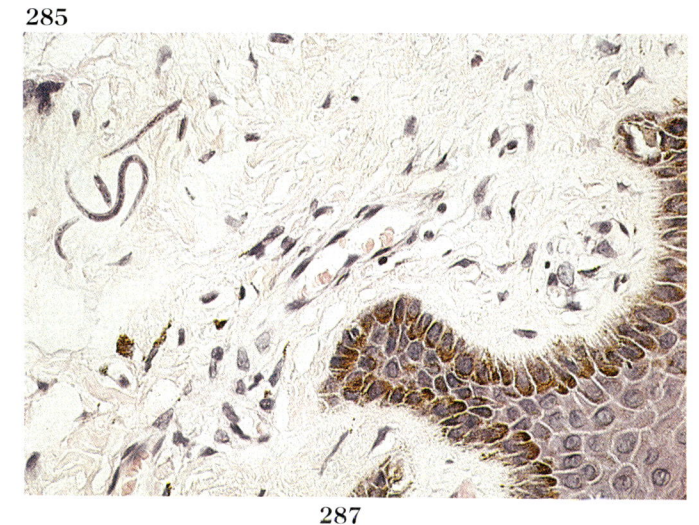

286 Papular dermatitis in onchocerciasis Early onchocerciasis is characterised by lesions in two main sites, the skin and the eye. A pruriginous condition, commonly called 'craw craw' in Africa, involves irregular, broad areas of the skin where small papules form around the microfilariae.

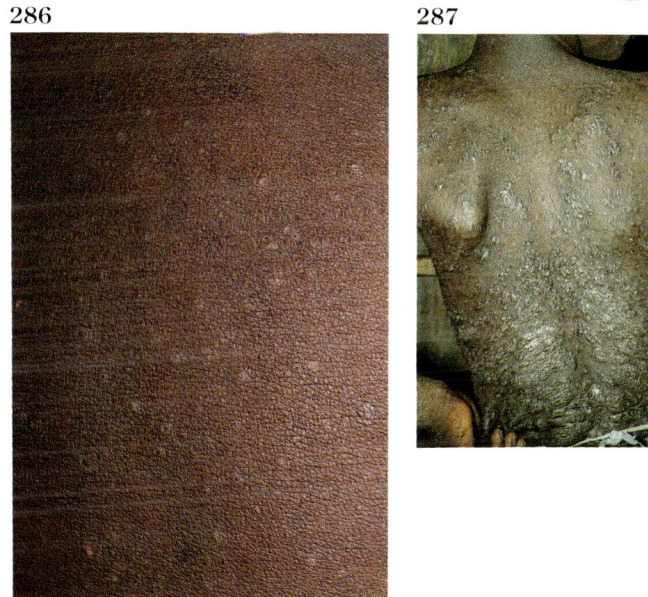

287 'Elephant' skin Thickening and wrinkling of the skin give rise to the 'lizard' or 'elephant' skin appearance.

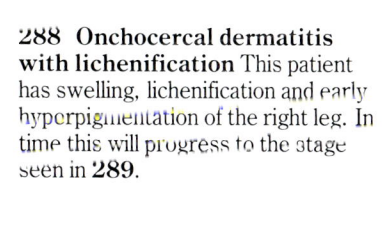

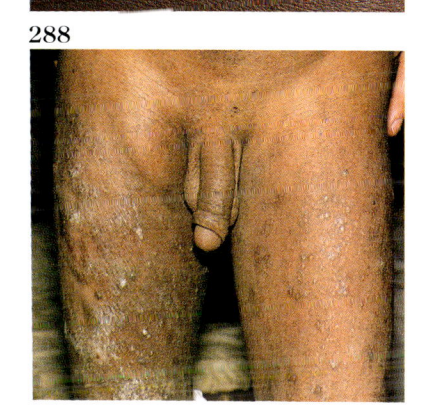

288 Onchocercal dermatitis with lichenification This patient has swelling, lichenification and early hyperpigmentation of the right leg. In time this will progress to the stage seen in **289**.

289 Advanced Sowda This is a peculiar and quite common feature of onchocerciasis in Africa. It is characterised by hyperpigmentation, usually of one of the lower limbs, and is often accompanied by inguinocrural lymphadenopathy.

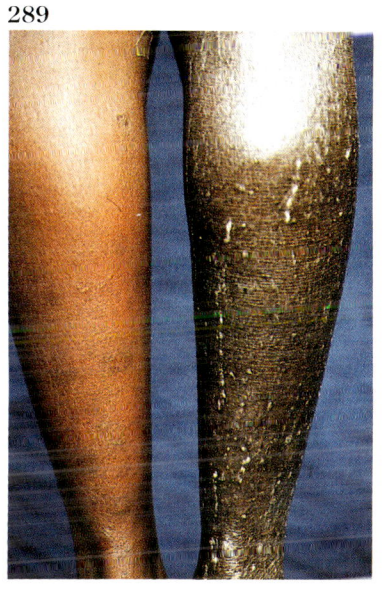

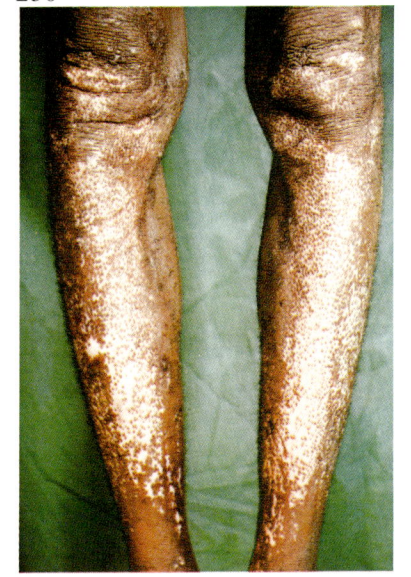

290 Depigmentation Pretibial atrophy and depigmentation in a patient with late (burnt-out) onchocerciasis. This condition is sometimes called 'leopard skin'.

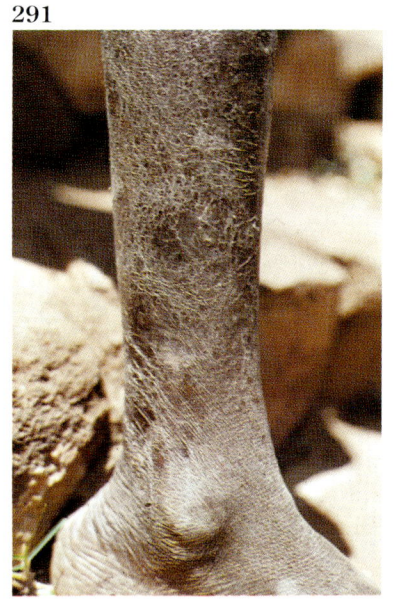

291 'Tissue paper' skin In chronic infections atrophy of the skin may occur resulting in a 'tissue paper' appearance.

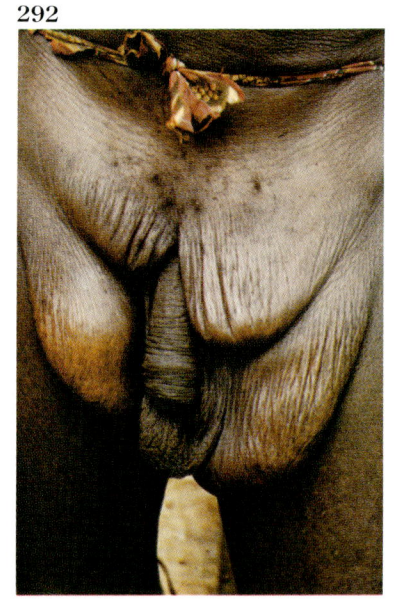

292 'Hanging groin' Involvement of the inguinocrural glands can result in an appearance described as 'hanging groin'.

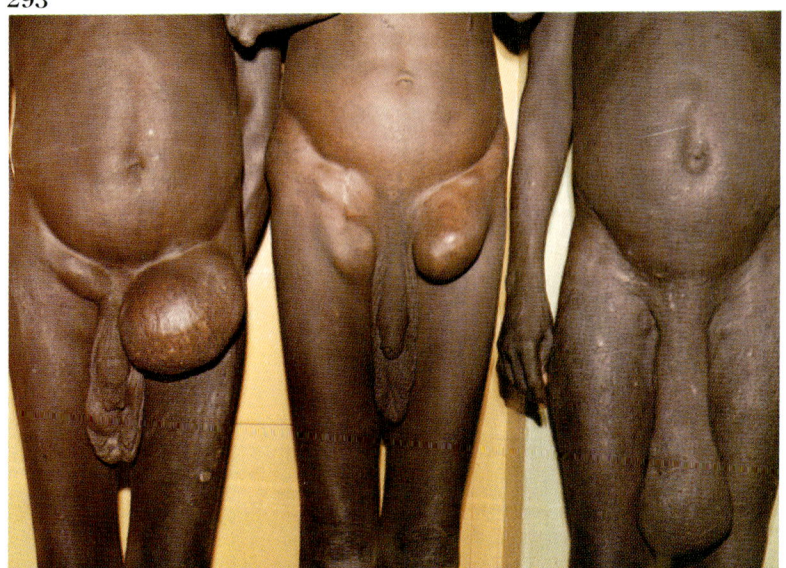

293 Hanging groin and scrotal elephantiasis

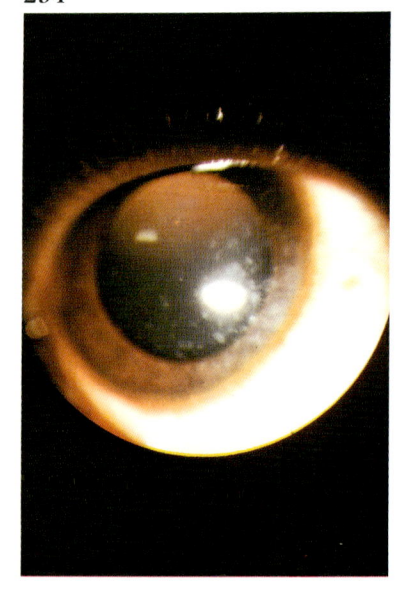

294 Early corneal involvement The tissue reaction associated with dead microfilariae in the cornea gives rise to a number of 'snowflake'-like opacities, as seen in the figure. This punctate keratitis may clear with time.

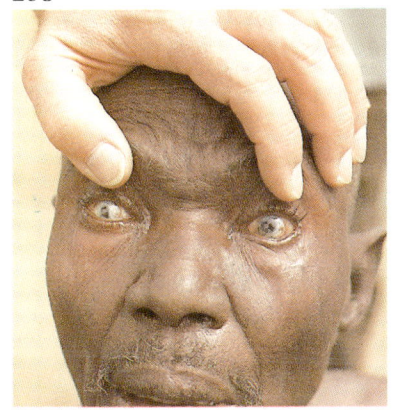

295 Sclerosing keratitis Heavy microfilarial infection of the cornea leads to the development of progressive, sclerosing keratitis which commonly produces blindness, as seen in this African patient.

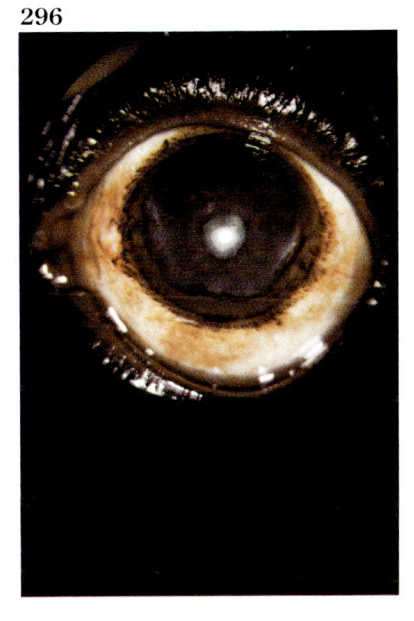

296 The cornea in sclerosing keratitis

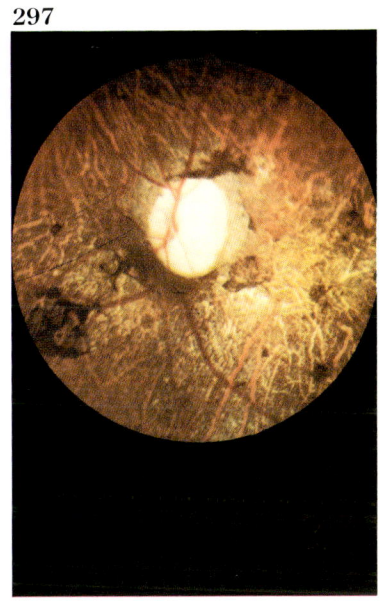

297 Optic atrophy A variety of choroidoretinal lesions may follow damage by microfilariae to the anterior segment of the eye, and finally optic atrophy may develop, as seen in this eye.

298 Abandoned village near the Volta River High blindness rates in some areas have resulted in the depopulation of entire villages, as seen here.

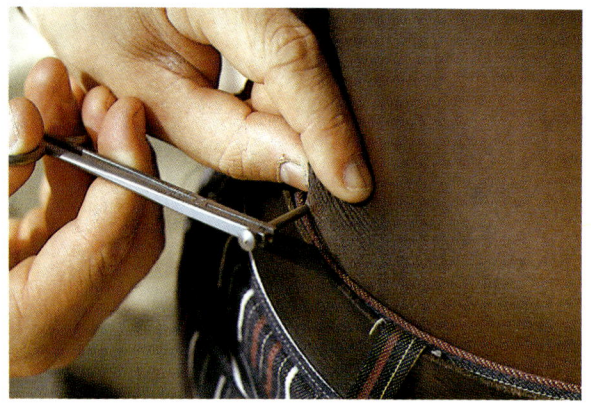

299 & 300 Skin snip technique A tiny but standard-sized piece of skin, often from the back of the shoulders, iliac regions or calf, is snipped off and placed in a drop of saline on a microscope slide under a cover slip where it is left for several minutes at room temperature.

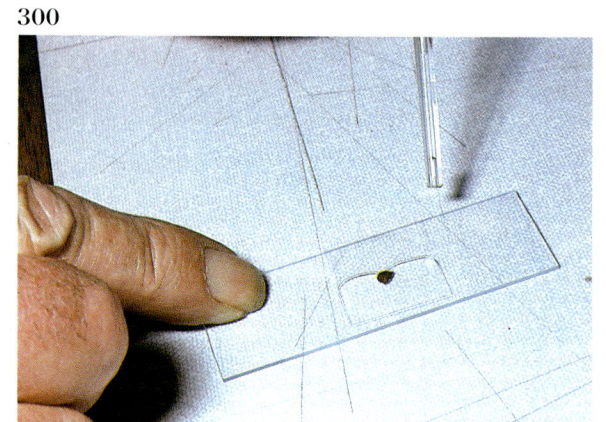

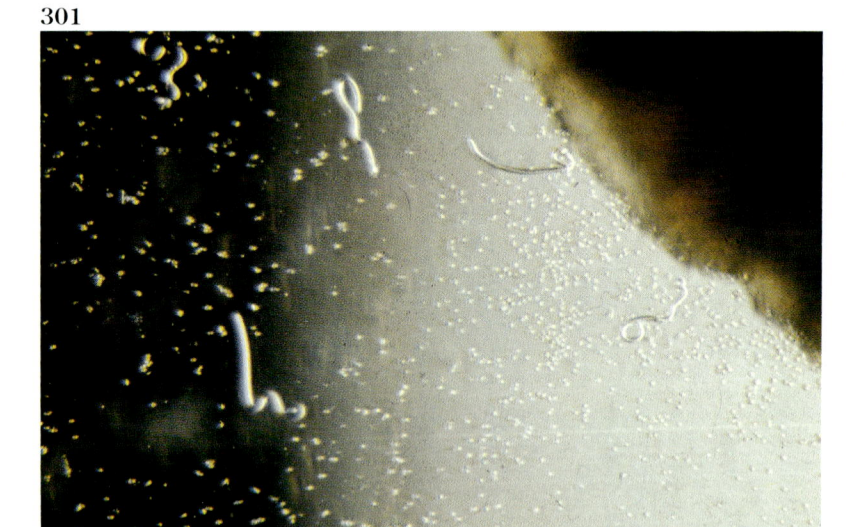

301 Living microfilariae of *O. volvulus* After some time, actively moving microfilariae emerge from the skin into the surrounding saline where they can be counted ($\times 600$).

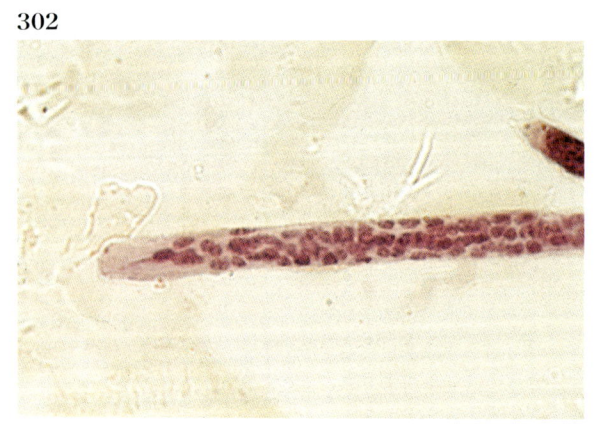

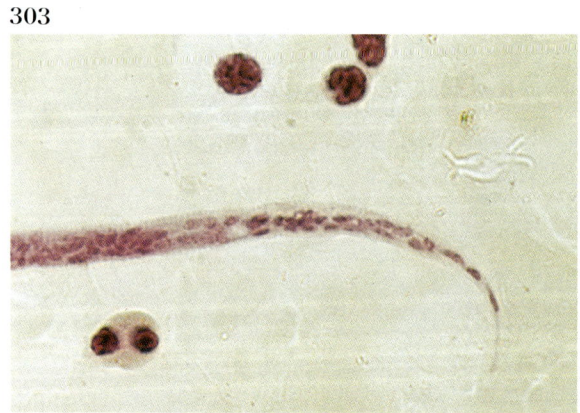

302 & 303 Microfilariae in skin snips *O. volvulus* head (**302**) and tail (**303**). ($\times 1\,150$) (cf. **250-256, 307, 308.**)

304 Slit lamp examination of the eye Slit lamp examination often reveals numerous microfilariae in the anterior chamber of the eye. They are best sought in the inferior medial quadrant.

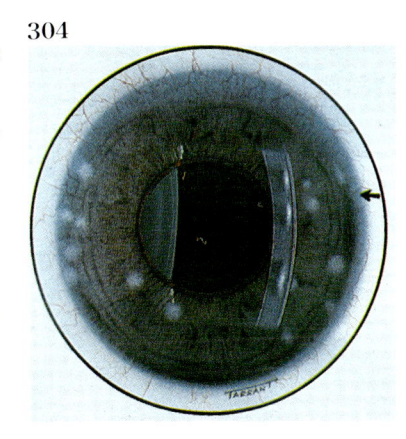

305 Onchocercal blindness in Guatemala In Central America, onchocerciasis ('Erisipela de la costa') is characterised by an erythematous appearance of the face or upper trunk. It occurs in heavily infected young people, usually under 20 years of age. Purplish tinged plaques or papules may be observed in Central America, usually in patients of an older age group. This condition is known as 'mal morado'.

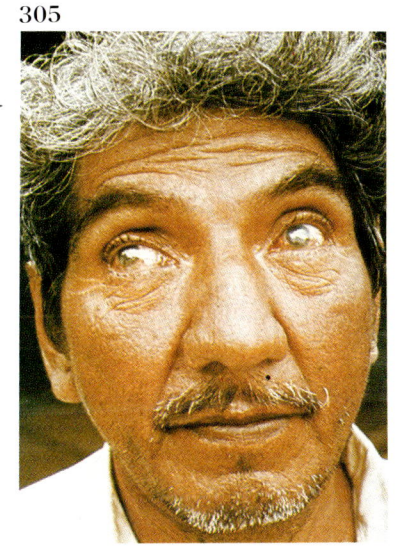

306 Nodulectomy Serious eye changes can be prevented in some early cases by excising the nodules containing the adult worms, thus preventing the continuing production of the microfilariae which are the actual pathogenic agents in this disease. Nodulectomy has been widely employed in Central and South America.

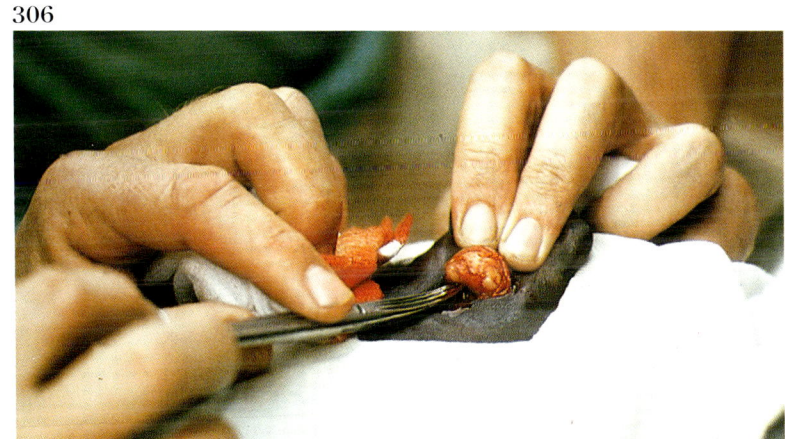

Other Filariases

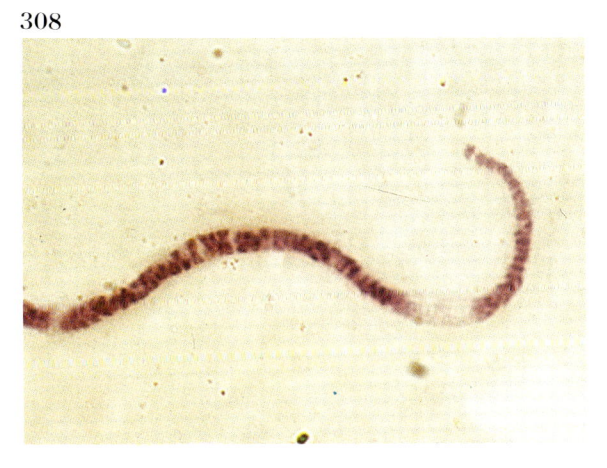

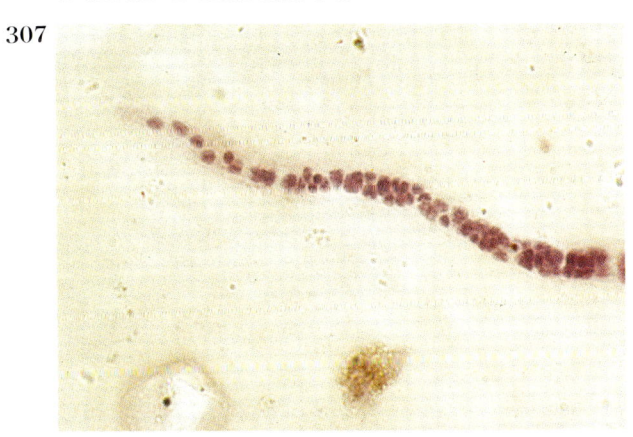

307 & 308 Microfilariae of *M. streptocerca* This skin-dwelling, unsheathed microfilaria must be distinguished from that of *O. volvulus* (**302 & 303**) in African patients. For this a stained preparation should be examined, e.g. with haematoxylin. *M. streptocerca* produces few pathogenic effects. It is transmitted by *Culicoides grahami*, also infects chimpanzees, and is only known in Africa. Head (**307**), tail (**308**). ($\times$ *1 150*) (cf. **250-256, 302 & 303**.)

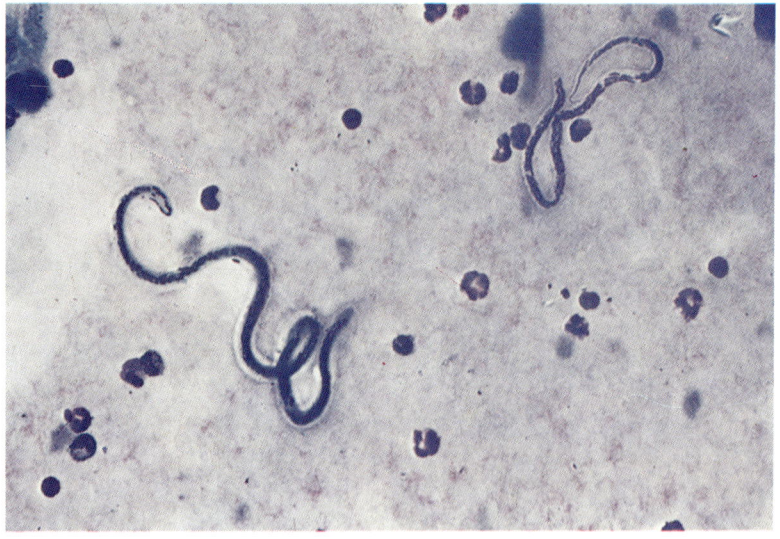

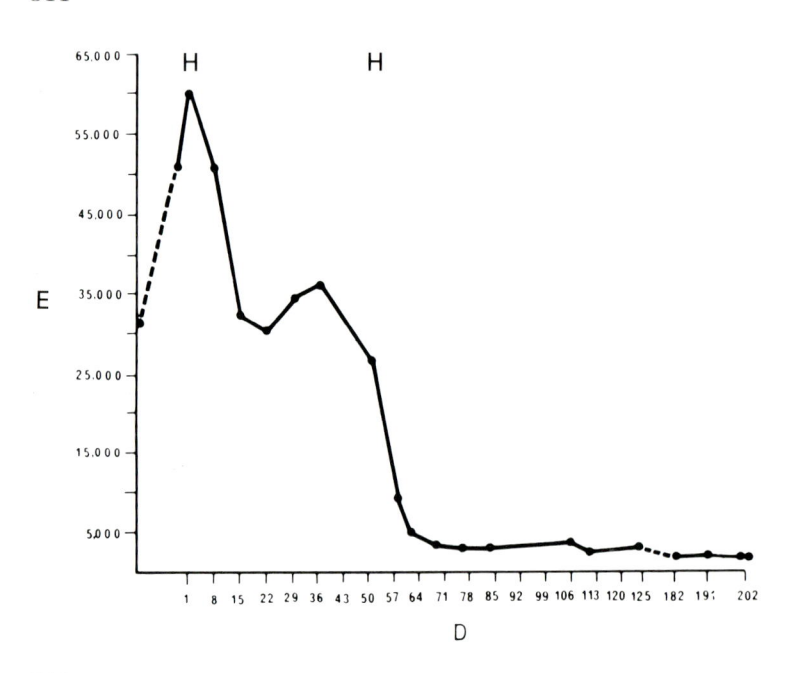

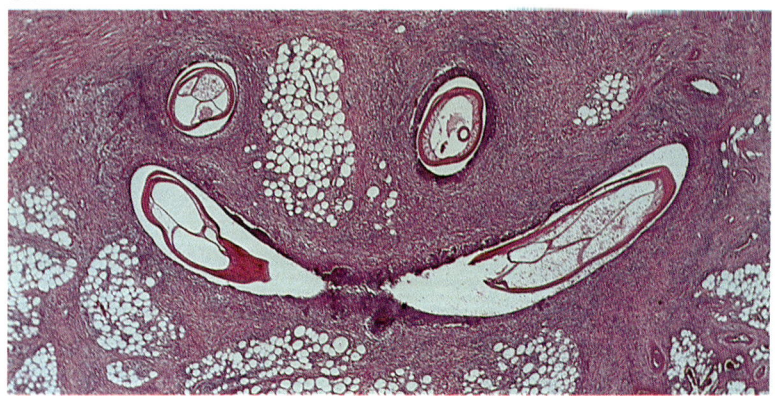

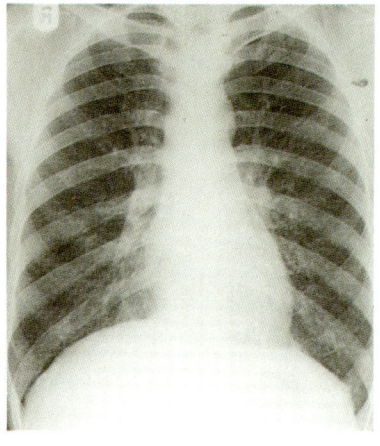

309 Microfilaria of *Mansonella ozzardi* This unsheathed microfilaria (right) is found in the blood in parts of South America and the Caribbean. The microfilaria is readily distinguished from the larger and sheathed microfilaria of *W. bancrofti* (left) which also occurs in parts of South America. Vague symptoms of various types have been attributed to infection with the parasite, which is also transmitted by *Culicoides* spp. (× 500)

310 Eosinophilic lung This is a peculiar allergic reaction to filarial infections that may be of human or animal origin. It occurs principally in SE Asia and particularly affects Indians. The condition is characterised by nocturnal cough and bronchospasm, with transient shadows in the lungs.

311 Eosinophilia in zoonotic filariasis Eosinophilia is very marked and the condition responds well to specific filaricides. A typical leucocyte response to healing with diethylcarbamazine is shown.
H = diethylcarbamazine (Hetrazan);
E = eosinophils/cu mm; D = days.

312 *Dirofilaria repens* in retrobulbar tissues The adult of this filarial worm has been found in the eyelids and retrobulbar tissues of the eye of patients in Europe. *D. repens* is normally a parasite of dogs. (*H&E* × 10)

Part II
Soil-mediated Helminthiases

Soil-transmitted helminthic infections are of two types: the hookworms which undergo a cycle of development in the soil, the larvae being infective; and a second group of nematodes which merely survive in the soil as eggs that have to be ingested in order for the cycle to continue. The geographical distribution of the hookworms is limited by the requirements of the developing larvae for warmth and humidity. Generally speaking, the second type can occur not only in the tropics and subtropics, but also in temperate regions. All these helminthiases provide an index of the level of hygiene and sanitation in a community since they depend for their dispersal on the indiscriminate deposition of faecal material on the ground, the use of untreated night soil as an agricultural fertiliser and similar unsophisticated human habits. In temperate as in other areas, those infections that are spread directly, i.e. through the ingestion of eggs, are common in microenvironments which favour such spread, for example, homes for mentally subnormal people, refugee camps, orphanages. The provision of adequate sewage disposal facilities virtually excludes these diseases.

The hookworm infections are transmitted through soil-dwelling infective larvae that penetrate the skin. Faecal contaminated soil in the neighbourhood of human habitations or on farmland is the source of infection for the barefooted inhabitants. Conversely, the use of footwear greatly reduces the prevalence of hookworm infection. Such people as rubber tappers in Malaya and farmers planting rice paddies commonly acquire infection from contaminated soil. Larvae of a number of animal hookworm species do not mature in man but the invasive larvae produce a transitory skin eruption as they migrate (cutaneous larva migrans). Visceral larva migrans may be due to infections with eggs of the dog or cat roundworm (*Toxocara canis*, *T. cati*). The larvae of these worms also do not mature in man but may set up inflammatory reactions in the viscera, especially the liver, or in the eye.

Generally speaking, the degree of harm done to the host is related to the worm burden in these infections. Hookworm disease results when large numbers of adult worms are present and the loss of blood due to the worms cannot be balanced because the host's diet is deficient in iron and other essential components. Moreover, multiple intestinal helminthic infection is the rule in many areas. Heavy infections with *Ascaris* may result in intestinal obstruction. *Trichuris* infection of the large bowel can lead to rectal prolapse in infants.

THE HOOKWORM INFECTIONS
Ancylostoma duodenale and *Necator americanus*

313-327 The eggs of helminths *Schistosoma haematobium* (**313**), *S. mansoni* (**314**), *S. japonicum* (**315**), *Fasciola hepatica* (**316**), *Ascaris lumbricoides* (**317**), *Ascaris* (infertile) (**318**), *Paragonimus westermani* (**319**), *Diphyllobothrium latum* (**320**), Hookworm (**321**), *Trichuris trichiura* (**322**), *Enterobius vermicularis* (**323**), *Hymenolepis nana* (**324**), *H. diminuta* (**325**), *Taenia* (**326**), *Clonorchis sinensis*, *Opisthorchis felineus*, *Heterophyes heterophyes* (**327**). (× 430) (See **Table IX** for classification. The eggs of the last three species are very difficult to distinguish.)

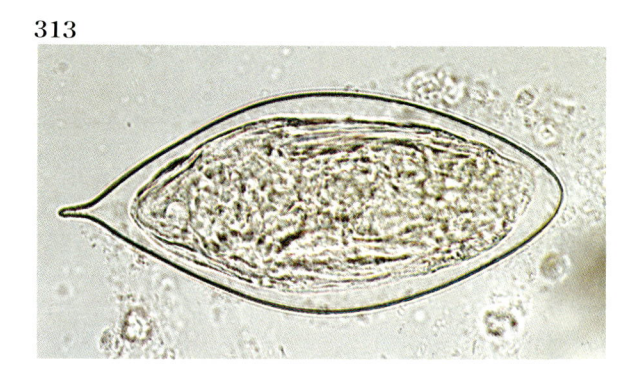

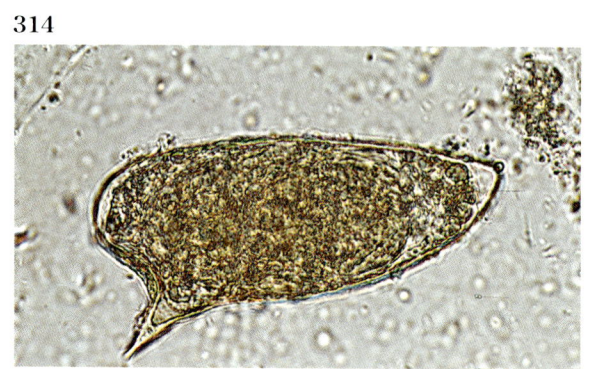

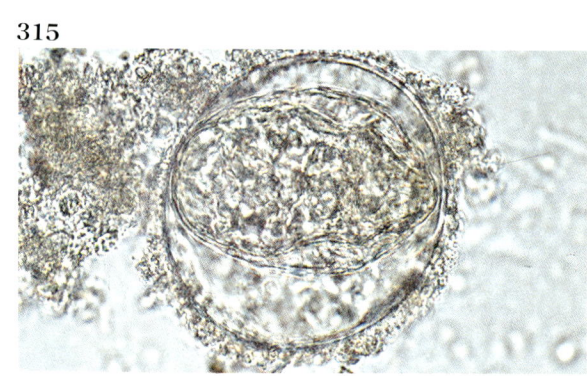

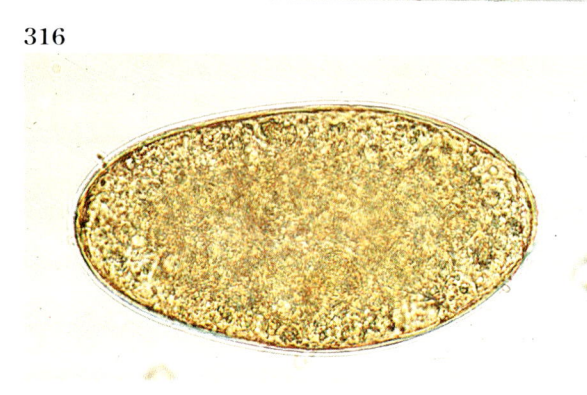

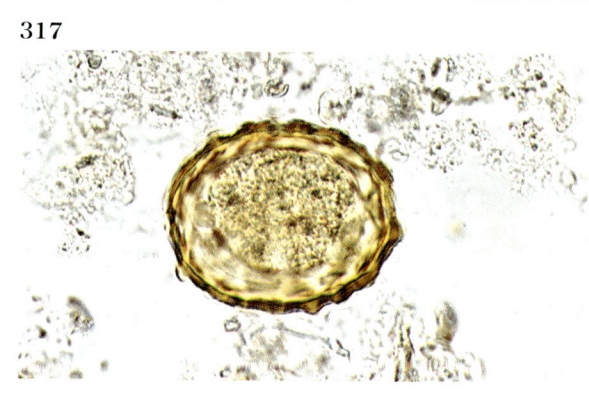

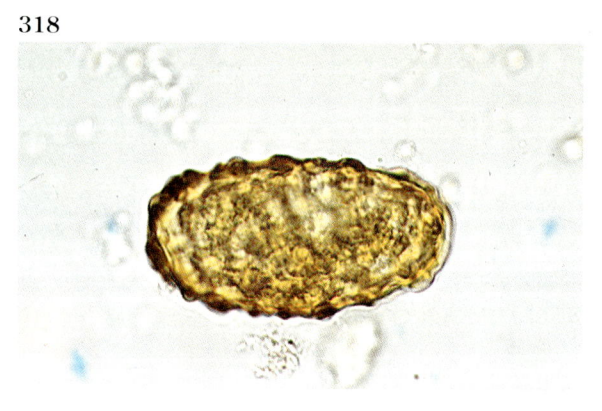

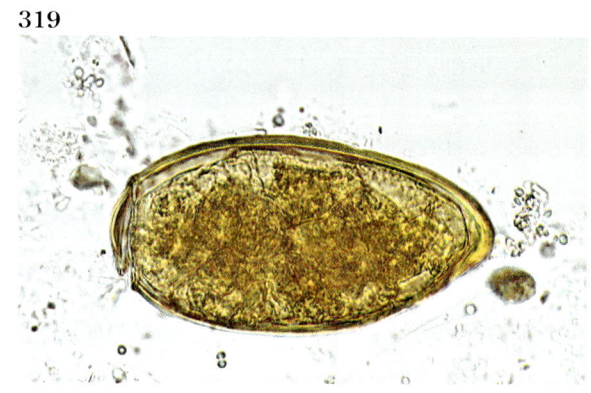

320

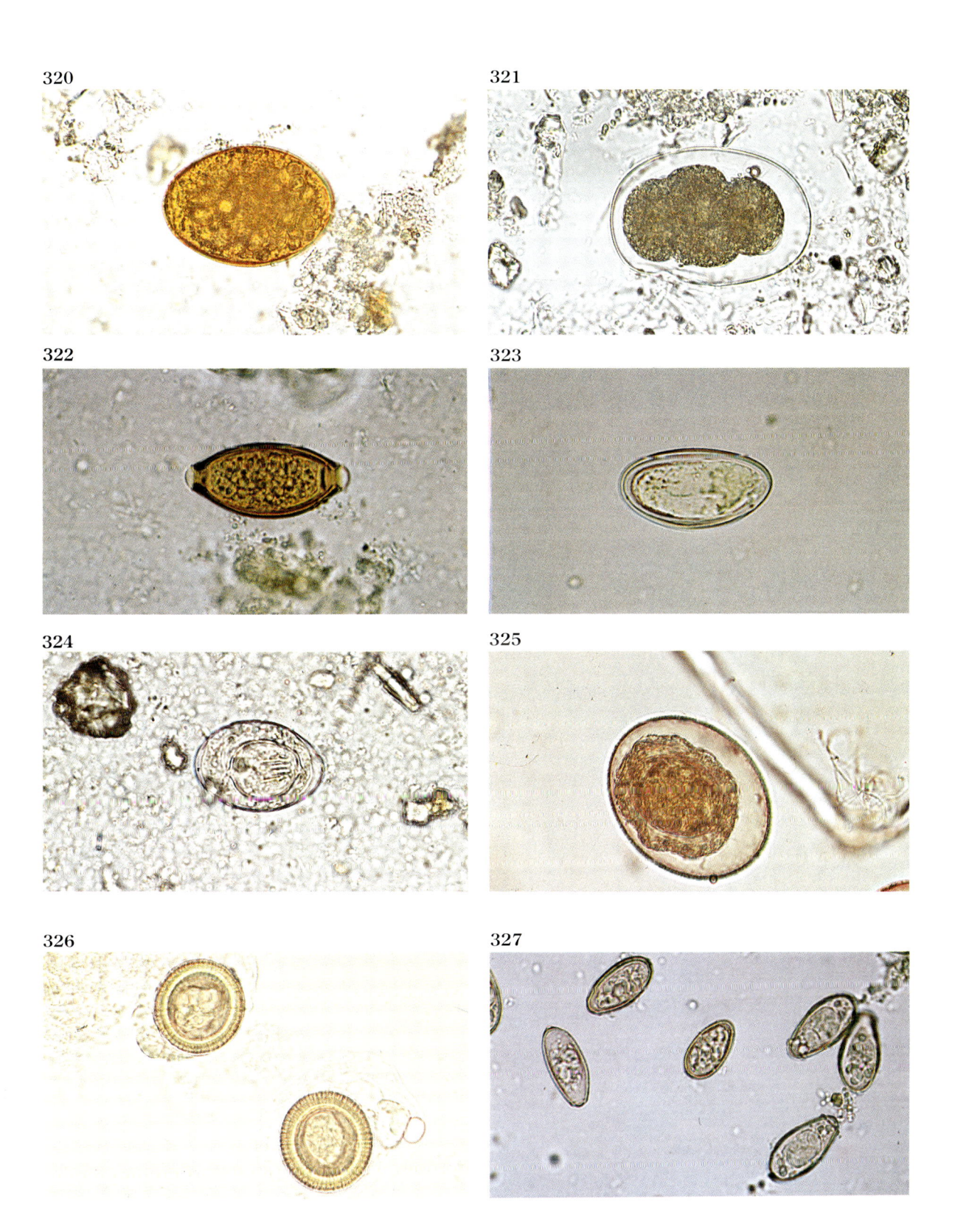

321

322

323

324

325

326

327

85

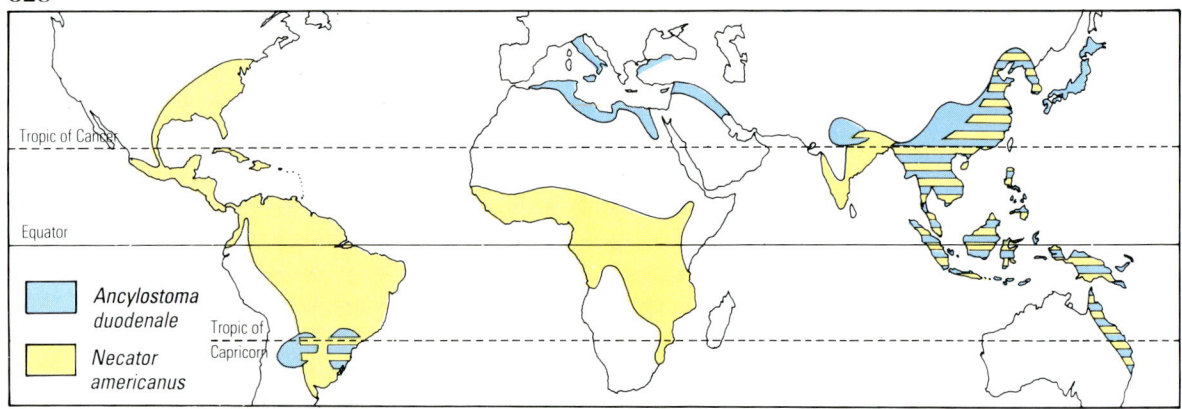

328 Distribution of hookworm infection The common hookworms of man are *A. duodenale* and *N. americanus*. It is estimated that 1000 million persons are infected with hookworm (about a quarter of the world's population). Usually one species predominates in any one locality. The map shows the approximate areas in which one or other species dominates. Since the larvae can only develop in warm moist soil the distribution of the parasite is limited by climatic conditions.

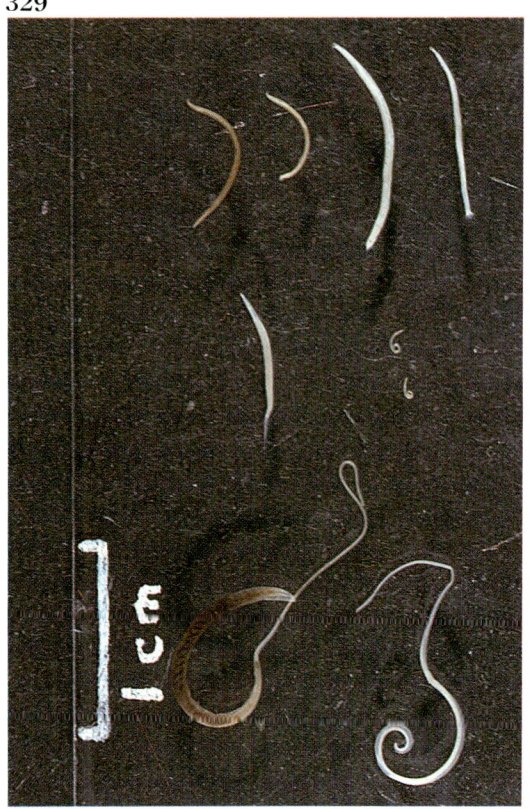

329 Comparative size of nematodes

First row	*N. americanus* ♀ ♂	*A. duodenale* ♀ ♂
Second row	*E. vermicularis* ♀	*T. spiralis* ♀ ♂
Third row	*T. trichiura* ♀ ♂	

330-334 Identification of adult hookworms *A. caninum* (**330**) (× *400*), *A. duodenale* (**331**) (× *630*), *A. ceylanicum* (**332**) (× *670*), *N. americanus* (**333**) (× *470*), *A. duodenale* (**334**) (× *470*). The different species may be distinguished by the characteristic morphology of the head capsule (**330-333**) and male bursa (**334**), seen here in scanning electro-micrographs. The male bursae are distinguished by the numbers and pattern of the 'rays'.

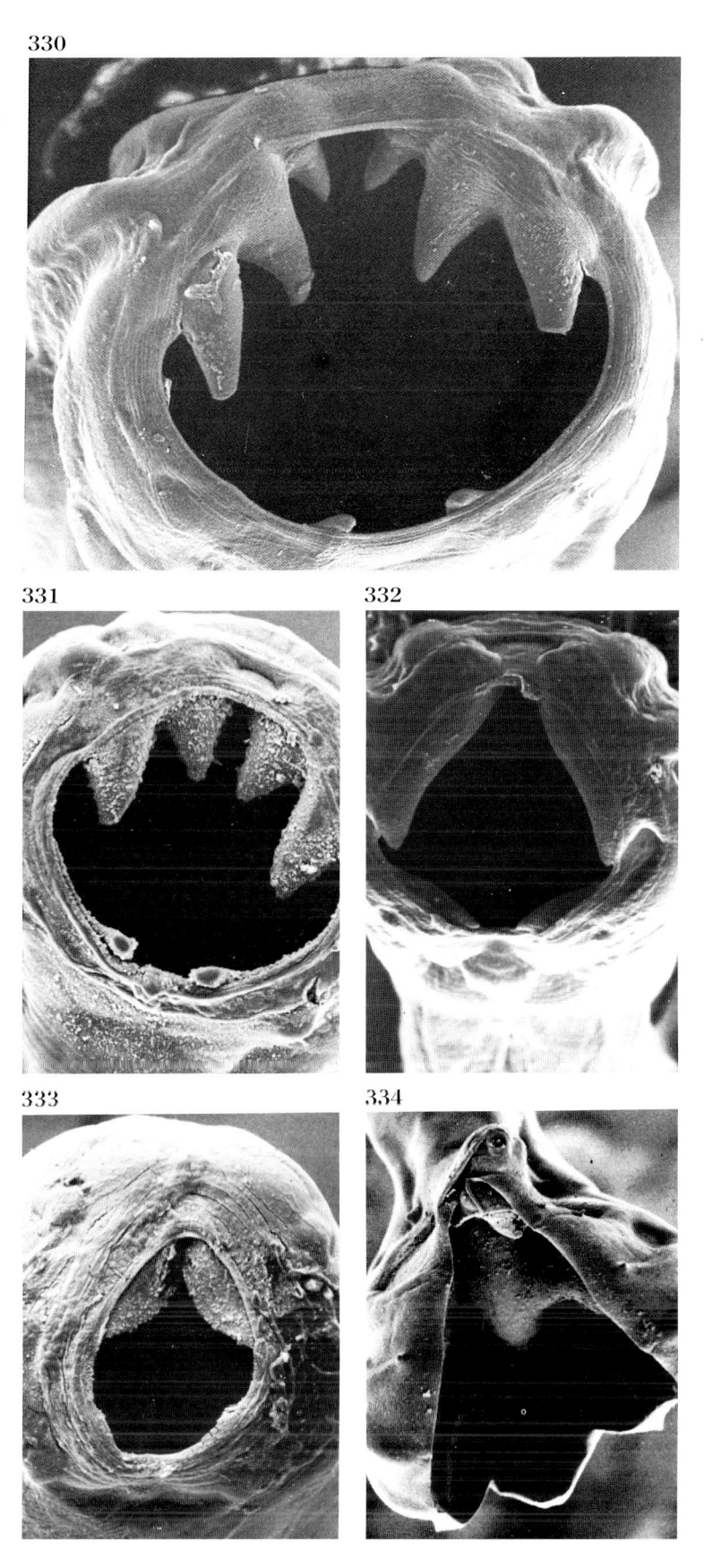

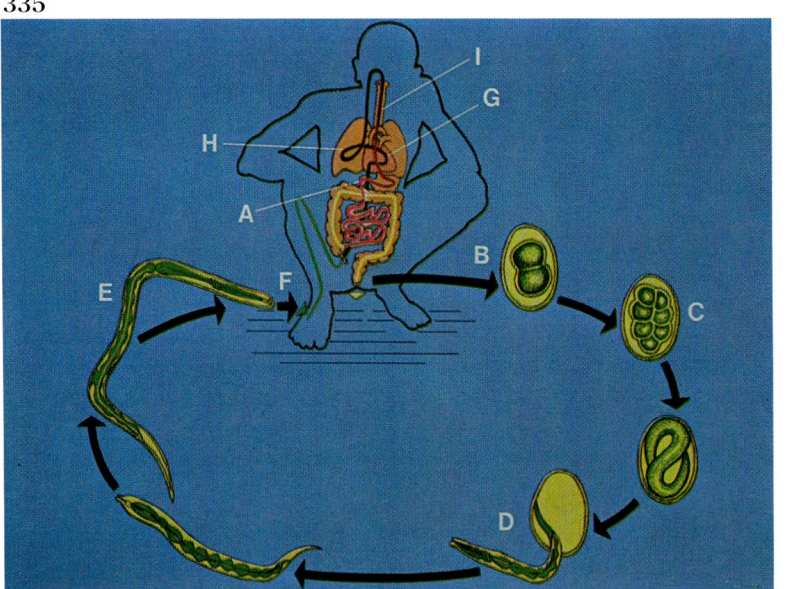

335 Life cycle of *N. americanus* and *A. duodenale* Adults are attached to the walls of the jejunum (A) by the buccal capsule. Females lay large numbers of eggs which are passed out with the faeces (B). They mature through four- and eight-segmented stages (C) to larvae which hatch in the soil (D). There they feed on bacteria and undergo two moults to produce filariform, infective larvae (E). These penetrate the skin of a new host (F), usually on the feet. They migrate into venules, entering the right heart (G) and lungs (H). Here they grow before penetrating from the capillaries into the alveoli. They enter the trachea (I), then the pharynx, are swallowed and pass into the small intestine (A) where they mature. (*See also* **321, 329–340**.)

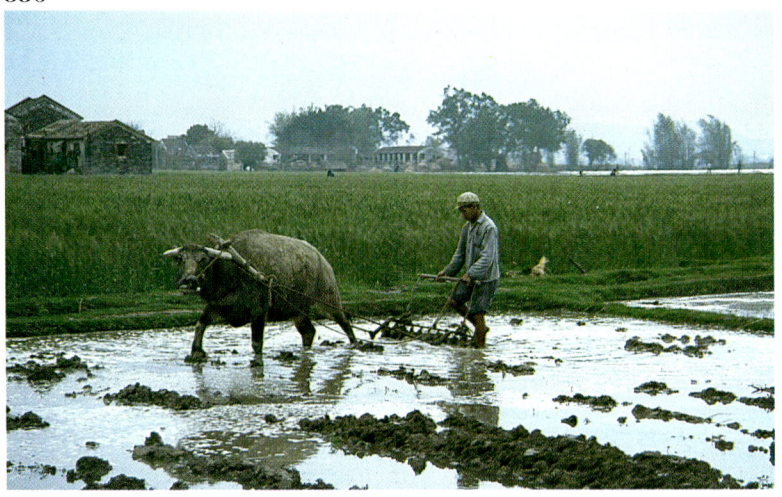

336 Ecology of geohelminth infection In tropical and subtropical areas, wet soil, such as that found at the edges of rice fields, rubber plantations and the surroundings of villages in areas of high rainfall, supports the maturation of hookworm larvae from eggs deposited by indiscriminate defaecation. This limits their geographical distribution. In contrast, the well-protected eggs of nematodes with a direct cycle of transmission (*Ascaris lumbricoides, Trichuris trichiuria*) can survive in drier conditions even at freezing temperatures. (*See also* **424**)

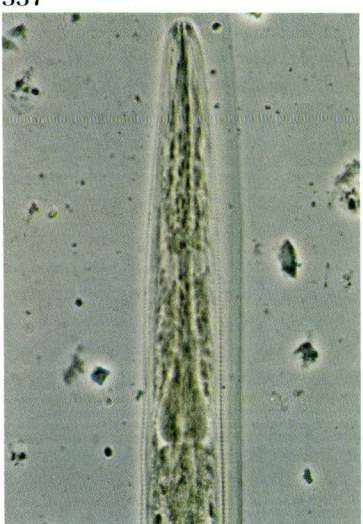

337 Filariform larva of hookworm Eggs (**321**) passed in the faeces hatch into rhabditiform larvae in damp soil; they feed and undergo two moults to produce an infective sheathed filariform larva. (× *350*)

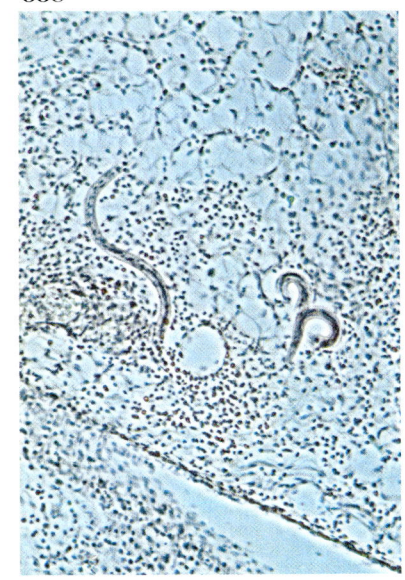

338 Larvae of hookworm in lung of dog The infective larvae penetrate bare skin, usually of feet or legs and, if they are in their correct host, enter the blood stream, to reach the lungs. The larvae then penetrate into the bronchioles, pass into the pharynx and are swallowed. They become attached to the small intestine and mature to adults. (× *100*)

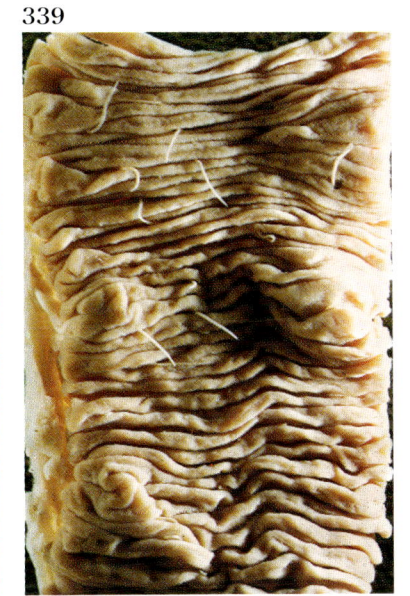

339 Adult hookworms *in situ* The worms are about 1 cm long and characteristically curved. They are attached by their buccal capsules to the villi of the small intestine. (*natural size*)

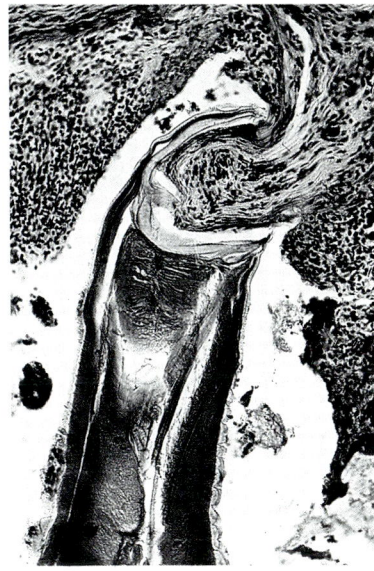

340 Section of adult *A. duodenale in situ* The hookworm feeds by sucking blood from the intestinal mucosa. It has been estimated that a single *A. duodenale* can withdraw as much as 0.2 ml a day while *N. americanus* withdraws 0.05 ml. (*H&E × 20*)

Reproduced with permission from the Armed Forces Institute of Pathology, Washington, D.C. (A.F.I.P. N 33818).

341 Clinical picture of gross hookworm disease Severe anaemia is the classical feature of hookworm disease. This results from high hookworm loads and low daily iron intake. The patients usually complain of lassitude and shortness of breath, while oedema and ascites also occur. This young woman with a heavy load of *N. americanus* in Costa Rica had a haemoglobin level of only 1.7 g/100 ml.

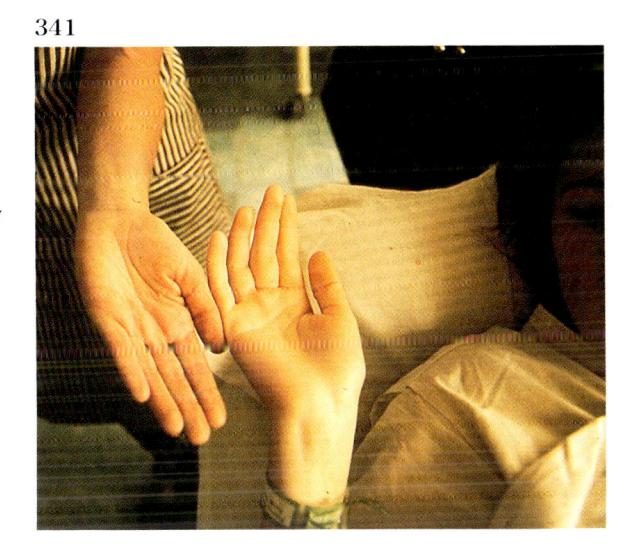

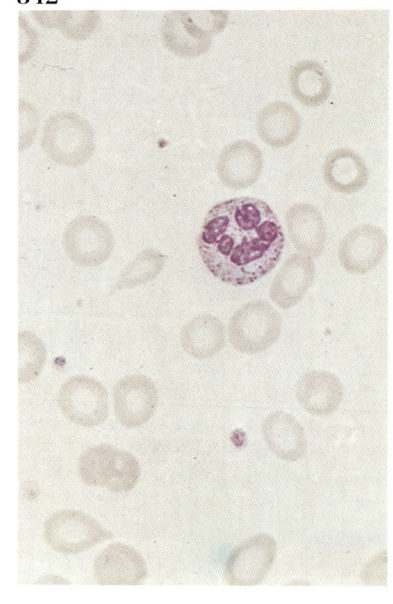

342 Blood film from a patient with hookworm anaemia The typical anaemia resulting from severe hookworm infection is of the iron deficiency type with a low MCHC and low serum iron. (× 900)

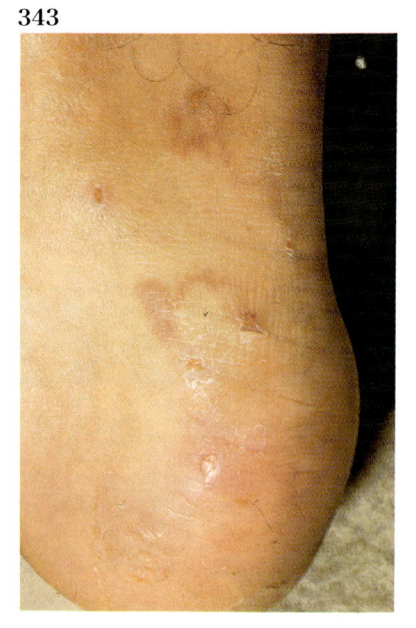

343 'Creeping eruption' due to larvae of dog hookworms Infective larvae of various species of animal hookworms (e.g. *A. braziliense, A. caninum, A. ceylanicum*) frequently fail to penetrate the human dermis. They migrate through the epidermis leaving typical serpiginous tracks known also as 'creeping eruption'.

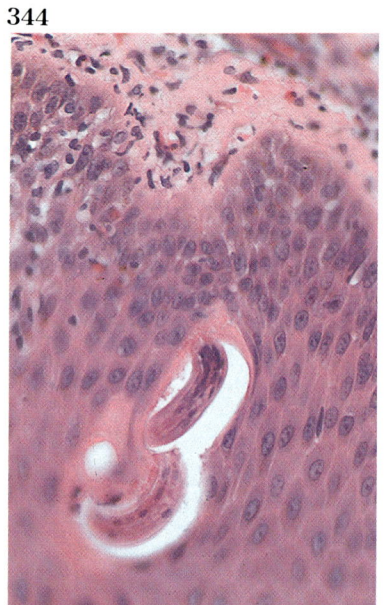

344 Larvae of dog hookworm epidermis of human foot (*H&E* × 400)

Strongyloidiasis

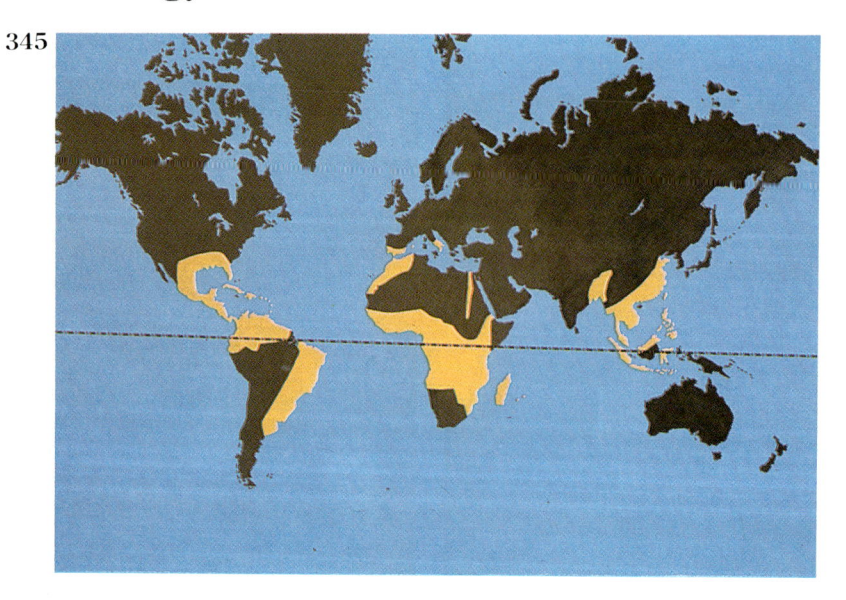

345 Distribution of strongyloidiasis

346 Life cycle of *Strongyloides stercoralis* This tiny nematode has two generations, one free-living and the other parasitic. I. *The parasitic generation*. Males are rare and the females are probably parthenogenetic, living in the mucosal glands of the small intestine (A). Eggs usually hatch in these glands into larvae which are passed in the faeces (B). These rhabditiform larvae can develop into filariform larvae (C) in the ground, the infective filariform larvae then penetrating the skin of a new host (D). The rest of the cycle in man is as in hookworm infections.
II. *Free-living generation*. Rhabditiform larvae (B) may develop into free-living males and females (E) which lay eggs (F) that hatch in the soil into rhabditiform (G), then infective filariform, larvae (H). These too can penetrate the skin (D) and recommence a parasitic cycle in man.
III. *Auto-infection*. Rhabditiform larvae (B) can mature into filariform larvae in the intestine, and these can directly penetrate the perianal skin, causing auto-infection.
IV. *Hyperinfection*. Rhabditiform larvae may penetrate the intestinal mucosa causing massive auto-infection, usually in people with diminished immune responsiveness (cycle not illustrated here).

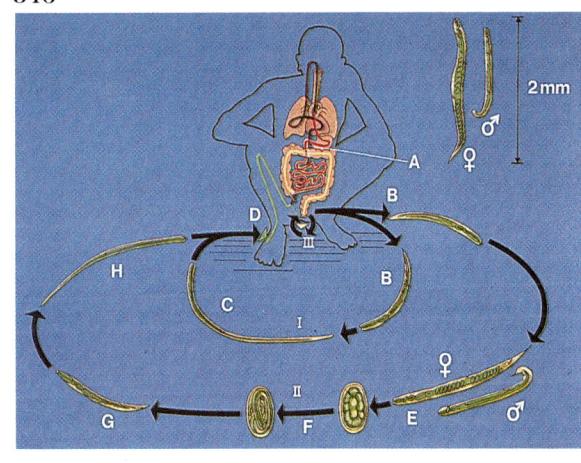

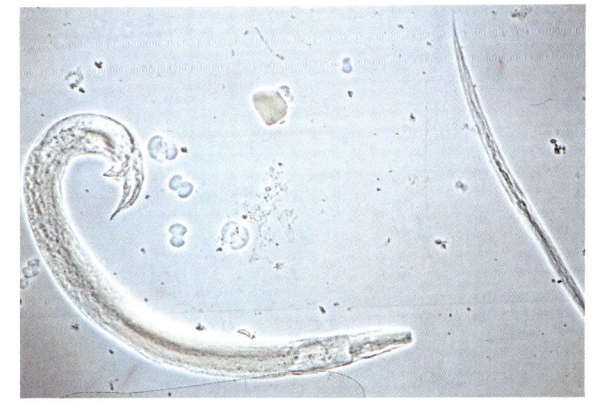

347 Rhabditiform larvae of *S. stercoralis* in faeces The figure shows rhabditiform larvae which are usually the only stages seen in faeces. Eggs, which are rarely seen, resemble those of hookworm but contain maturing larvae ($\times 80$) (See **357**.)

348 Adult male and free-living larva in soil ($\times 65$)

349 Sections of parasitic female and eggs embedded in jejunal mucosa Free-living females (about 1 mm long) are smaller than the forms found in the intestine (up to 2.2 mm). Males are normally only found in the soil and are about 0.7 mm long. The parasitic females lying in the intestinal mucosa may reproduce parthenogenetically, the eggs filtering through to the intestinal lumen or first hatching in the mucosa ($\times 180$)

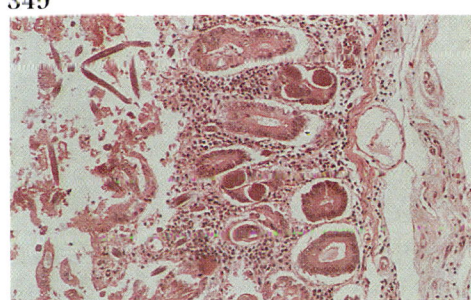

350 Migrating larvae of *S. stercoralis* in skin Auto-infection can lead to severe 'creeping eruption' which usually occurs on the back. This may occur many years (30 or more) after initial infection. Deep migration of the larvae may be associated with an 'eosinophilic lung' type of syndrome.

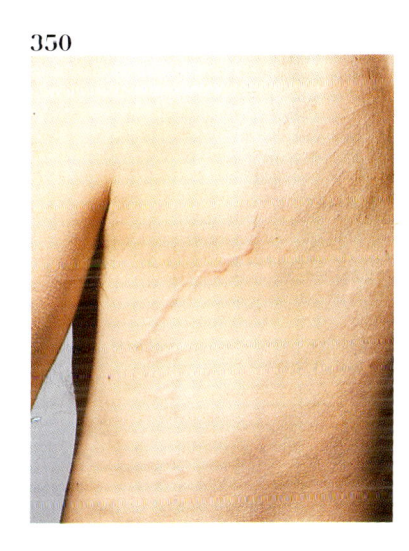

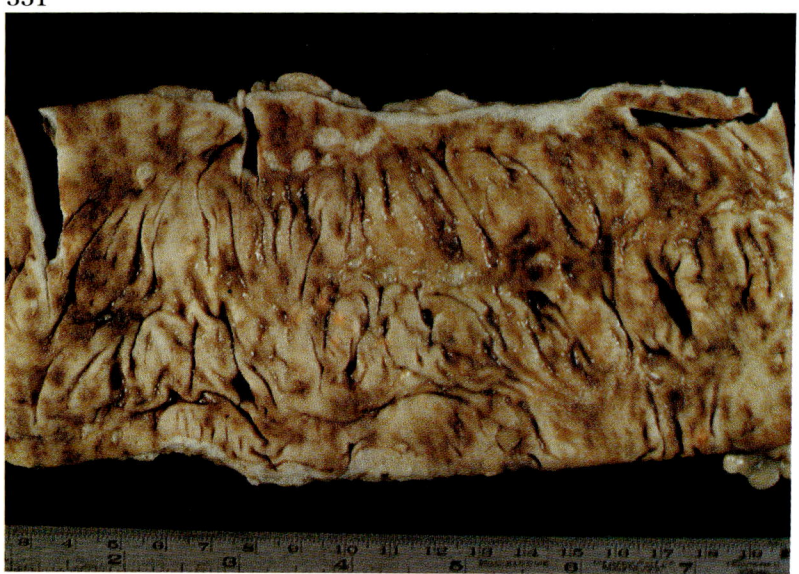

351 Post-mortem appearance of colon The incidental administration of steroids and immunosuppressive agents such as HIV in patients with AIDS may greatly enhance infection with *S. stercoralis*, which may even be fatal as in this case. Note the multiple ulcerations and thickening of the wall of the colon.

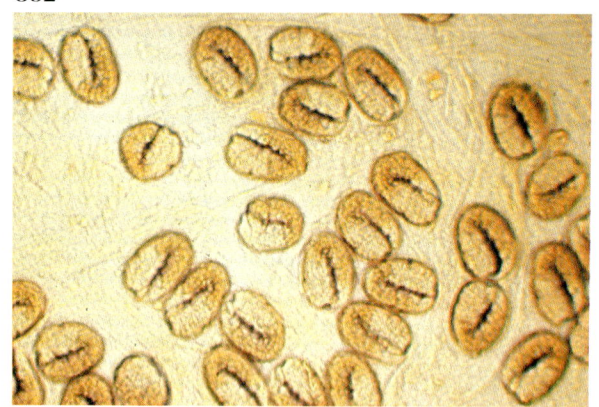

352 Eggs of *Strongyloides fülleborni* in faeces *S. fülleborni*, a common intestinal nematode in African and Asian primates, is found in man in a number of countries, including Zambia where 10 per cent of human *Strongyloides* infections may be caused by this species. Massive infections with a nematode apparently indistinguishable from *S. fülleborni* cause an often fatal illness in infants in the west of Papua New Guinea, a country from which monkeys are absent. This condition, known as 'swollen belly sickness', is characterised by respiratory distress, abdominal distension and generalised oedema. Very heavy egg loads, such as are seen here, occur in such cases (× 300).

Other phasmid nematodes of man

353 Head capsule of adult *Ternidens deminutus* In some areas such as East and Central Africa infection commonly occurs with a hookworm-like parasite of monkeys, *T. deminutus*, which also infects monkeys in Asia. The adult worm, which is about 1 cm long, is found at any level in the small and large intestine and normally infection is asymptomatic. (× 95)

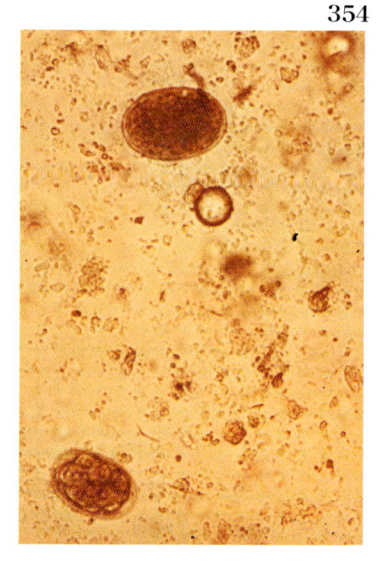

354 Eggs of *T. deminutus* and hookworm compared The eggs (top) are usually mistaken for those of hookworm, but the adults passed accidentally during hookworm therapy are distinctive. (× 125) (See also **321**, and **491-496** for *Angiostrongylus*.)

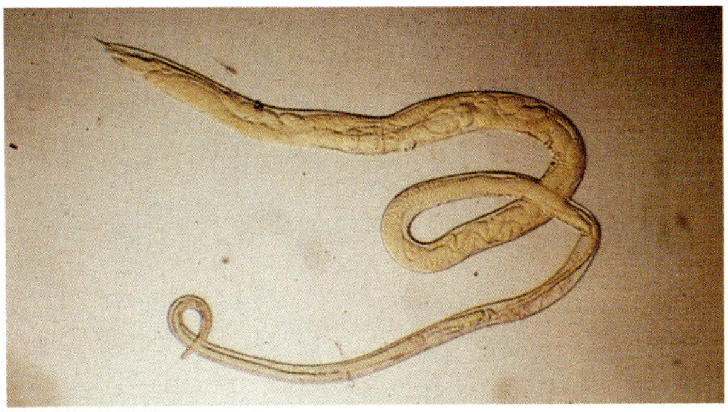

355 Adult male *Trichostrongylus* Various species of *Trichostrongylus* inhabit the digestive tract of herbivores, burrowing into the mucosa, like hookworms, to obtain their nutrition. They have been encountered infrequently in man but in many different countries and, in one Iranian town, they were said to be present in 70 per cent of the population. They are readily distinguished from human hookworms, firstly by their smaller size and more slender shape. The male bursa is different in form from that of *A. duodenale* (**334**). (× 100).

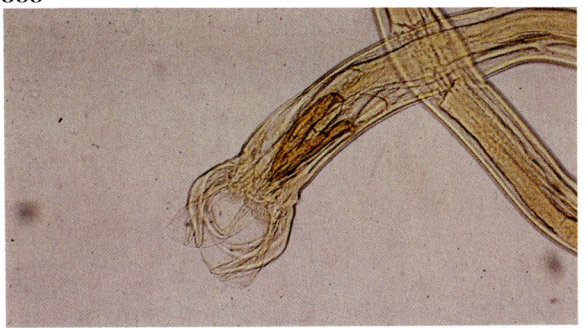

356 Adult female *Trichostrongylus* The head of this tiny, very slender worm (about 0.5 cm long) lacks the distinct buccal cavity of the human hookworms (**330-333**). (× 50)

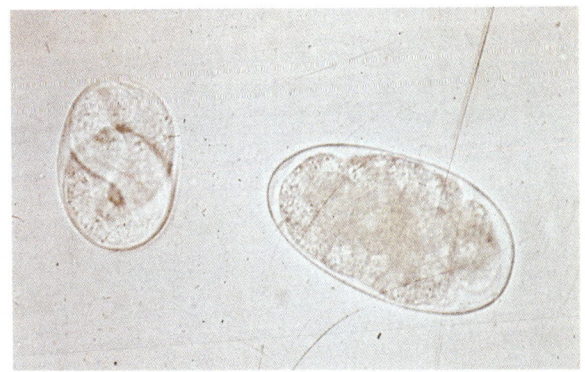

357 Eggs of *Trichostrongylus* and *S. stercoralis* in faeces The hookworm-like egg of the *Trichostrongylus* (right) is much larger (about 60 × 40μm) than that of *S. stercoralis* which contains an embryonic larva ready to hatch. (× 320)

INFECTION WITH *ASCARIS* AND RELATED NEMATODES

Ascariasis

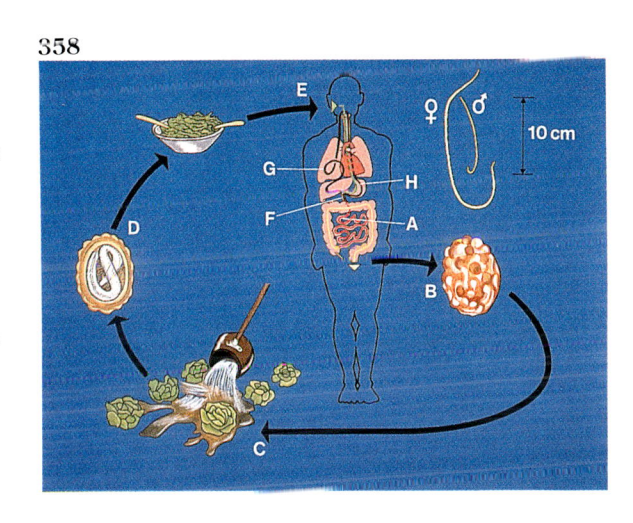

358 Life cycle of the roundworm, *Ascaris lumbricoides* Adult worms live in the small intestine (A) where they lay large numbers of eggs (B) that are passed out with the faeces. In the soil they can readily contaminate vegetables, for example, when night-soil (C) is used as fertiliser. The larvae develop inside the eggs (D) which are swallowed when they are present in uncooked food (E). The eggs enter the jejunum where the larvae hatch, penetrate the mucosa, and are carried through the hepatic circulation to the heart and lungs (G). There they grow, moulting twice before escaping from the capillaries into the alveoli. They again enter the stomach (H) via the trachea and oesophagus, and thence pass to the small intestine where they grow to adulthood. (*See also* **317** & **318**)

93

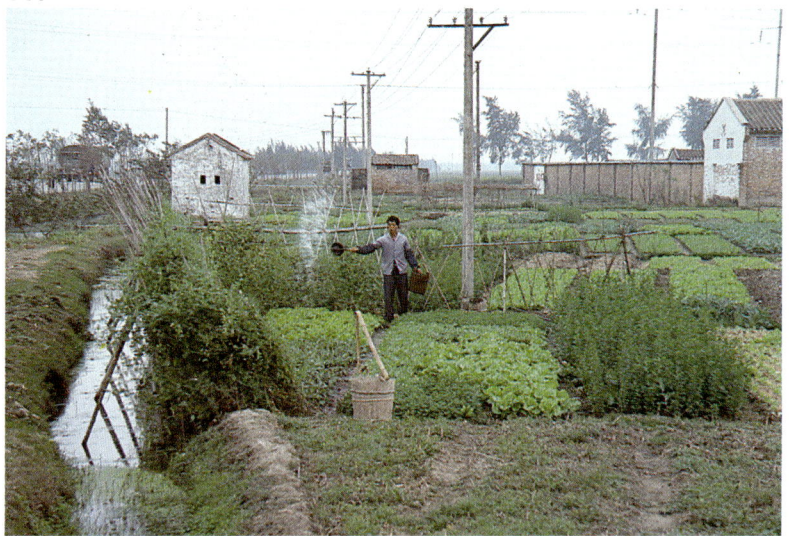

359 Ecology of infection with *Ascaris* and *Trichuris* The use of fresh night-soil to fertilise green leaf vegetables which are then eaten without adequate washing is a sure way to maintain the transmission of these roundworms. Their prevalence in a community is a good indicator of the standards of personal hygiene and sanitation. Since their eggs can survive even in a cold climate, their distribution is global.

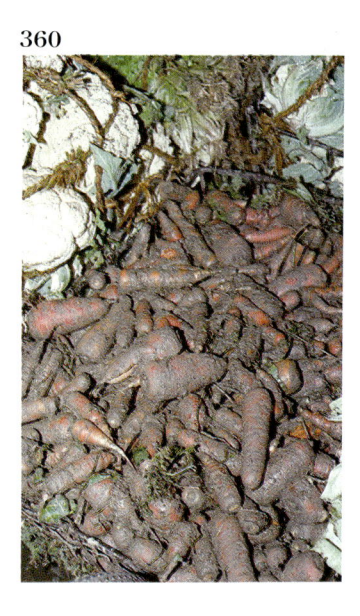

360 Vegetables in an Eastern market These carrots are likely to be heavily contaminated with helminth eggs, as well as protozoal cysts, but the parasites will be destroyed when the vegetables are cooked.

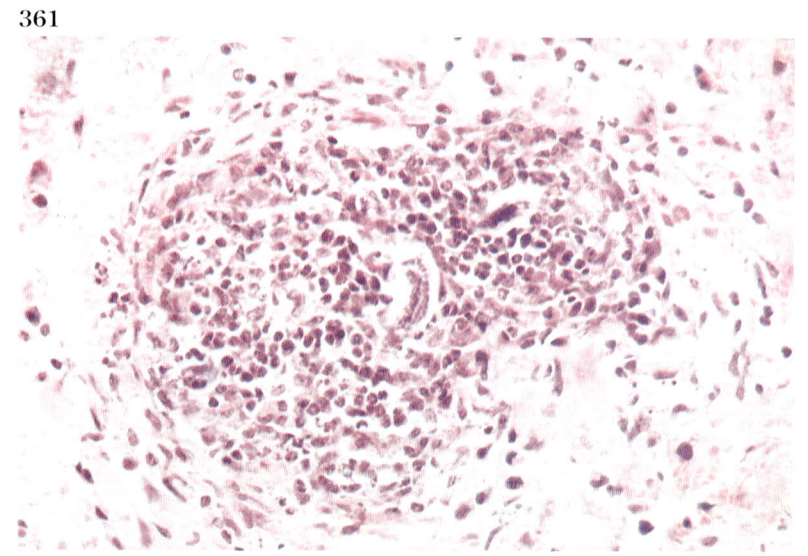

361 *Ascaris lumbricoides* larvae migrating in lung The figure shows a section of a larva in the interstitial tissue of the lung. This stage is associated with eosinophilia, and pneumonitis may accompany heavy infestations. ($\times 128$)

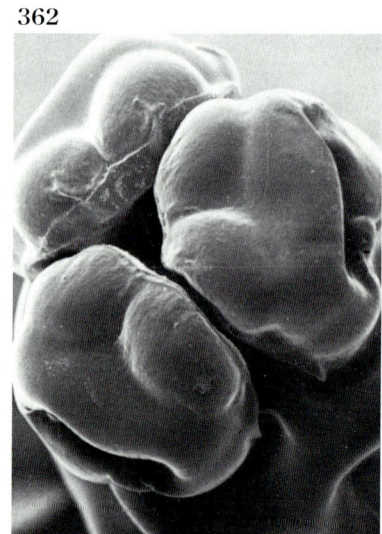

362 Head of adult This scanning electron micrograph shows the typical head structures. ($\times 110$)

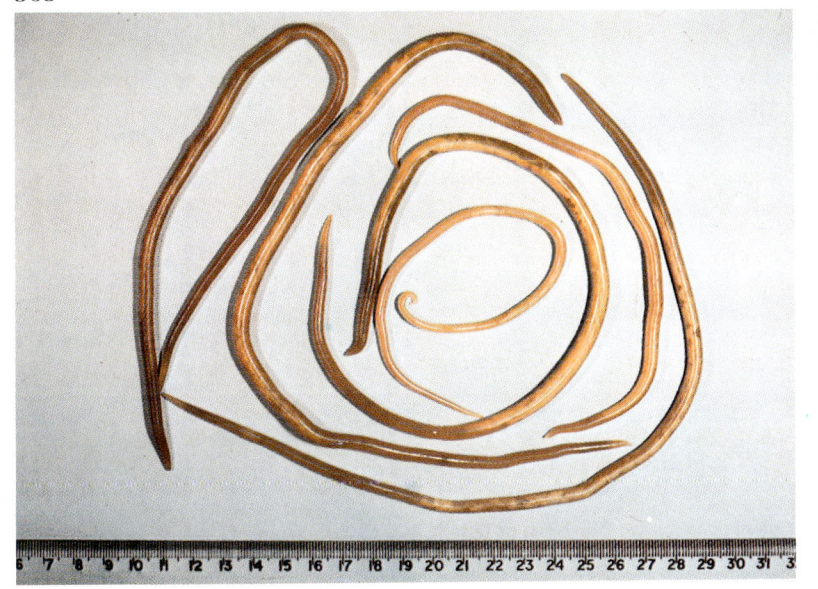

363 Adult *Ascaris* They mature into adult roundworms in the small intestine. The adult males are about 15 to 30 cm long, and females 20 to 35 cm.

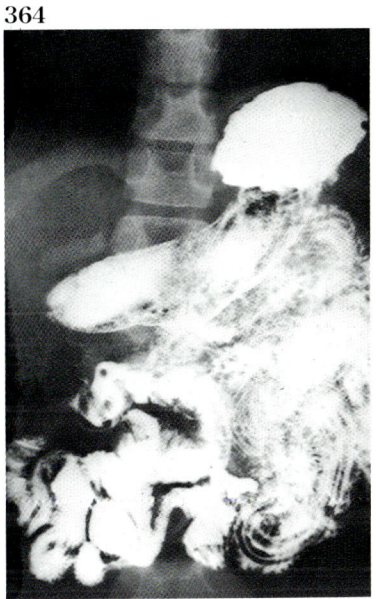

364 *A. lumbricoides* seen in X-ray The adults may be seen as filling defects in patients having barium meals for investigation of intestinal symptoms.

365 Obstruction due to roundworms Heavy infections, especially in children, may lead to intestinal obstruction. Volvulus is an additional complication in this intestine from a two-year-old child.

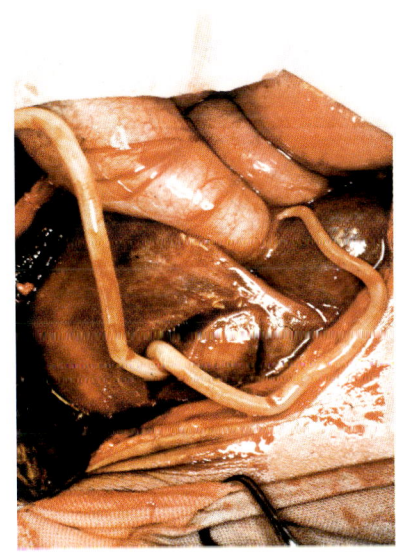

366 Adult roundworms migrating in liver The adult worms have a marked tendency to penetrate any available hole in their vicinity and may escape through abdominal fistulae following operations such as appendicectomy. They may also block such organs as the common bile duct, and the appendix itself.

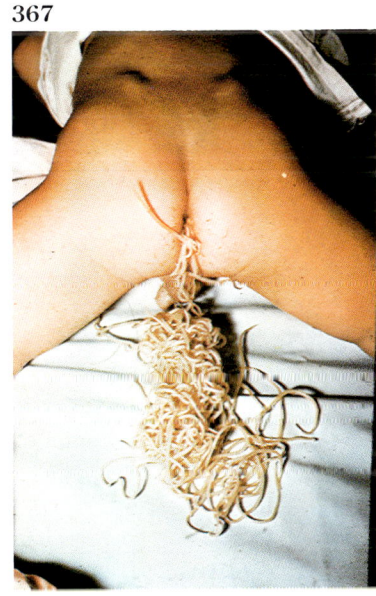

367 Massive *Ascaris* infection in child A large bolus of roundworms expelled following anthelminthic treatment.

Toxocariasis

Visceral larva migrans results from accidental infection of man with eggs of the ascarid roundworm of the dog *Toxocara canis* and cat *T. cati*. The life cycle in the animal host is the same as that of *Ascaris* but the invasive larvae in man become arrested in various tissues where they are gradually phagocytosed. In the process they induce marked eosinophilia and local tissue reaction. The liver and eye are the most common sites involved.

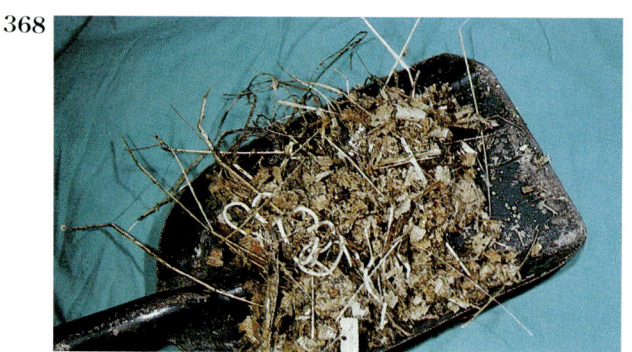

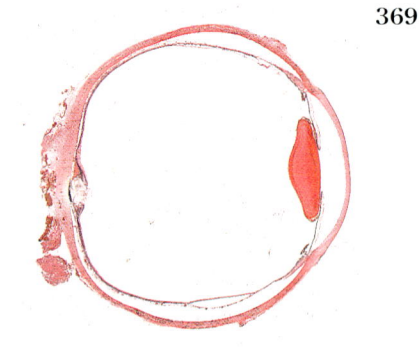

368 Adult *Toxocara canis* The worms seen here were from a puppy following anthelminthic therapy. The adults are about 10 cm long and similar in general appearance to *A. lumbricoides*. Uncontrolled contamination of soil by dogs and cats is common everywhere. Like those of *Ascaris*, the eggs of *T. canis* and *T. cati* can survive even in a cold climate.

369 Longitudinal section of human eye Invasion of the eye produces a retinoblastoma-like mass which may lead to blindness. Sometimes the eye is mistakenly enucleated.

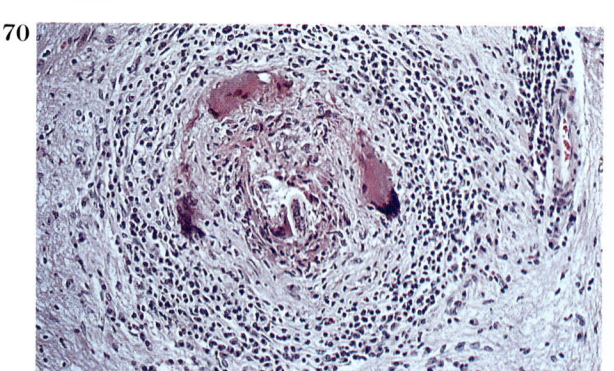

370 Larva of *T. canis* in human brain The larva is seen in the centre of the granuloma formed by mononuclear cells, eosinophils and multinucleated giant cells. (*H&E × 120*)

371 Migrating larva in human kidney In this section a larva is seen in the kidney surrounded by an inflammatory exudate and fibroblasts. (*H&E × 300*)

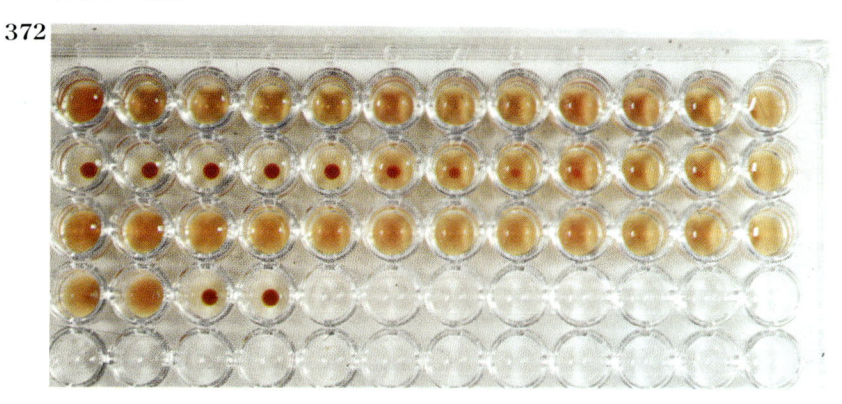

372 Serological diagnosis The diagnosis is supported by a positive serological response to *Toxocara* antigen such as the CFT. (Top row is a negative control serum; second row - positive response at 1/64 from a patient with visceral larva migrans; third row - negative serum from another patient with suggestive symptoms; fourth row - complement control.)

TRICHURIASIS

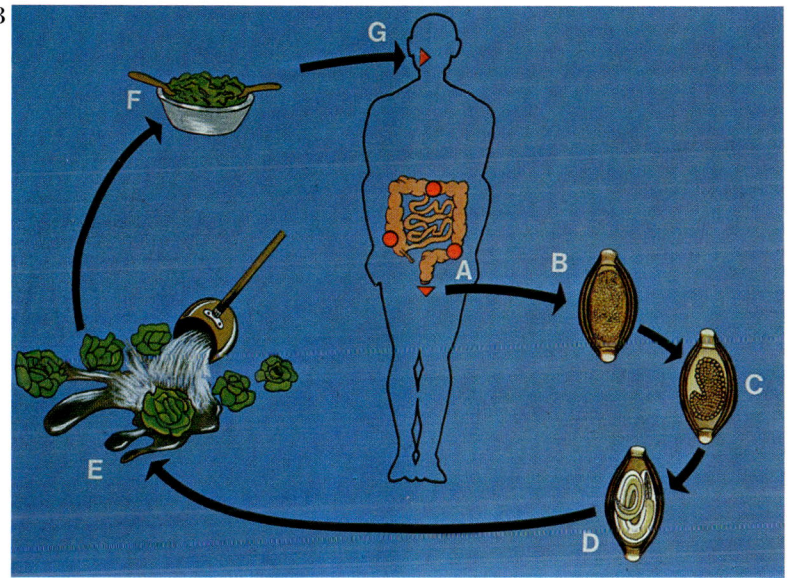

373 Life cycle of the whipworm, *Trichuris trichiura* Adults inhabit the caecum (A) and sometimes the colon and rectum where they are attached to the mucosa. Eggs passed with the faeces (B) mature in the soil to larvae (C & D) which remain in the eggs. Eggs can readily contaminate vegetables, e.g. when night-soil is used as fertiliser (E) or sanitary habits are otherwise primitive, and are then swallowed in uncooked food (F & G). The eggs hatch in the small intestine and the developing larvae pass directly to their attachment sites in the large intestine (A). Females commence egg-laying after about three months. (*See also* **322 & 329**)

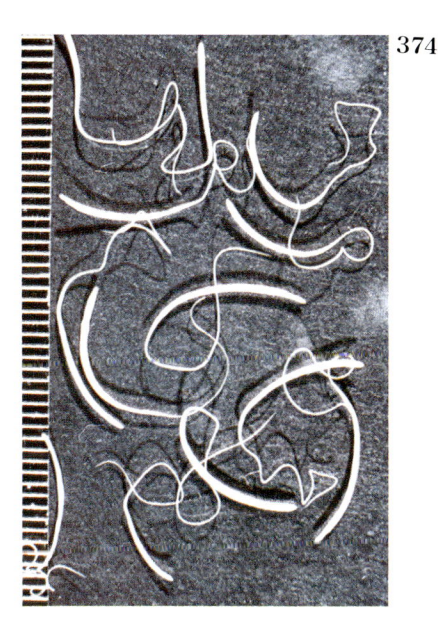

374 & 375 Adult morphology, females and males Three to ten days after the eggs are ingested, the young worms pass down to the caecum where the whip-like anterior portion becomes entwined in the mucosa. The adult worms are about 3 to 5 cm long, the females being slightly larger than the males which are coiled.

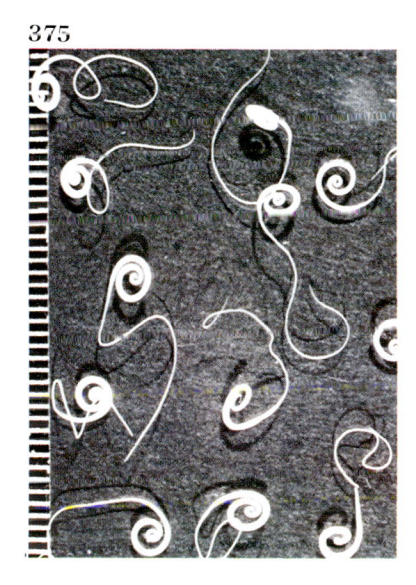

376 Whipworms *in situ* The adult worms are readily seen in this figure of the caecal mucosa.

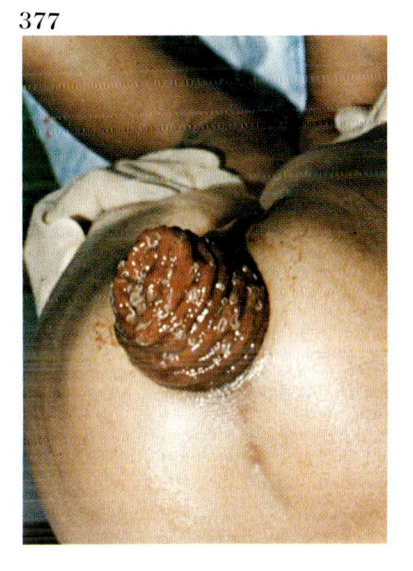

377 Rectal prolapse Heavy infections in infants and young children may cause rectal prolapse following chronic bloody diarrhoea with abdominal pain.

(For Capillariasis *see* **596-598**.)

Part III
Snail-mediated Helminthiases

With the exception of angiostrongyliasis, which is a nematode infection transmitted accidentally to man in the course of its complex life cycle in rodents, the important group of snail-transmitted helminths that infect man are all trematodes (flukes) which undergo a complicated cycle involving various species of land or aquatic snails. The three common schistosome infections of man are responsible for a vast amount of general ill health and contribute in certain areas to the heavy mortality rate found among adolescents and young adults. Since infection occurs by penetration of the skin by water-dwelling infective stages (cercariae), transmission tends to increase in parallel with the increase of land utilisation by irrigation. Hence schistosomiasis is a positive obstacle in the way of agricultural and economic development in many parts of the developing world.

The intestinal liver and lung flukes have a somewhat more complicated life cycle in that the cercariae develop a resting stage (the metacercariae) which, in turn, must be ingested by man in order to infect him. As the metacercariae are found usually on various water plants, on fish or on crustaceans, infection with these worms tends to be localised to areas where particular local eating habits bring man and the metacercariae together. Thus clonorchiasis is restricted to parts of SE Asia where raw fish is commonly ingested, fasciolopsiasis where, for example, water caltrops and water chestnuts are eaten uncooked, and paragonimiasis where the appropriate crustaceans form part of man's diet in one culinary delicacy or another. Many of these flukes are primarily parasites of animals other than man, for example, *Fasciola hepatica* is essentially a parasite of sheep that infects man when he eats watercress or other aquatic plants from contaminated, wet pastures. They are thus zoonoses and, like many zoonoses, are relatively uncommon, with notable, highly localised exceptions. In certain villages in northeast Thailand, for example, *Fasciolopsis buski* has been found to infect nearly 100 per cent of the population and *Opisthorchis viverrini* 90 per cent. An idea of the numbers of human infections with these trematodes is given in **Table XI**.

SCHISTOSOMIASIS

378 Life cycle of human schistosomes The schistosomes provide a classical example of the life cycle of trematodes. The three common parasites of man, *Schistosoma haematobium*, *S. japonicum* and *S. mansoni* have a similar life cycle. Eggs passed in urine (*S. haematobium*, A) or faeces (*S. japonicum*, B, *S. mansoni*, C), hatch in aggregations of water such as ponds, lake edges, streams and canals. From the eggs miracidia (D) hatch into the water where they penetrate into suitable snails. In the snails they develop two generations of sporocysts (not shown here), the second of which produces fork-tailed cercariae (E). These penetrate the skin (F) when a new host comes into contact with contaminated water. Once through the skin, the cercariae shed their tails and become schistosomulae which migrate through the tissues until they reach the portal venous system of the liver (G). There males and females (H) copulate before settling down in pairs in the venous system of the liver. From there *S. haematobium* usually migrates to the venous plexus of the bladder (I) and other species (including the geographically localised *S. intercalatum* and *S. mekongi*) to the rectum (J) where spiny eggs are laid. The eggs penetrate into the bladder or rectum from which they reach the exterior. Eggs laid by worms in the liver itself lead to local fibrotic changes and cirrhosis. (See also 313-315, 381-383, 385-393, 397, 407, 416, 431 & 432.)

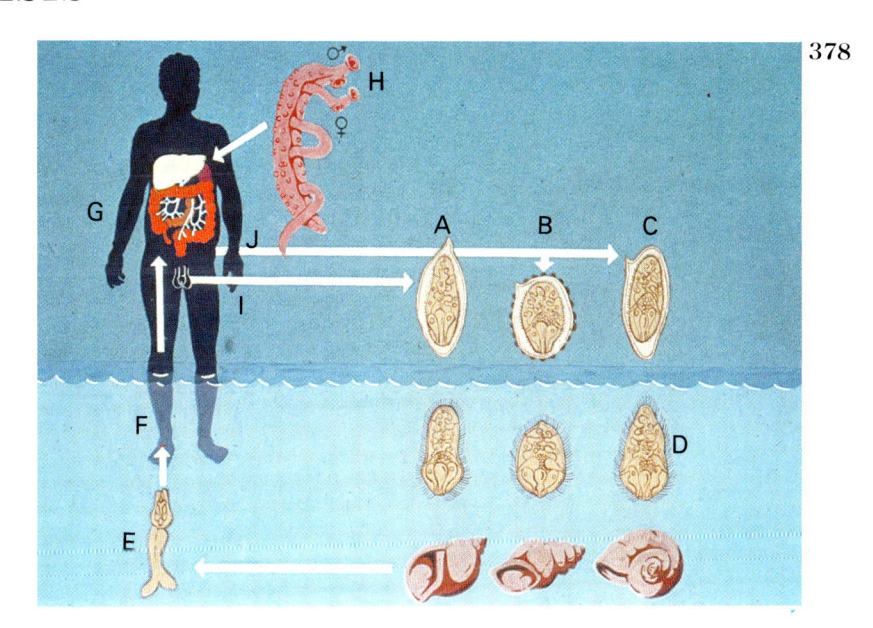

379 Distribution of *S. mansoni* The distribution of schistosomiasis is regulated both by the presence of susceptible snail intermediate hosts and human sanitary habits. *S. mansoni* occurs in Africa, the Middle East, some Caribbean islands, and in parts of South America. It was introduced from the Old World into the New World where potentially susceptible species of *Biomphalaria* were already present.

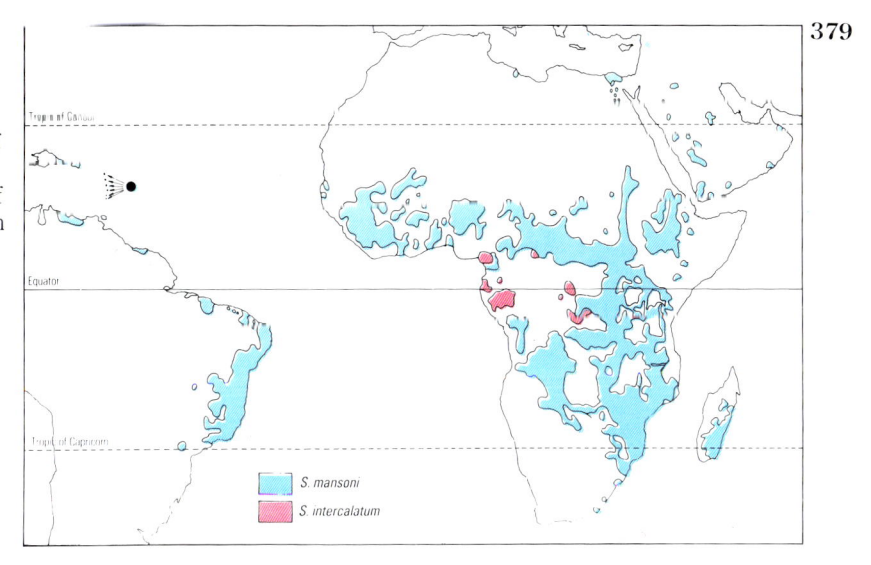

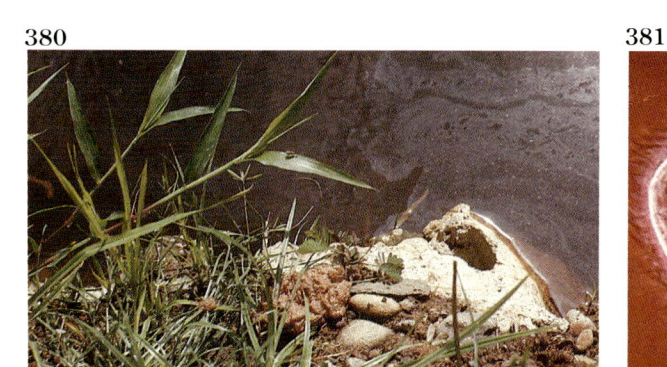

380 Ecology of intestinal schistosomiasis Human faeces deposited at the edge of a pond in which snail hosts of *S. mansoni* were breeding. Eggs enter the water to hatch and perpetuate the cycle of transmission.

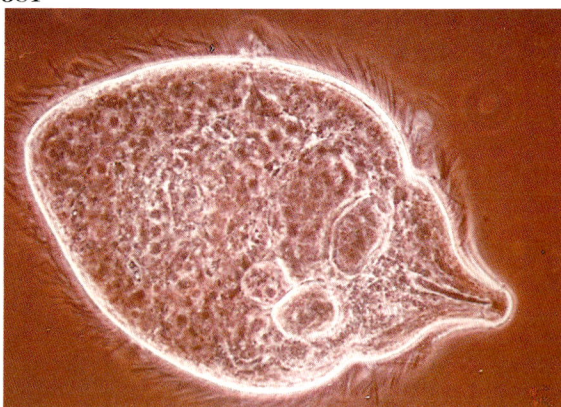

381 Hatched miracidium of *S. mansoni* The three common species of schistosomes infecting man have easily recognisable eggs although those of *S. haematobium* may be confused with *S. intercalatum* (**431**). Miracidia can often be seen inside mature eggs. ($\times 600$)

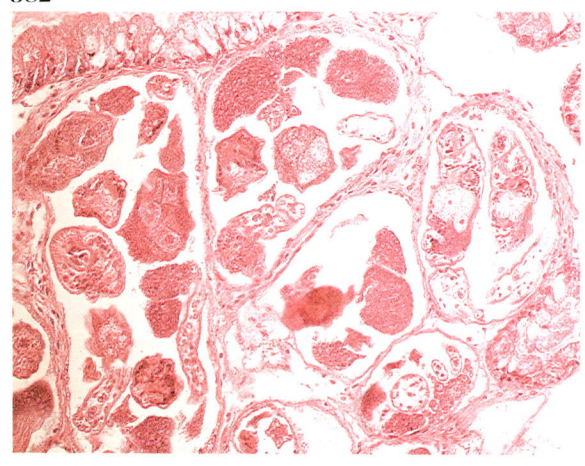

382 Section of 'mother' sporocyst in the hepatopancreas of a snail The cycle in the snail is of variable duration depending on the species of parasite, host and environmental conditions, but it is usually only one month. Cercaria develop in the second generation ('daughter') sporocysts. The figure shows several coils of the sporocyst in the hepatopancreas and sections of cercaria. (*Acetic carbol fuchsin* $\times 130$)

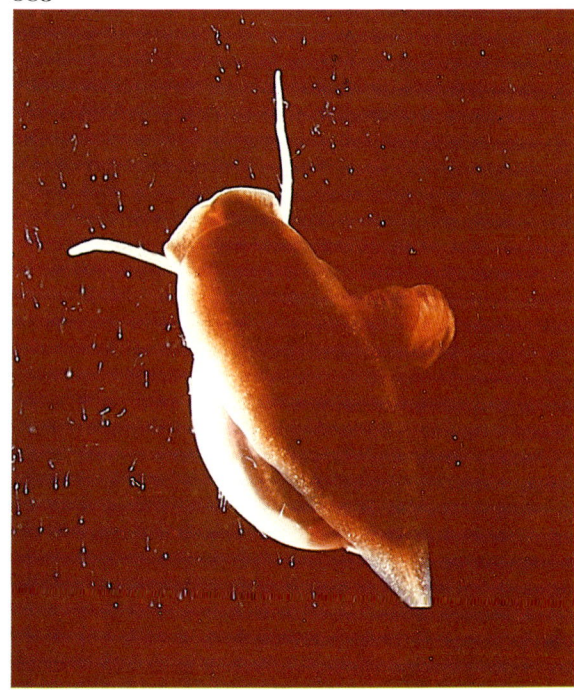

383 A snail 'shedding' living bifurcate cercaria of *S. mansoni* Once snails start to 'shed' cercariae, they continue to do so during daylight hours for up to as much as 200 days. A heavily infected snail may shed 1 500 to 2 000 cercariae a day. ($\times 6$)

384 Site of human infection with *S. mansoni* These women and their children became infected by cercariae while washing clothes in contaminated water. The provision of a piped water supply to the village drastically reduced the amount of transmission.

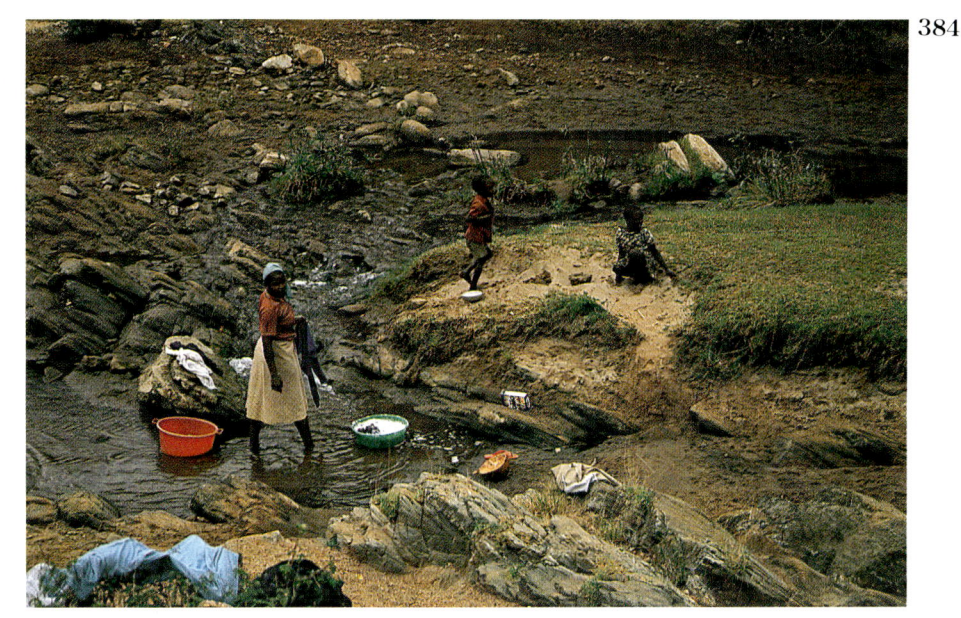

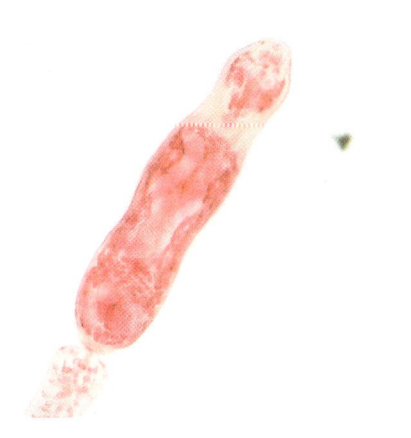

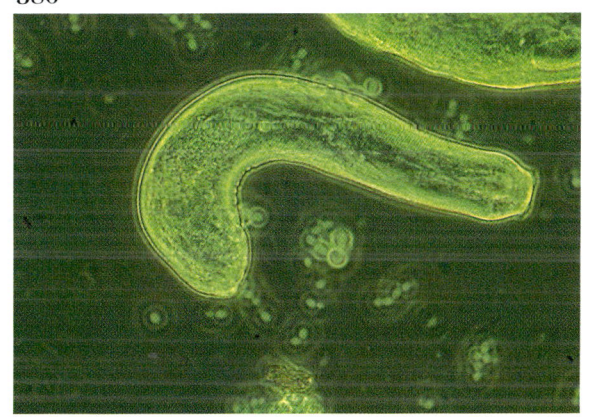

385 Head of cercaria The apical and ventral suckers of the future schistosomule are clearly seen in this preparation. (*Mayer's haemalum* × 350)

386 Schistosomule of *S. mansoni* (*phase-contrast* × 350)

387 Living male and female *S. mansoni* The slender female normally lives within the gynecophoral groove of the male. (× 15)

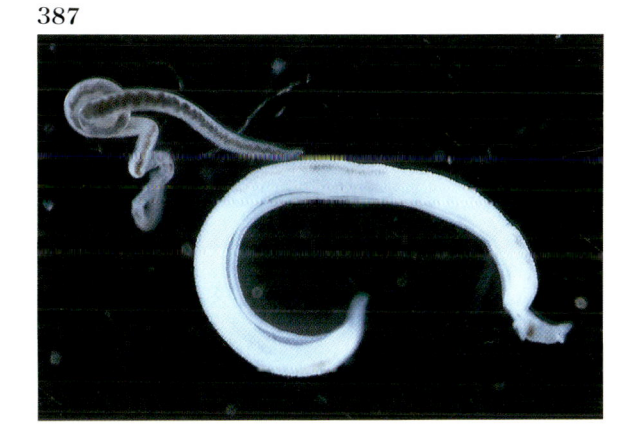

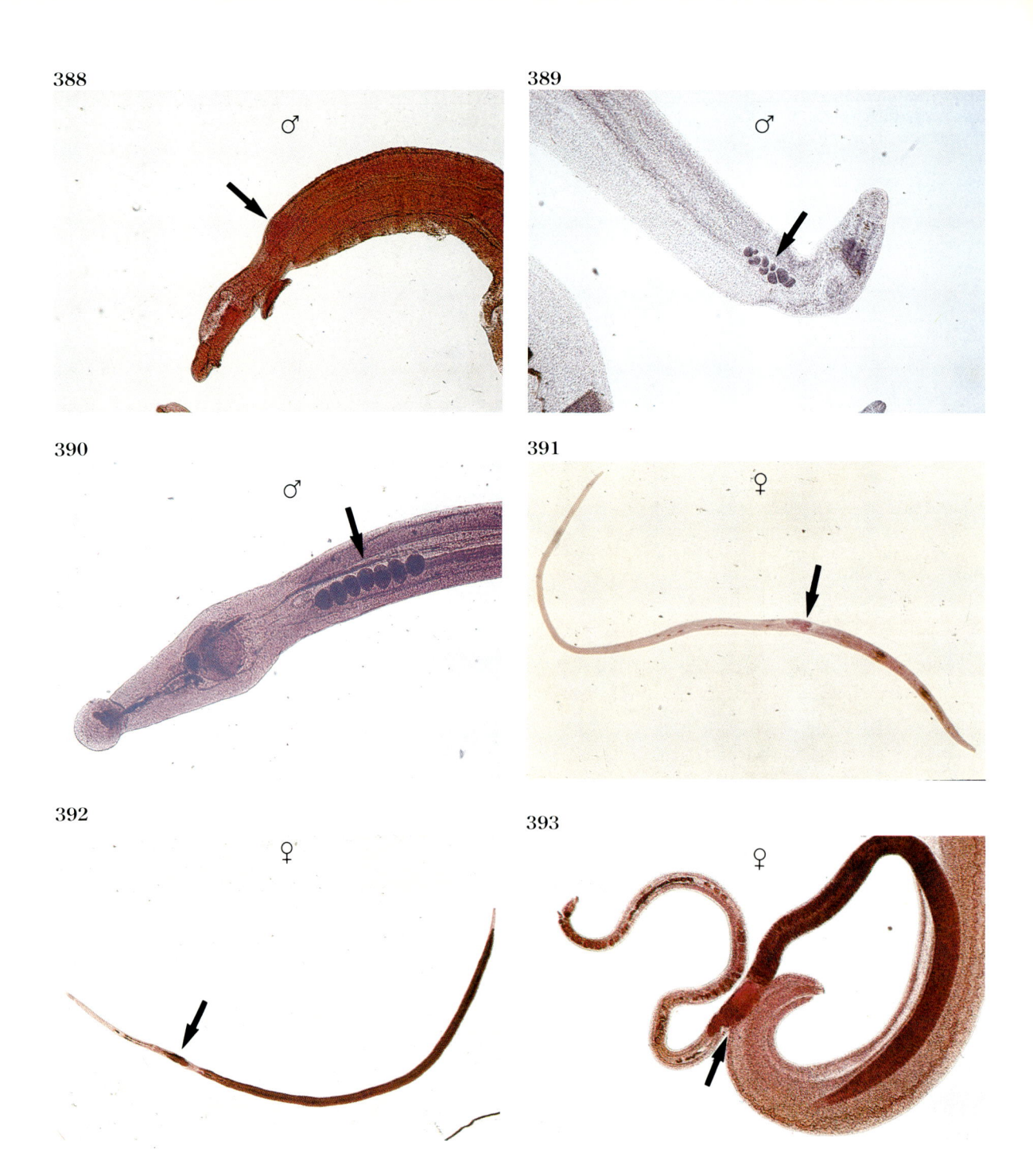

388–393 Morphology of adult schistosomes Mature males and females live in copulating pairs. The common species are recognised by the characters shown in the figures. Testes of males: *S. haematobium* (**388**); *S. mansoni* (**389**); *S. japonicum* (**390**). Ovaries of females: *S. haematobium* (**391**); *S. mansoni* (**392**); *S. japonicum* (**393**). ($\times 25$)

394 Dermatitis from avian cercariae in a Japanese patient Penetration of the skin by cercariae may give rise to an itchy rash known as 'cercarial dermatitis'. This is occasionally seen in countries free of human schistosomiasis due to invasion by the cercariae of avian schistosomes which are otherwise non-pathogenic to man.

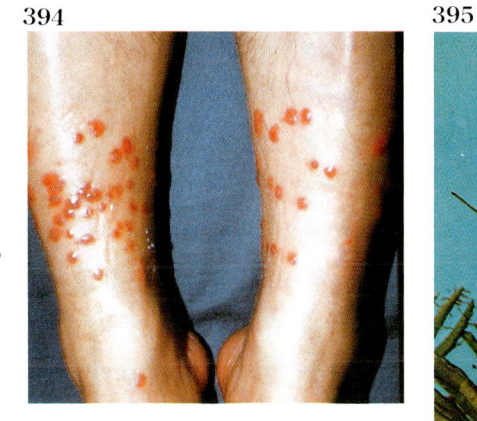

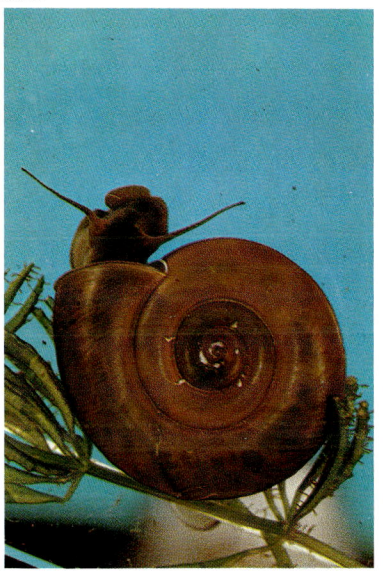

Schistosoma mansoni

395 Intermediate host of S. mansoni The snail intermediate hosts of S. mansoni are various species of *Biomphalaria* (× 4) (See also **Table XII**.)

396 Sampling snail populations A scoopful of *Biomphalaria sudanica*, a host for *S. mansoni* in Lake Victoria.

397 Adult S. mansoni in portal tract Male and female schistosomes lodge *in copula* in the portal tract, mesenteric or vesical plexuses. The figure shows a cross-section of a male and female *S. mansoni* in a branch of the portal vein. (H&E × 40)

398 Granuloma surrounding egg of S. mansoni in liver Eggs (**314**) may lodge ectopically in any tissues, where they cause characteristic granulomas. It has been suggested that toxic substances associated with the ova trigger the fibrotic process. In histological sections the ova are seen in the portal and periportal regions. All types of reaction may be present from acute eosinophilic cellular infiltration (as seen here) to the dense collagenous deposition which leads to periportal fibrosis (*see also* **408**). (H&E × 120)

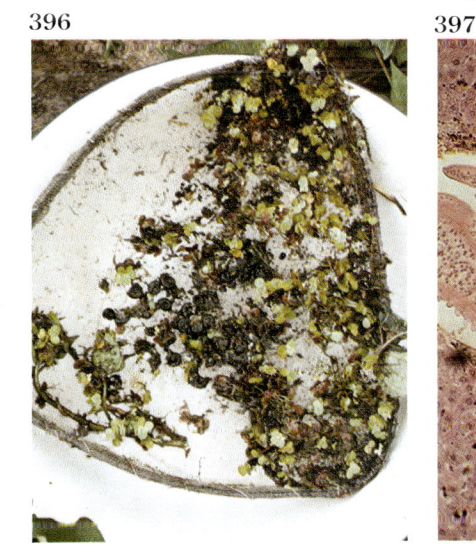

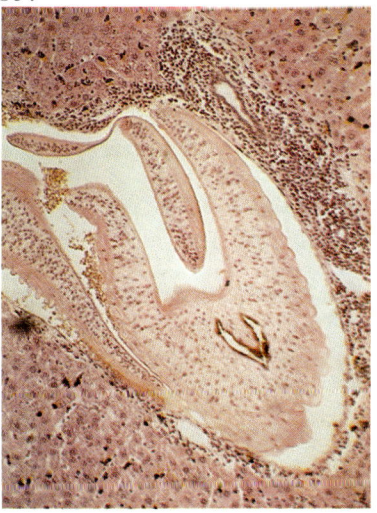

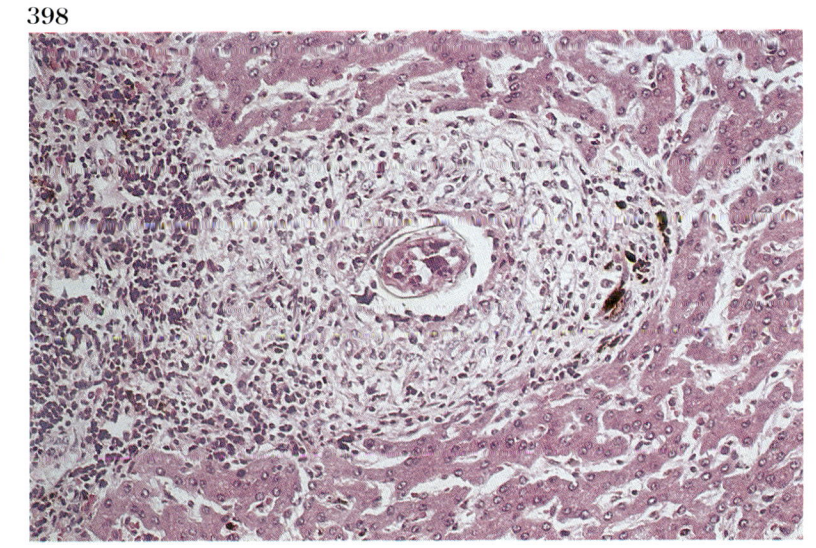

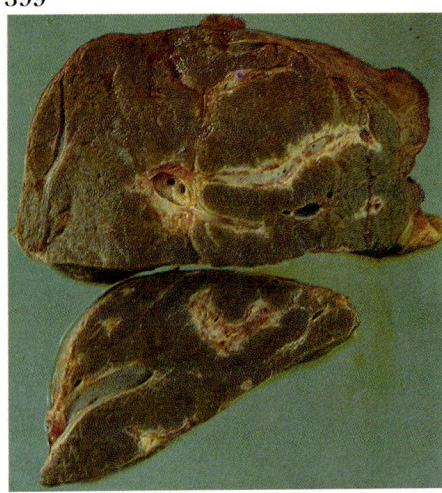

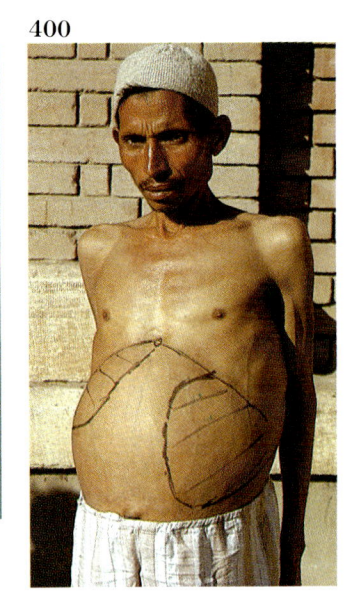

399 Periportal fibrosis of the liver Periportal fibrosis ('pipestem fibrosis') is the classical pathological hepatic lesion. The white areas, which may be round, oval or stellate, are due to the terminal fibrotic reaction originally caused by the presence of the ova in and around the portal venous radicles.

400 Egyptian splenomegaly The combination of enlarged, irregularly fibrosed liver and greatly enlarged spleen is commonly called 'Egyptian hepatosplenomegaly'.

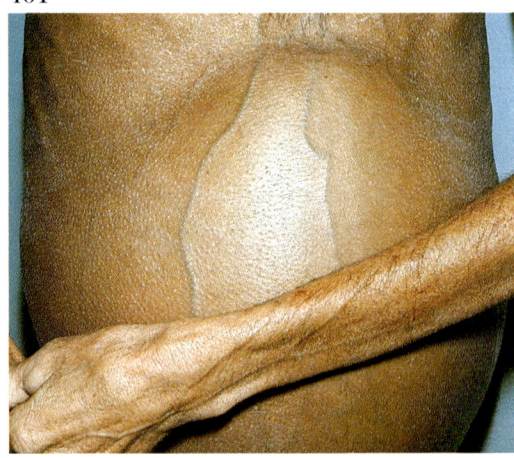

401 Ascites secondary to chronic portal hypertension in a Brazilian The classical clinical feature of chronic *S. mansoni* infection is portal hypertension. The opening up of a secondary, circulatory shunt leads to the development of varices in the oesophageal and gastric veins, ascites and gross splenomegaly.

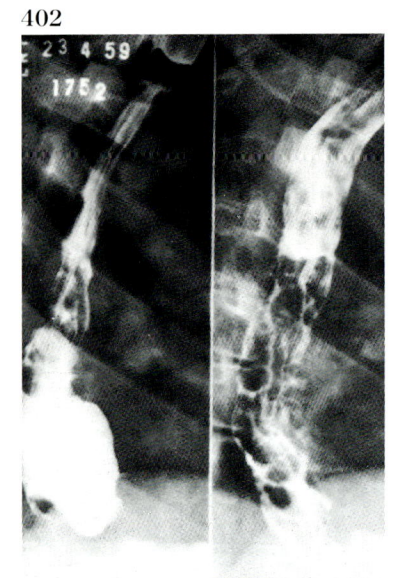

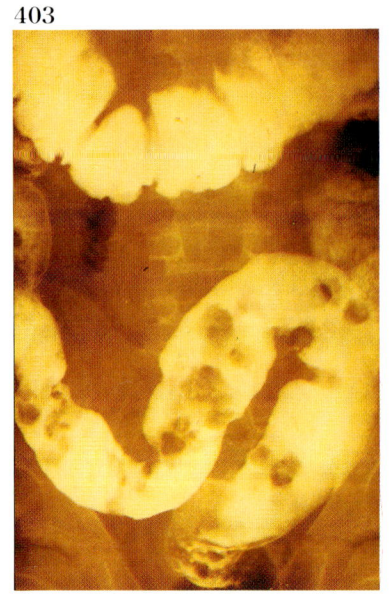

402 X-ray of oesophageal varices Oesophageal varices like those shown on this X-ray can rupture, leading to a fatal haematemesis.

403 X-ray of colonic polyposis In the early stages of *S. mansoni* infection diarrhoea is a common complaint. Extensive polyposis of the colon sometimes occurs. This lesion is reversible with antischistosomal drug therapy.

404 & 405 Sigmoidoscopic view of colonic polyps Four views of polyps in the descending colon.

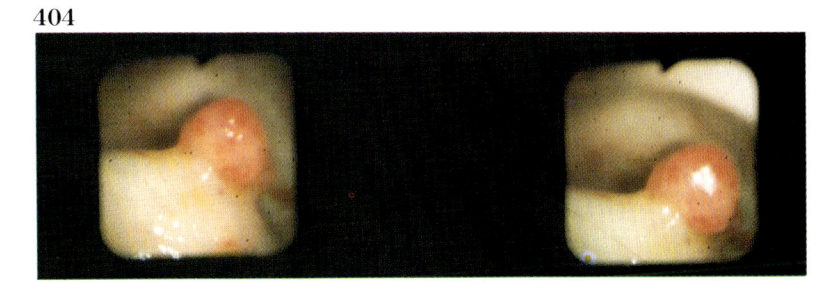

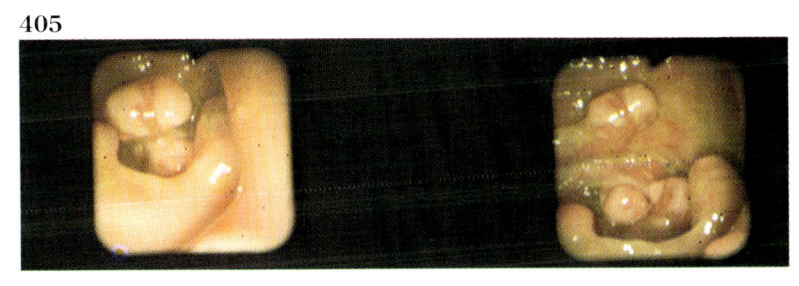

406 Polyposis of colon at post-mortem Massive polyposis of the colon with fatal intestinal haemorrhage occurred in this Egyptian farmer.

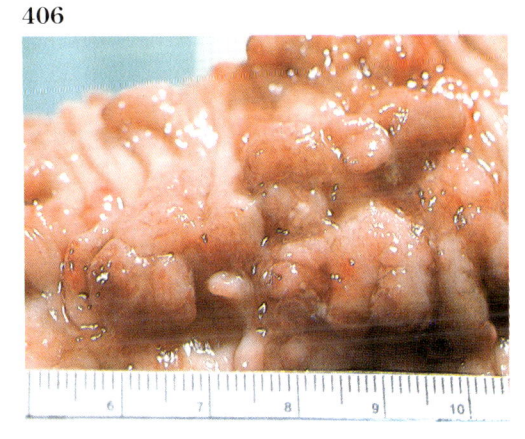

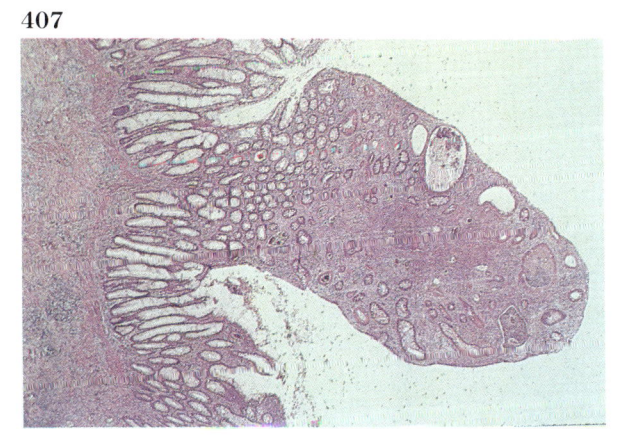

407 Biopsy showing *S. mansoni* eggs in a colonic polyp Diagnosis is usually confirmed by demonstrating eggs of *S. mansoni* in the stool. However, intestinal biopsy through a proctoscope or sigmoidoscope is also an effective means of finding eggs and establishing a definitive diagnosis of *S. mansoni* infection. It may also be positive in patients with *S. haematobium* or *S. japonicum*. (*H&E* × 25)

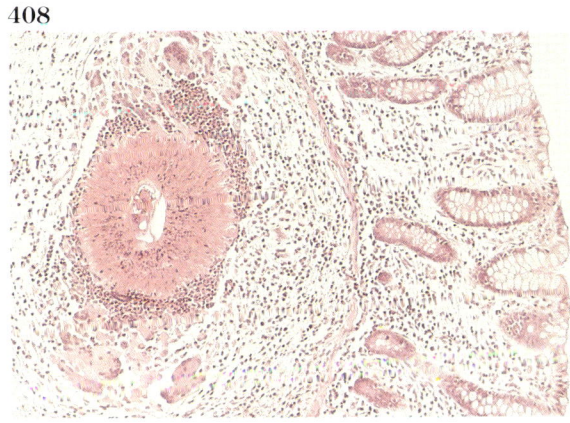

408 Hoeppli reaction The eosinophilic material surrounded by a fibrotic granuloma around this dead ovum in the colon is known as a Hoeppli reaction. (*H&E* × 95)

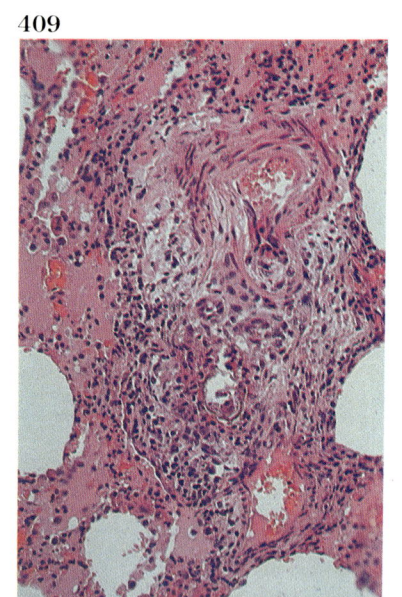

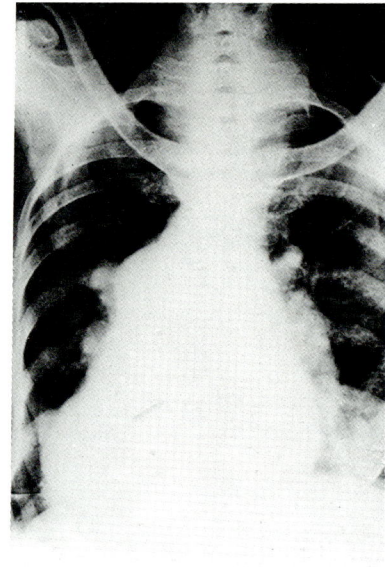

**409 Ectopic infection—
S. mansoni infection of lung** When the lungs are affected, typical eggs may appear in the sputum. Such ectopic lesions usually contain large numbers of ova in necrotic material surrounded by eosinophils, and multi-nucleated giant cells. (H&E × 100)

410 X-ray of 'cor pulmonale' Eggs that reach the lungs by metastatic blood spread lead to periarteritis. This is followed by fibrosis of the pulmonary arterioles with pulmonary hypertension and, finally, enlargement of the right heart, i.e. cor pulmonale.

Schistosoma haematobium

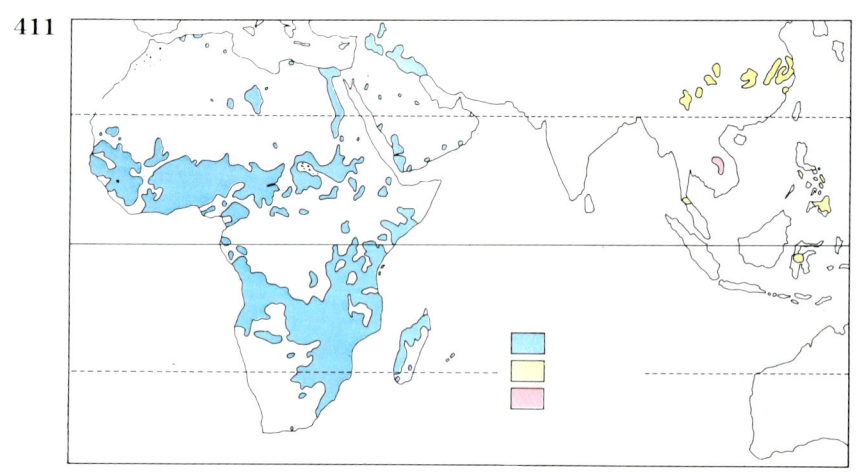

411 Distribution of S. haematobium, S. japonicum and S. mekongi. S. haematobium is found in Africa and the Middle East. S. japonicum is endemic in the Far East, SE Asia and the Philippines, while S. mekongi is limited to parts of Laos, Kampuchea and south Thailand bordering the lower Mekong River basin.

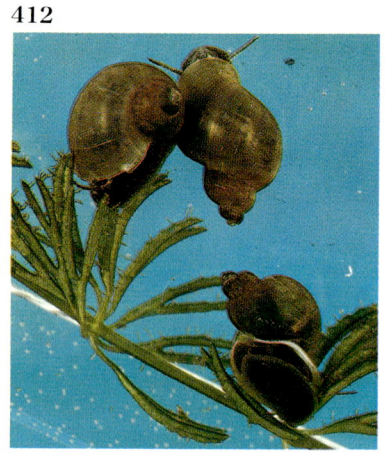

412 Intermediate hosts of S. haematobium The intermediate hosts of S. haematobium are species of Bulinus. (× 4) (See also **Table XII**.)

413 Ecology of *S. haematobium* infection Increased land use through the development of irrigation projects, as in Egypt, the Sudan and Kenya, may result in an increasing incidence of *S. haematobium* transmission through *Bulinus* snails breeding in the irrigation canals which are favourite swimming places for children. In the village near this canal 62 per cent of children from two to six years were infected.

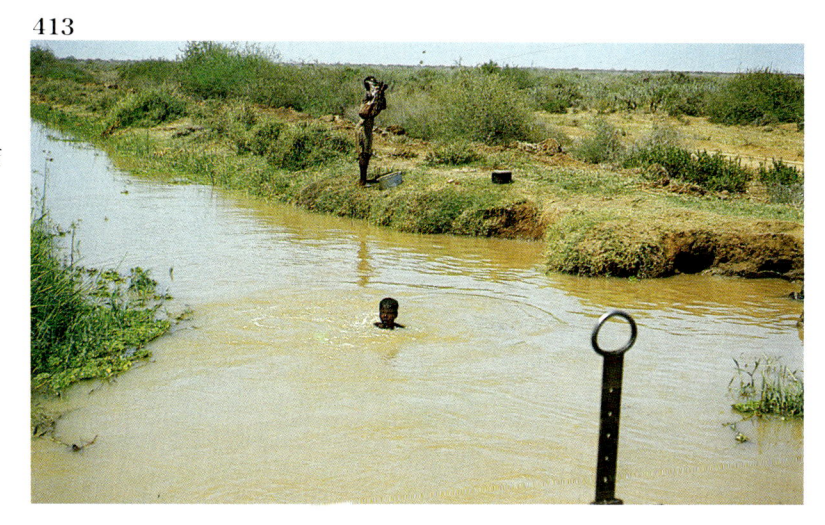

414 Haematuria Often best seen at the end of urination, haematuria is a characteristic early clinical feature of infection with this parasite. Typical, terminal spined eggs of *S. haematobium* (*see* **313**) may be found in the centrifuge deposit.

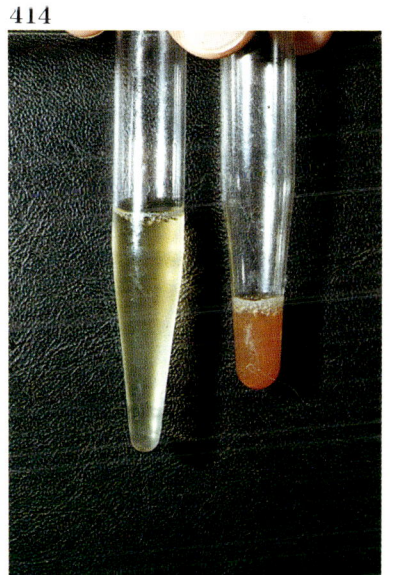

415 Village survey for urinary schistosomiasis A simple and effective technique is to collect urine samples in plastic bags which are then hung up at an angle to allow eggs to deposit in a corner. The eggs can be simply removed with the aid of a syringe and needle for microscopy or a miracidial hatching test.

416 Eggs in section of bladder Schistosome ova laid by female worms in the vesical plexus are retained in the vesical tissues and later become calcified. (H&E × 50)

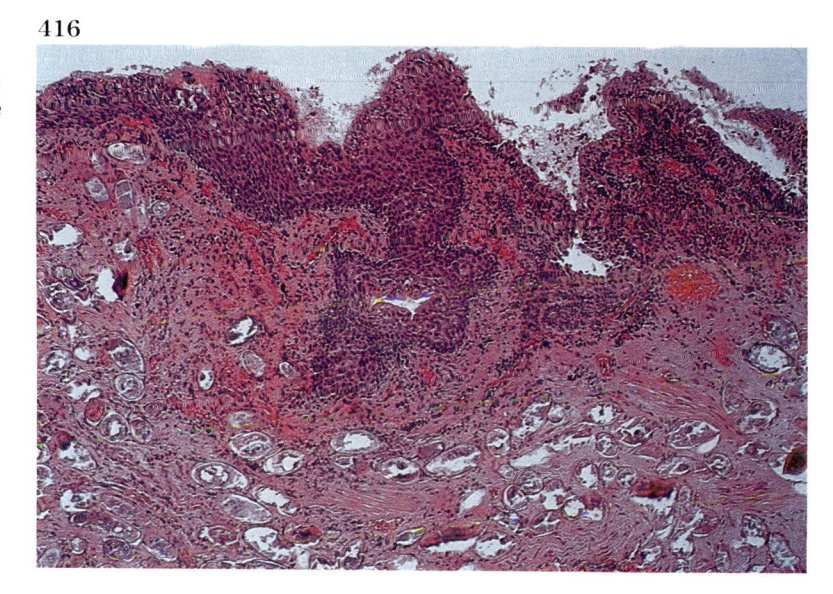

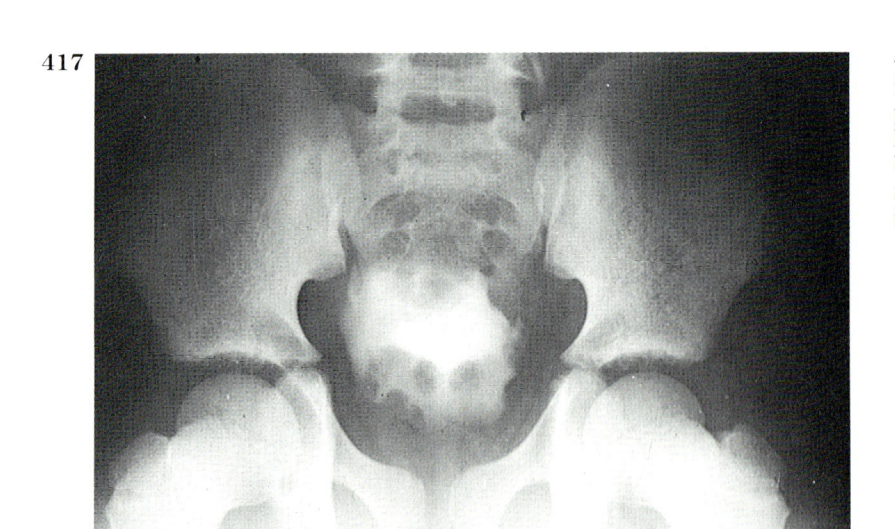

417 X-ray of bladder in early infection Active, proliferating, papillomatous or granulomatous lesions are responsible for the nodular bladder-filling defects seen radiologically in the early stages of the infection.

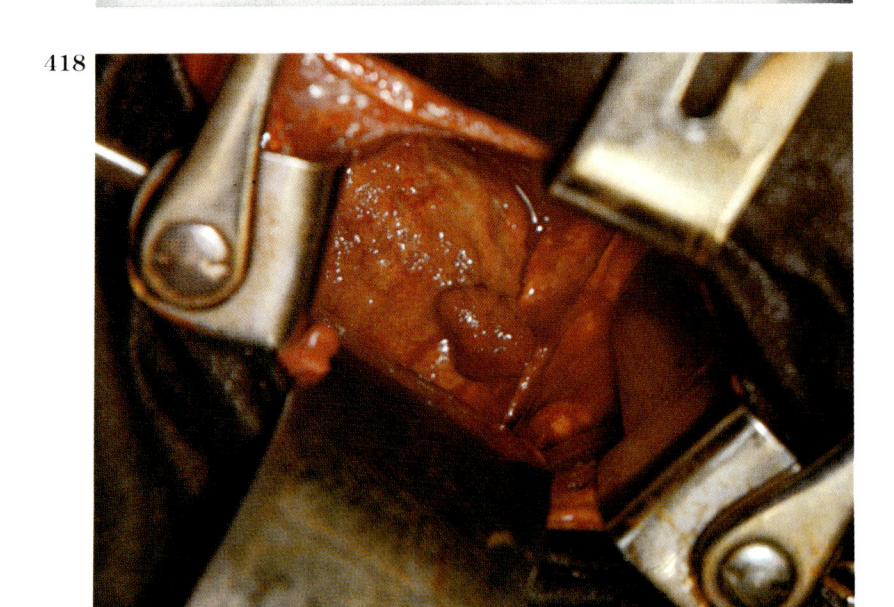

418 Nodules due to *S. haematobium* The appearance of a nodular lesion in the vesical wall as seen at open operation is well shown here.

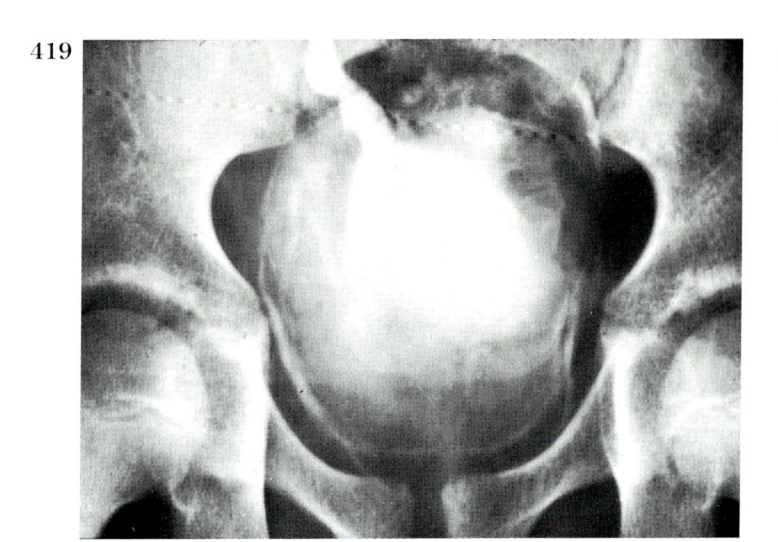

419 X-ray of bladder with calcification Widespread fibrosis and eventually calcification of the bladder wall result in this 'fetal-head' appearance.

420 X-ray of dilated ureters Gross tortuosity and dilatation of the ureters result from stenosis of the ureteric orifices due to calcification.

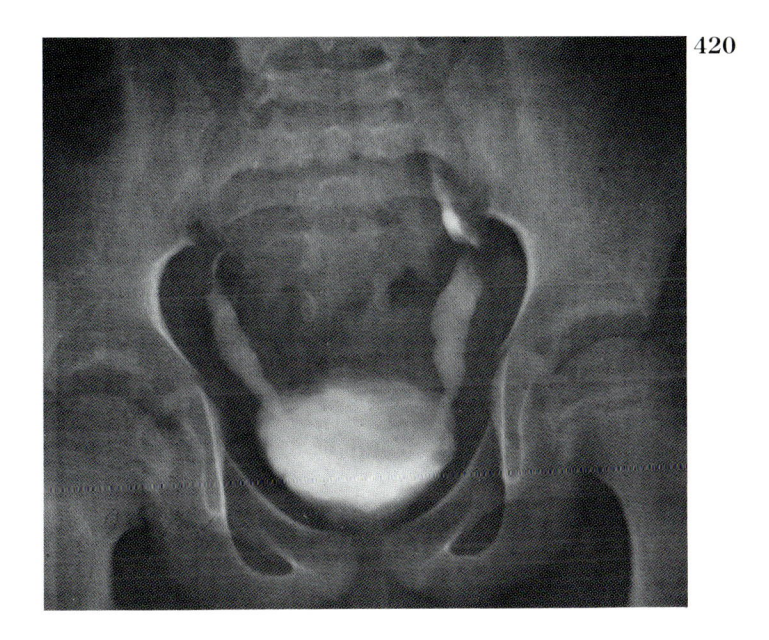

421 X-ray of kidney showing persistent hydronephrosis Unilateral and bilateral hydronephrosis due to vesical and ureteric destructive lesions are not uncommon in haematobium infection. Hydronephrosis due to *S. haematobium* infection in children is often reversible with adequate antischistosomal drug treatment. In this six-year-old the lesion persisted despite therapy. The non-invasive technique of renography has replaced pyelography in the investigation of urinary tract lesions due to *S. haematobium*.

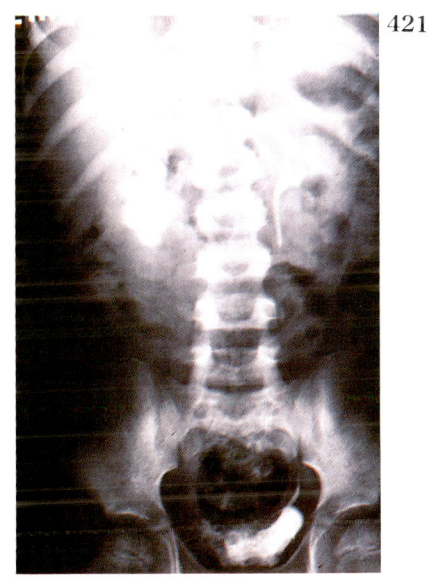

422 Squamous cell carcinoma of the bladder In areas where *S. haematobium* infection is intense, the incidence of vesical cancer is high. Squamous cell carcinoma is the type most commonly found, and ova of *S. haematobium* are often present in such tumours. Adenocarcinoma also occurs. (*H&E × 90*)

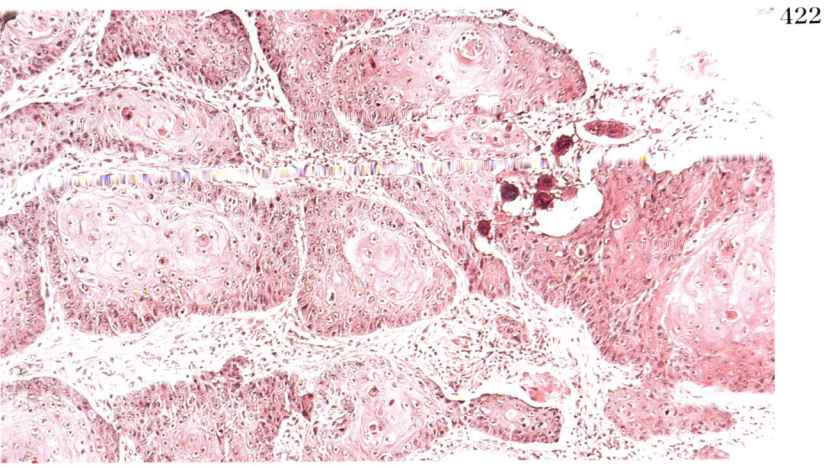

Schistosoma japonicum and S. mekongi

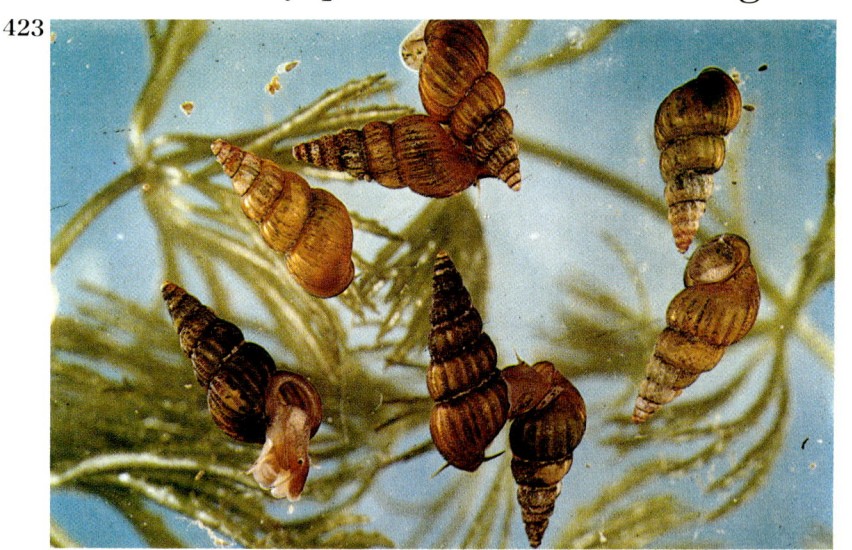

423 Oncomelania, intermediate host of S. japonicum Various species of the amphibious genus *Oncomelania* serve as intermediate hosts for *S. japonicum*. In the lower Mekong River basin, a river-dwelling snail, *Tricula aperta*, is the intermediate host for *S. mekongi*, a trematode closely related to *S. japonicum*. (× 4). (*See also* **Table XII**.)

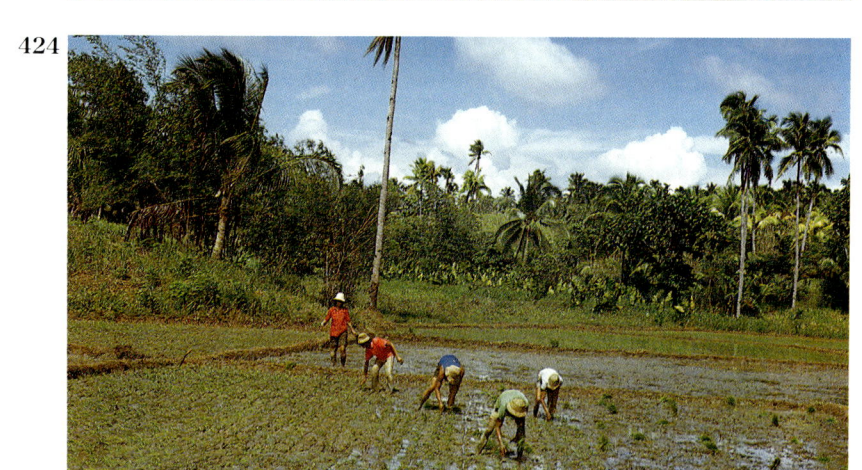

424 Ecology of S. japonicum and S. mekongi These infections are zoonoses. *S. japonicum* is found in a wide variety of vertebrate hosts, including domestic animals and bovines. Human infection frequently occurs in farm workers, for example, when planting rice in contaminated paddy fields as seen here (see also **336**). *S. mekongi*, on the contrary, is associated more with rivers. It is likely to increase as irrigation works in the lower Mekong River basin are extended. In some Kampuchean 'floating villages' up to 47 per cent of sampled villagers have been found infected with this parasite.

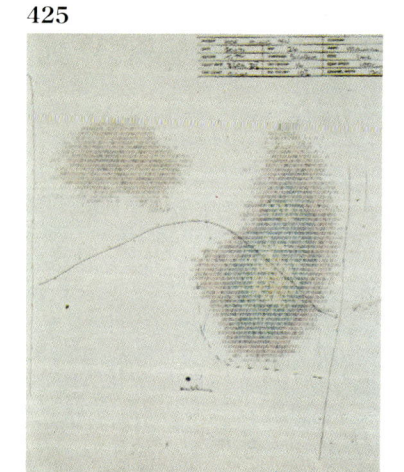

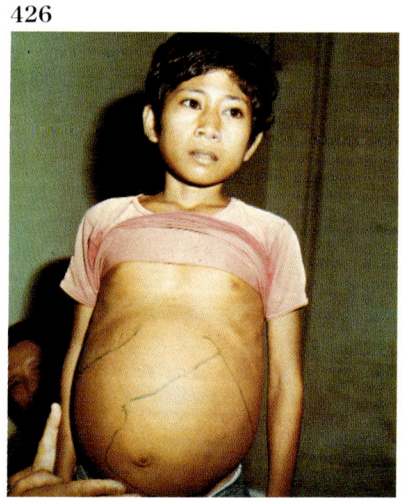

425 Radio-isotope scan of patient with S. japonicum infection Severe hepatic fibrosis and massive splenomegaly occur in *S. japonicum* infection, in the same manner as in *S. mansoni* (see **400** & **401**), often with ascites. *S. mekongi* may also produce severe changes like these. This Chinese patient was infected both with *S. japonicum* and *Clonorchis sinensis*.

426 Philippino boy with gross splenomegaly Advanced lesions due to *S. japonicum* may be seen in children and adolescents.

427 Eggs of *S. japonicum* in wall of colon The adult worms do not invade the vesical plexus, but usually inhabit the mesenteric plexus. The diagnosis of *S. japonicum* can usually be made by finding typical eggs in the faeces. However, it is commoner for eggs of *S. japonicum* to be deposited in ectopic sites than those of other schistosome species. (H&E × 150)

428 Ova of *S. japonicum* in spinal cord Schistosomal lesions in the spinal cord or brain may contain large numbers of ova in necrotic material, often surrounded by eosinophils. Patients with cerebral schistosomiasis usually present with epileptiform attacks. This post-mortem specimen shows marked cellular reaction including a multinucleated giant cell round a dead ovum in the spinal cord of a 24-year-old Japanese male. (H&E × 200)

429 Intradermal test In any type of schistosomiasis the diagnosis may be suggested in the absence of demonstrable ova by the response to an intradermal injection of a suitable antigen. This figure shows a typical response to antigen prepared from *S. mansoni*.

430 ELISA test This, the most sensitive test currently available, is of particular value in epidemiological surveys. Alkaline phosphatase-p-nitrophenyl phosphate was used as indicator in rows A–D of this plate and horseradish peroxidase in rows E–H, with different sera in each of the wells. A & E show a strong positive, B & F a weak positive and C & G a negative reaction. D & H are the buffer controls. Antigen detection and DNA probes to diagnose current infection are being actively pursued.

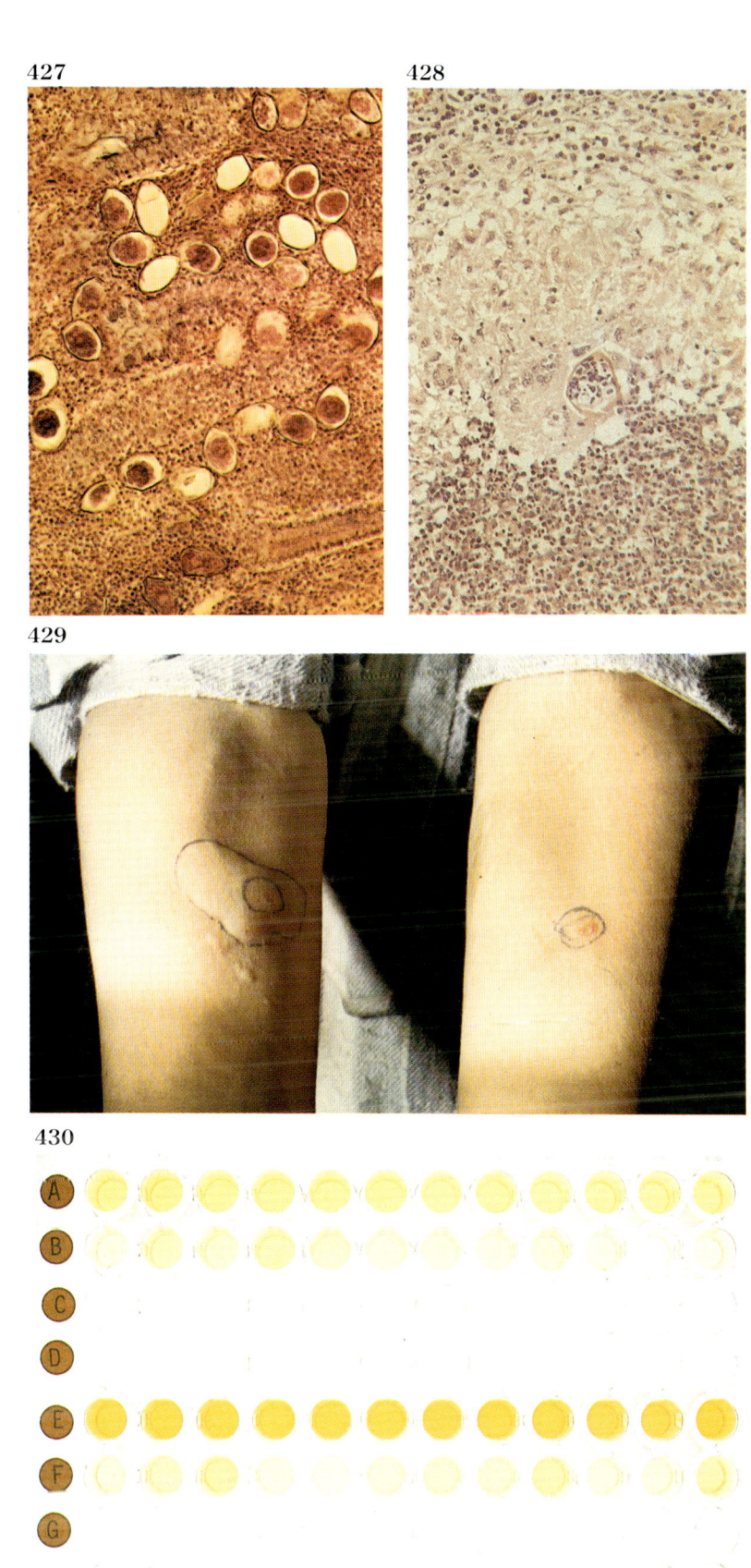

Schistosomes Found Uncommonly in Man

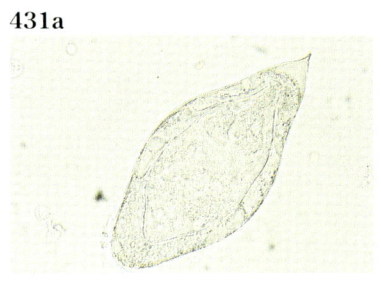

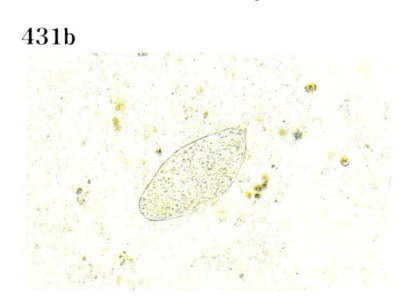

431 & 432 Eggs of unusual schistosomes seen in man The eggs of *S. intercalatum* (**431a**) are similar to those of *S. haematobium* but are found only in the faeces.
S. mattheei (**431b**), which occurs in sheep and cattle, has been found in man on rare occasions. ($\times 190$)
S. mekongi (**432a**) is easily mistaken for *S. japonicum* which is shown here for comparison (**432b**). ($\times 70$)

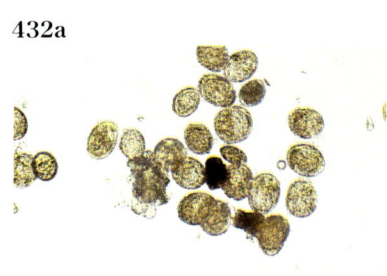

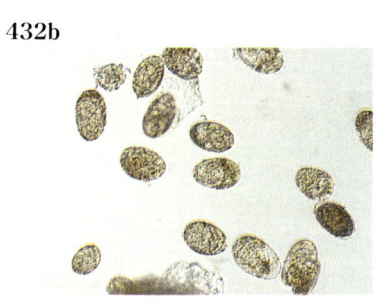

THE INTESTINAL FLUKES (*See* Tables XI & XII)

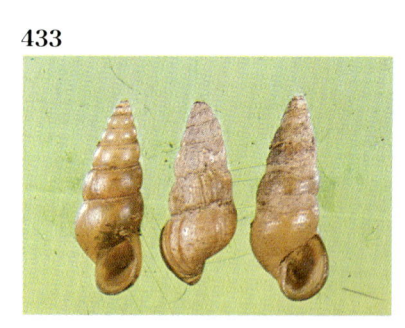

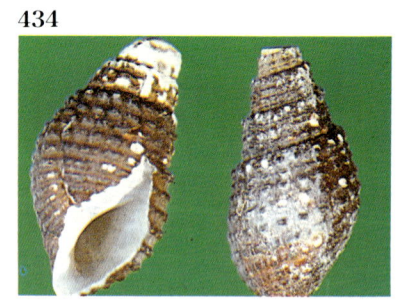

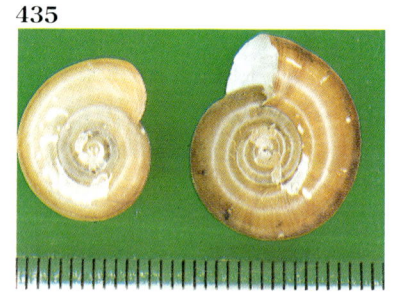

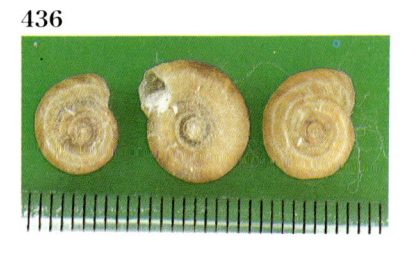

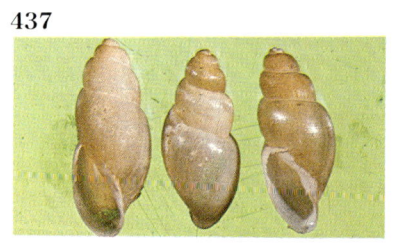

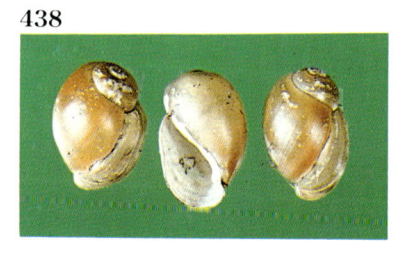

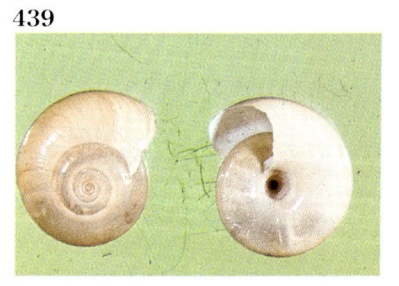

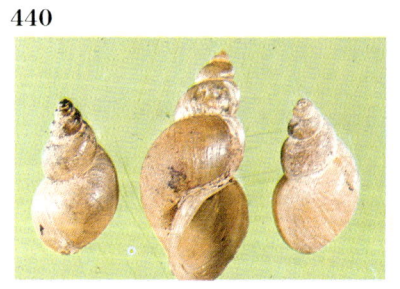

433-440 Snail intermediate hosts of trematode infections of man A number of the molluscs listed in **Table XII** are figured here: *Oncomelania nosophora* ($\times 3$) (**433**); *Thiara granifera* ($\times 1.5$) (**434**); *Biomphalaria glabrata* ($\times 3$) (**435**); *Biomphalaria sudanica* ($\times 1.5$) (**436**); *Bulinus (Bulinus) senegalensis* ($\times 3$) (**437**); *Bulinus (Physopsis) globosus* ($\times 1.5$) (**438**); *Segmentina* sp. ($\times 3$) (**439**); *Lymnaea truncatula* ($\times 3$) (**440**).

441 Comparative sizes of flukes
From left to right: first column—
S. mansoni ♂ and ♀; second column—
H. heterophyes; third column—
O. felineus, *C. sinensis*,
P. westermani; fourth column—
F. hepatica and *F. buski*.

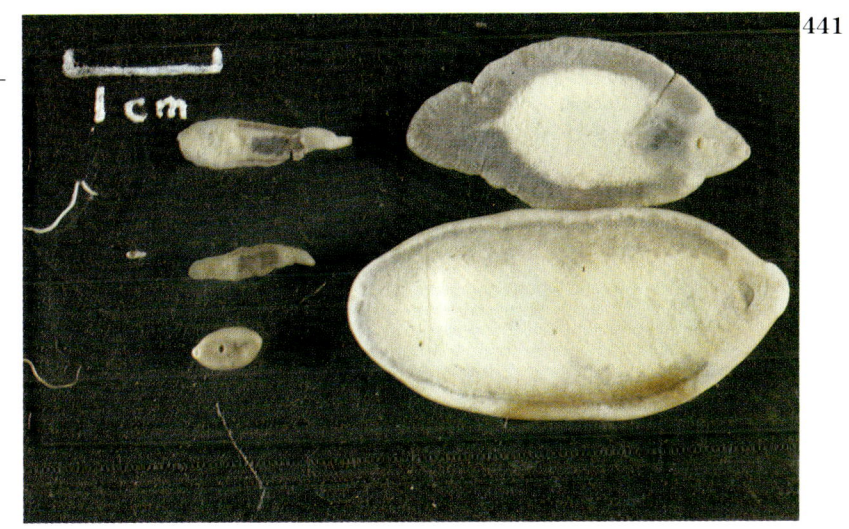

Fasciolopsiasis

442 Distribution of *Fasciolopsis buski* *F. buski* is limited to areas of the Far East. In certain localities, e.g. northeast Thailand, almost the entire population of some villages may be infected.

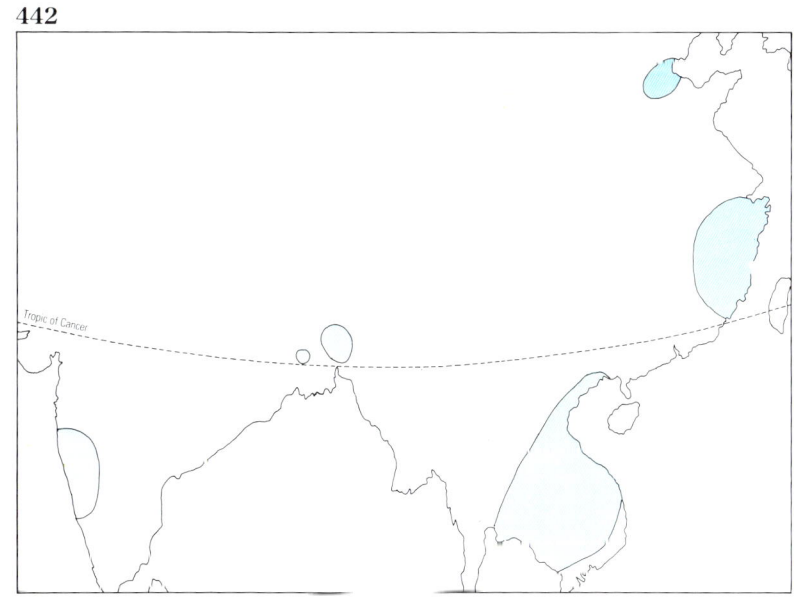

443 Egg of *F. buski* Miracidia, hatching from eggs passed in the faeces after shedding their ciliated coats, invade snails of various genera, including *Segmentina* and *Hippeutis*. The reproductive cycle in the snail differs from that of the schistosomes. After development through the sporocysts and two generations of rediae, cercariae emerge into the water. They then encyst on aquatic plants such as the water caltrop (**447**) and water chestnut (**463**). (× 200)

444 Metacercaria of *F. buski* The metacercaria of *F. buski* with its cyst wall. (× 200)

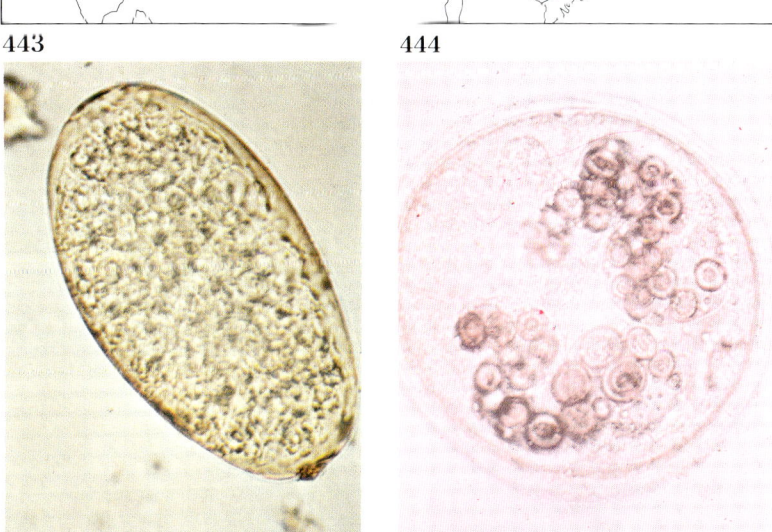

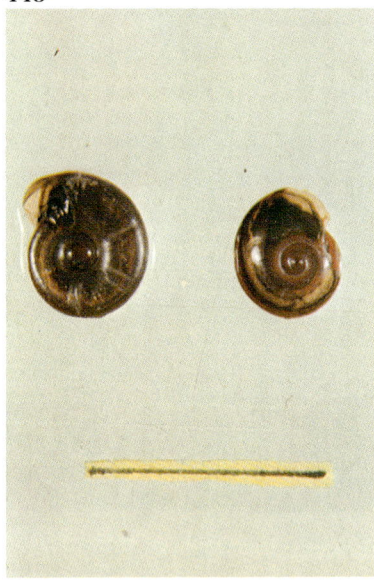

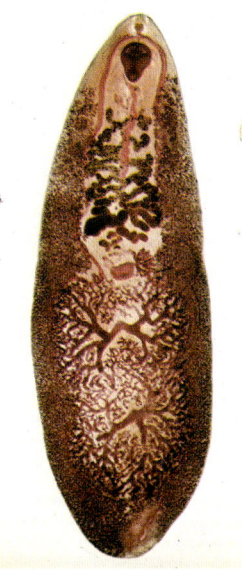

445 *Segmentina hemisphaerula*
This is the intermediate host of *F. buski*. (× 2)

446 Adult *F. buski* The adult *F. buski* is the largest parasitic trematode of man and may reach 7.5 cm in length. The pig is the main animal reservoir of infection for man. (*natural size*)

447 The water caltrop
'Plantations' of water caltrop are harvested in endemic areas. The characteristic fruits of this plant are commonly eaten raw, and the metacercariae are thus swallowed. In the digestive tract they attach to the mucosa of the upper part of the small intestine where they mature. Water chestnuts (**463**) commonly serve as a source of infection for children who peel the raw plants with their teeth, thus ingesting the attached metacercariae.

448 Adult *Heterophyes heterophyes* This is an uncommon but widely distributed, tiny trematode with a typical life cycle in brackish water snails, e.g. *Pirenella* (see **Table XII**). The cercariae encyst on fish such as the mullet and infect man when improperly cooked fish is eaten. The adult trematode shown here lives in the middle part of the small intestine. The eggs (*see* **327**) are very similar to those of *Clonorchis* and *Metagonimus*. (× 35)

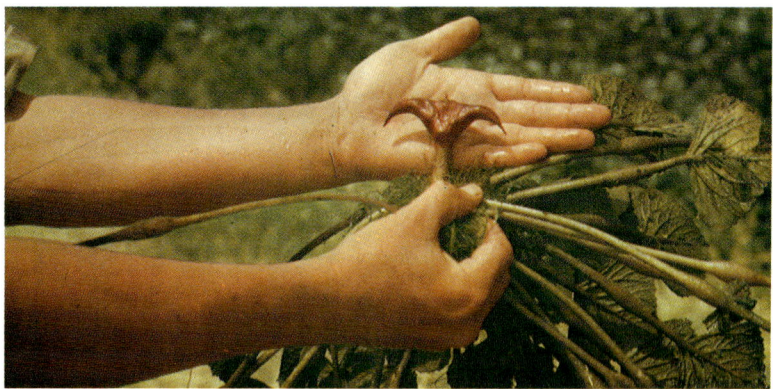

Uncommon Species

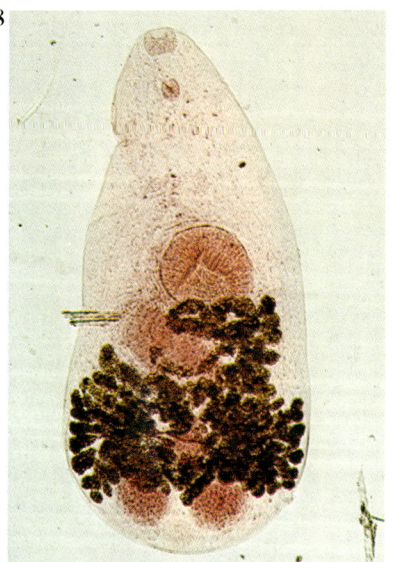

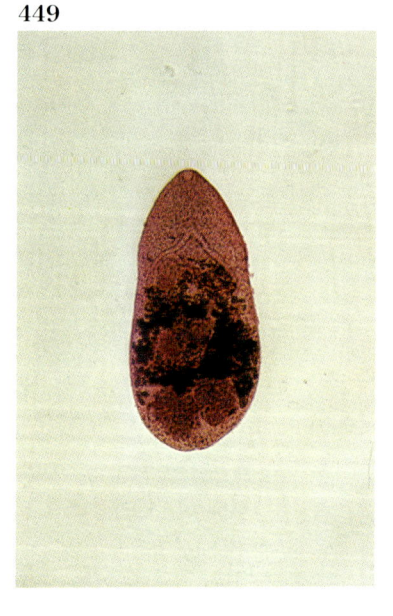

449 Adult *Metagonimus yokagawai* This is the most common heterophyid fluke of the Far East but is also found in the Mediterranean basin. The life cycle is similar to that of *Heterophyes* and the eggs of the two species can only be distinguished with difficulty. The adult worm shown here is also very small (1.4 × 0.6 mm) and lives in the upper and middle jejunum. Several genera of snails including *Semisulcospira* (see **Table XII**) are the first intermediate hosts for the species. The cercariae encyst on fish. (× 35)

450 Cyprinoid fish in an Eastern market The mullet and other fish living in fresh or brackish waters are common intermediate hosts for *H. heterophyes* and *M. yokagawai*. The metacercariae are attached under the scales or in the skin.

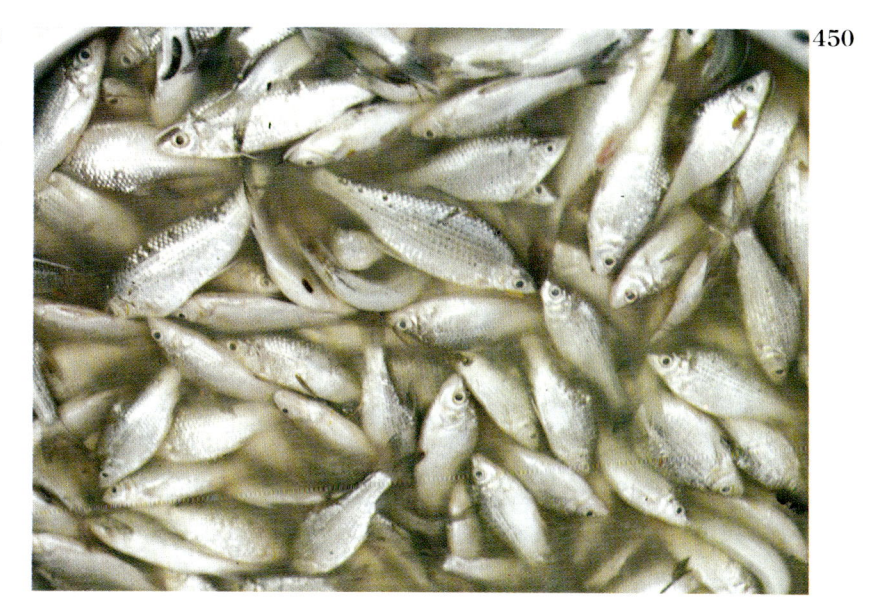

LIVER FLUKE INFECTIONS
Clonorchis sinensis
(Currently referred to as *Opisthorcis sinensis* by some authors)

451 Distribution map *C. sinensis* is also known as the Chinese or oriental liver fluke. It is found in man and also in other fish-eating mammals in the areas shown.

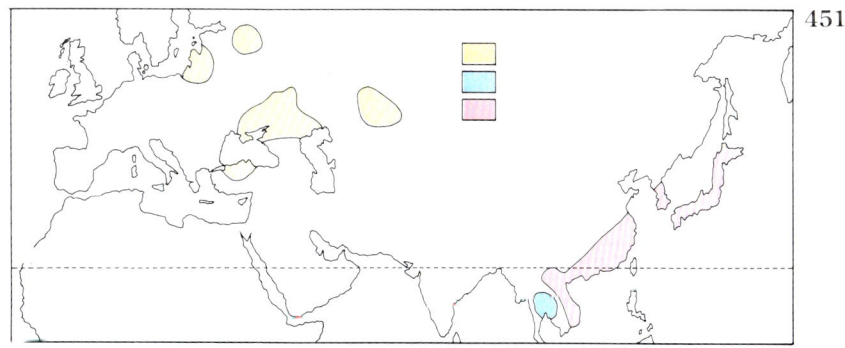

452 Life cycle of *C. sinensis* The adult flukes (a) living in the biliary tree produce eggs (b) which are passed in the faeces. When ingested by the snail host (c), miracidia (d) hatch from the eggs to produce sporocysts (e) where a single generation of rediae develop (f). Within these lophocercous cercariae develop (g) which leave the snails to enter various freshwater fish (h) where they encyst to form metacercariae (i). When the fish is eaten by a carnivore the young trematodes emerge and eventually pass up the common bile duct, finally reaching the smaller branches of the biliary tree where they mature. (See also **327**.)

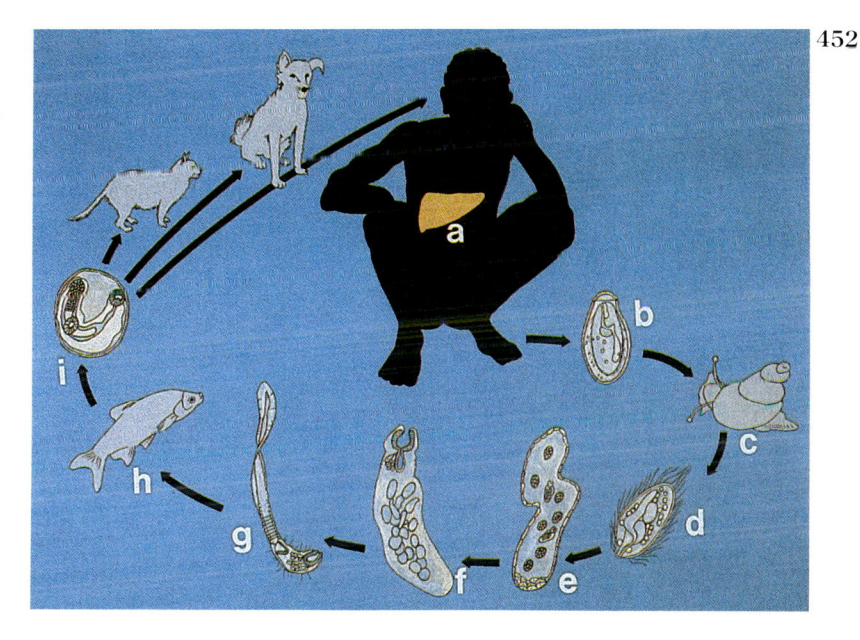

115

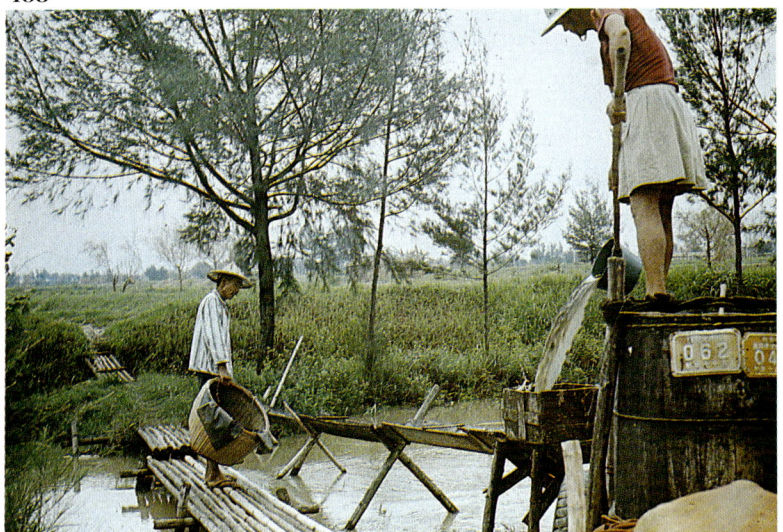

453 Ecology of *C. sinensis* infection Latrines used to be built over the edges of fishponds where faecal material containing helminth eggs would drop. This provided an ideal way of infecting cultivated fish and perpetuating the cycle of transmission. While this practice has been greatly reduced, it is still common practice to pour fresh night-soil into fishponds, as seen here.

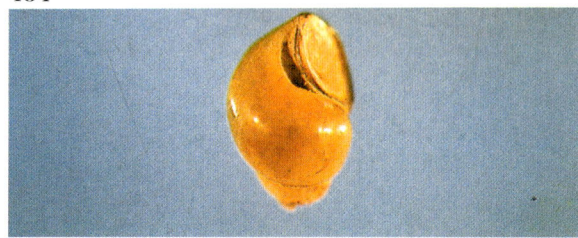

454 Intermediate host of *Clonorchis* *Bithynia funiculata* is one of the species of this genus in which *C. sinensis* will develop. Other molluscan genera (*see* **Table XII**) can serve as intermediate hosts. (× 3)

455 Cercaria of *C. sinensis* The lophocercous cercariae escape from the snail to encyst under the scales of various species of freshwater cyprinoid fish. (× 80)

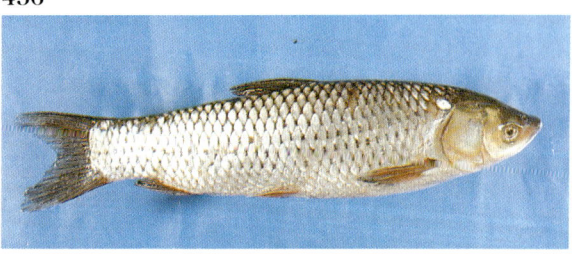

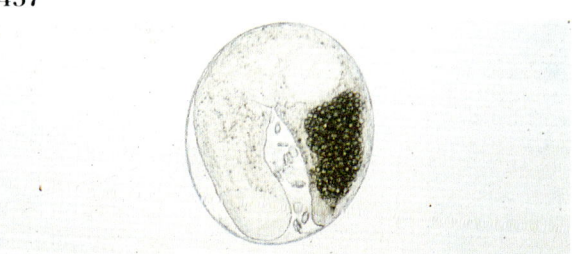

456 *Ctenopharyngodon idellus* This fish is a common host for metacercariae of *C. sinensis*.

457 Metacercaria in fish Man is infested by eating raw or incompletely cooked fish, a common delicacy among many Chinese. Metacercariae are thus ingested and excyst in the duodenum. (× 160)

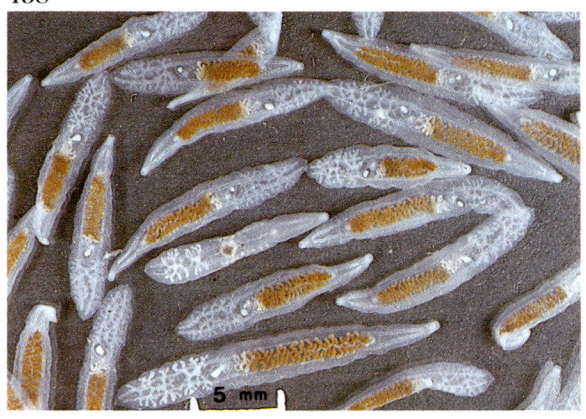

458 Adult *C. sinensis* The young worms migrate up the common bile duct to the liver. At maturity they may reach 2 cm in length. (x 2.5)

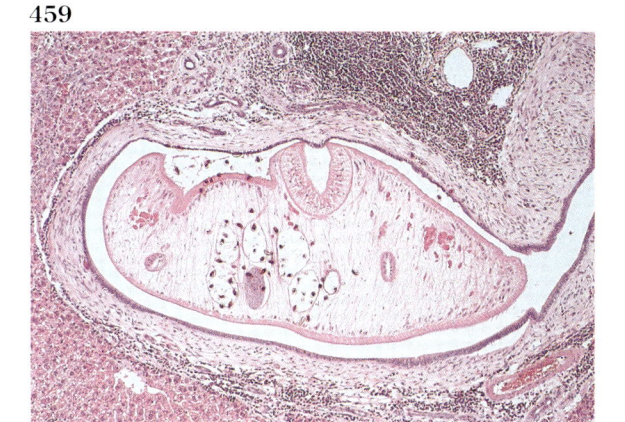

459 Section of *C. sinensis* in bile duct Direct mechanical damage and possibly toxic effects of the adult worms lead to fibrotic changes in the bile ducts. ($\times 25$)

460 Cholangiocarcinoma of the liver Severe chronic infection with *C. sinensis* may lead to marked pericholangitic fibrosis, and finally multifocal cholangiocellular carcinoma of the liver. In this case, metastases were widely distributed throughout the body. (*H&E* $\times 100$)

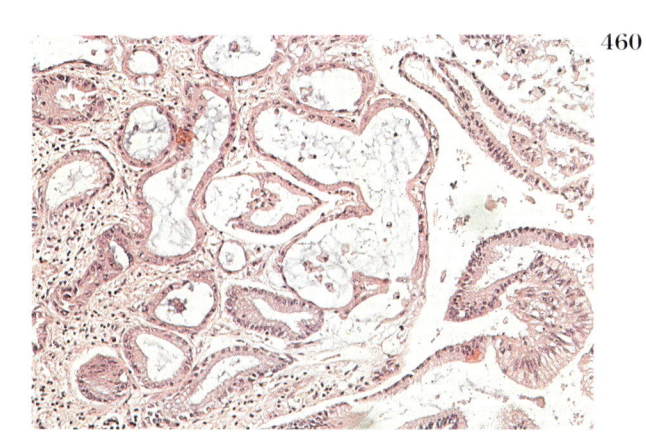

Opisthorchis felineus and *Opisthorchis viverrini*

The distribution is shown in **451**. *O. felineus* is common in domestic cats, dogs, and some other animals in Eastern and Southeastern Europe, and parts of the USSR. It is largely replaced by *O. viverrini* in the Far East. This occurs mainly in northeast Thailand where it infects up to 90 per cent of the population in some villages, a total of some 10 million. Cats as well as man serve as reservoirs of infection. The life cycles are similar to that of *C. sinensis*, snails of the genus *Bithynia* serving as intermediate hosts (*see also* **454**).

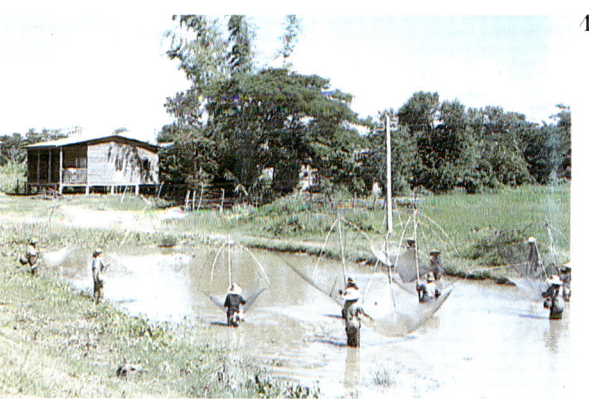

461 Ecology of *O. viverrini* Man is infected by ingesting the metacercariae in cyprinoid fish. The figure shows a typical village fishpond in northeast Thailand.

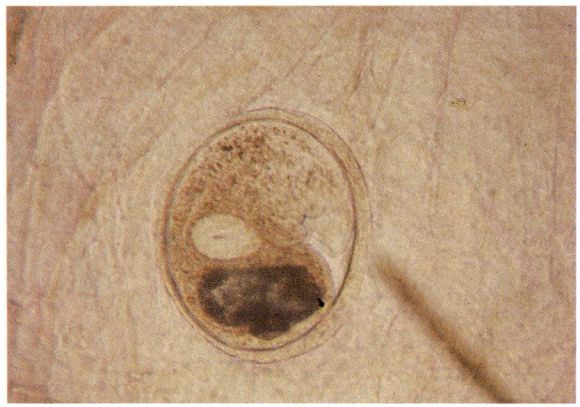

462 Metacercaria in fish Most infection is from uncooked fish. In northeast Thailand the fish sauce 'koipla' is the most important source. (× 350)

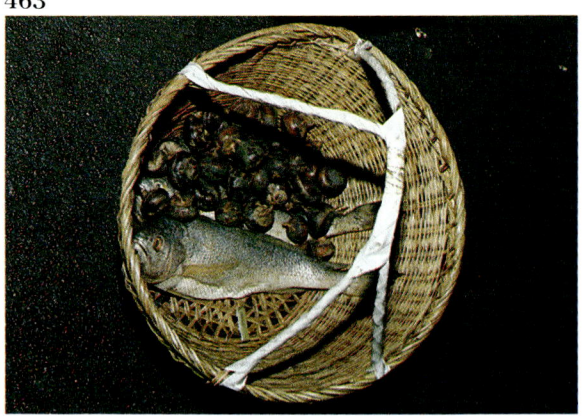

463 *Cyprinus carpio*, host for metacercariae of *O. felineus* These freshwater fish are often infected in the Far East and are a common source of infection in northeast Thailand. This shopper's basket also contains water chestnuts on which metacercariae of *F. buski* may encyst (*see* **443**).

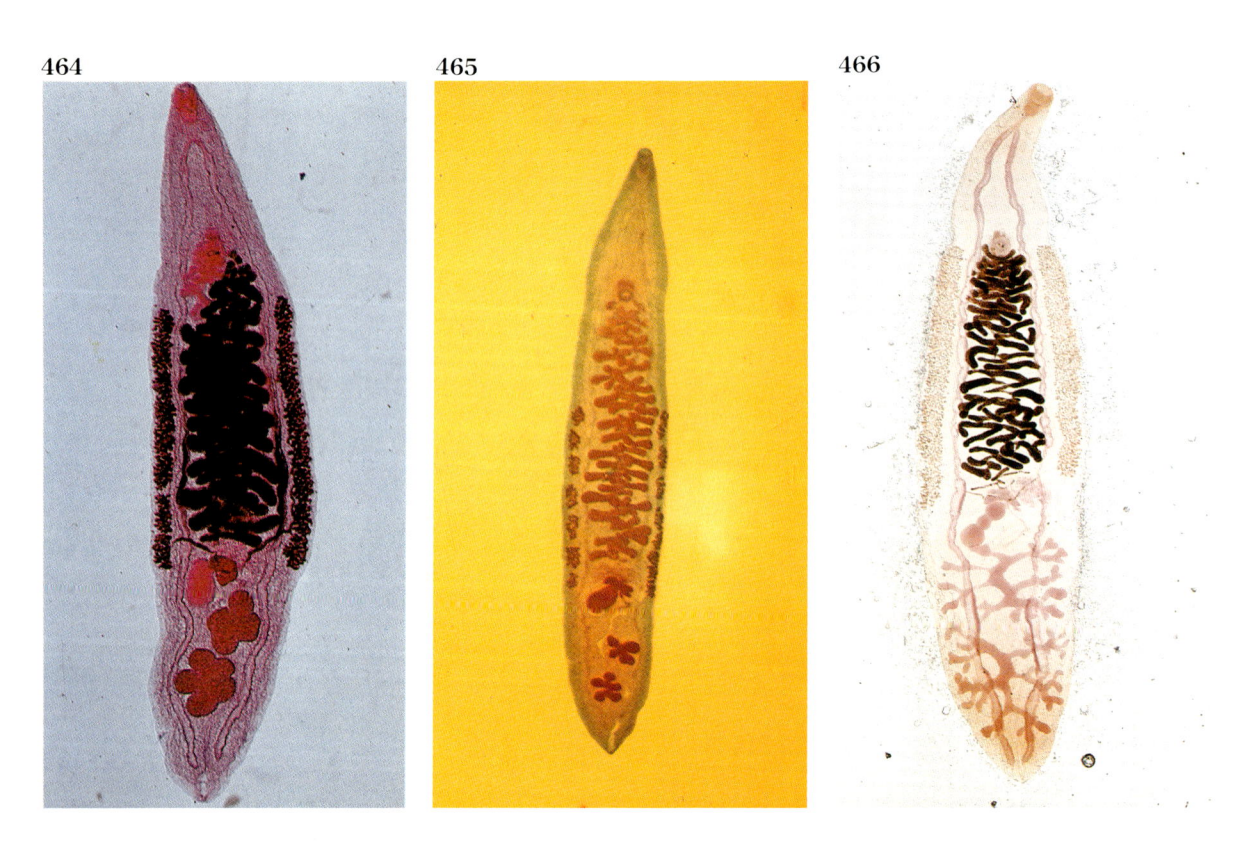

464-466 Adult flukes of *O. felineus*, *O. viverrini*, *C. sinensis* The adults of *Opisthorchis* which are similar to those of *C. sinensis*, live in the bile ducts and produce similar pathological changes. They can be distinguished by such structural details as the numbers, positions and shapes of the testes in the posterior parts of the worms (lower thirds in these figures). (× 9)

118

467

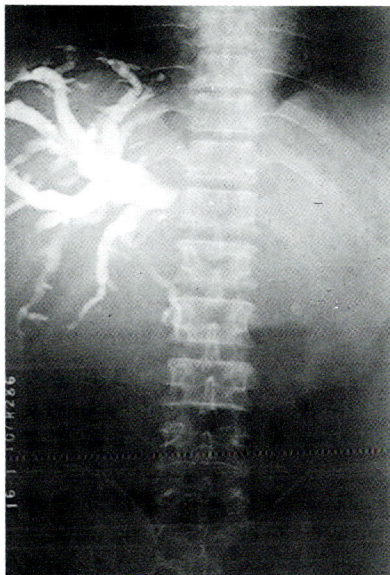

467 Cholangiogram of patient with clonorchiasis This X-ray shows dilatation of the main bile ducts and disorganisation of the biliary tree.

Dicrocoelium dendriticum

468 Adult *D. dendriticum* This trematode is very common in sheep and other herbivores in many countries and is occasionally found in man. The adult, which grows up to 1.5 cm long, lives in the biliary tract. The eggs are similar to those of the *Clonorchis* group (*see* **327**). (× 6)

468

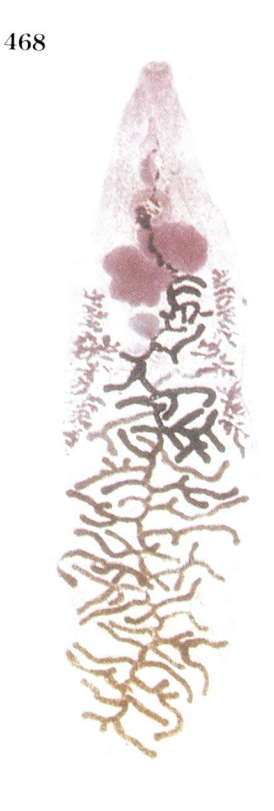

Fasciola hepatica and *F. gigantica*

469 Ecology of fascioliasis
Infection with *F. hepatica* is cosmopolitan in herbivores that graze in wet pasturage where the intermediate hosts, snails of the genus *Lymnaea*, are found. Man is most often infected by eating wild watercress on which metacercariae have encysted. *F. gigantica*, the common liver fluke of cattle in the Middle East, much of Africa and Asia, occasionally infects man.

470 Miracidia of *F. hepatica*
Motile miracidia hatch from eggs passed in faeces and infect snails of the genus *Lymnaea*. (× 150)

471 *Lymnaea swinhoei* This snail is a host for *F. hepatica* in parts of China. In England the usual intermediate host is *L. truncatula* (**440**). (× 6)

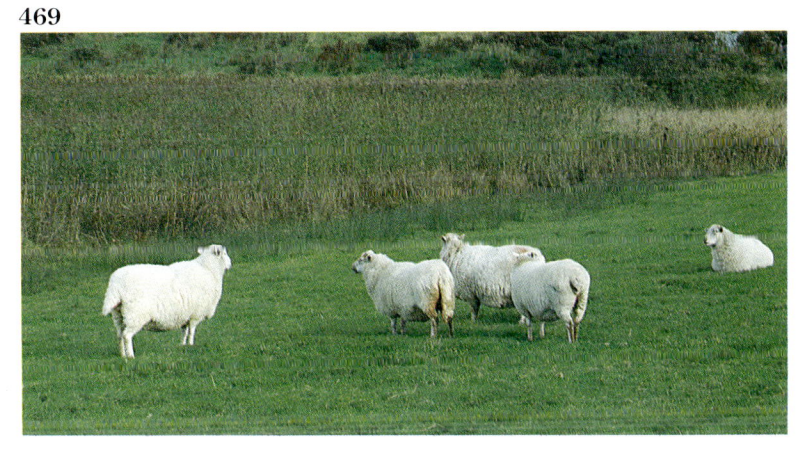

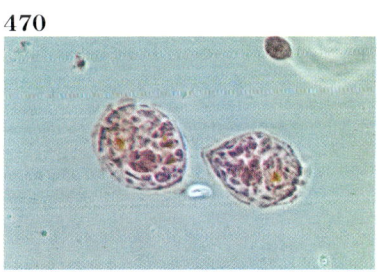

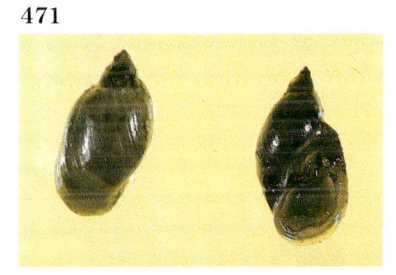

469

470

471

119

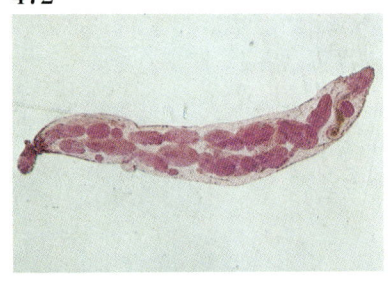

472 Redia from intermediate host These develop in the hepatopancreas with the formation of cercariae. (× 25)

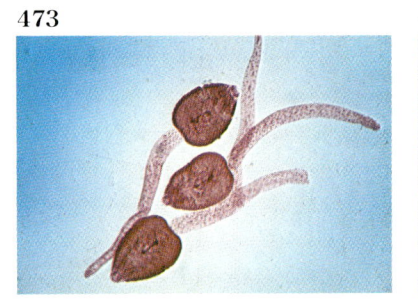

473 Cercaria of *F. hepatica* The cercariae, which have unforked tails, encyst on aquatic vegetation to form metacercariae. (× 60)

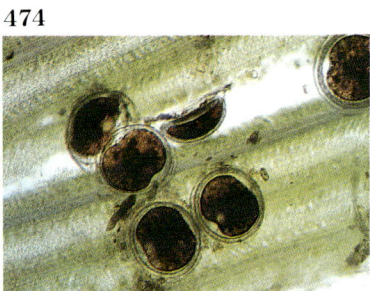

474 Metacercariae on grass These are found on grass or other moist herbage such as watercress. When the metacercariae are ingested, the cycle recommences. (× 60)

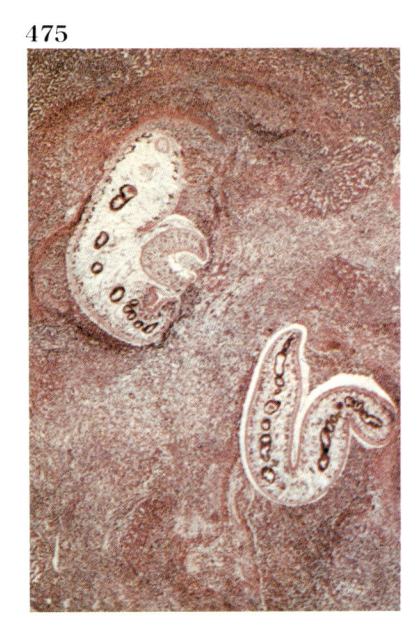

475 Migrating flukes in liver After being swallowed, the metacercariae pass through the intestinal wall and penetrate the liver capsule to enter the liver parenchyma. The figure shows a sheep liver with migrating, immature flukes. (H&E × 20)

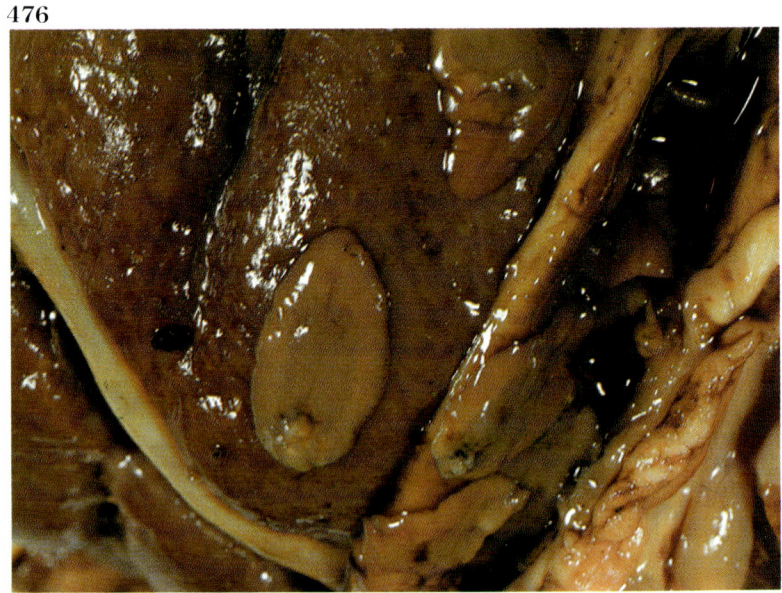

476 Adult flukes in bile ducts of a sheep liver The adult flukes penetrate into the bile ducts where they cause serious damage to the biliary tract. Eggs (**316**) are passed with the bile into the faeces. (*life size*)

477 Adult *F. hepatica* in section of liver The surface spines of the adult fluke produce mechanical damage in the biliary epithelium. (*H&E × 350*)

478 CAT scan of *F. hepatica* in human liver Using a contrast medium, cystic filling defects suggestive of this trematode infection could be visualised. They disappeared after therapy.

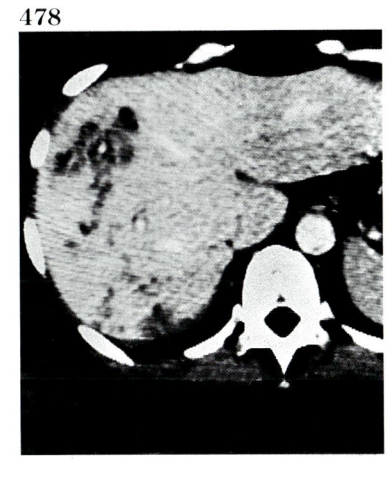

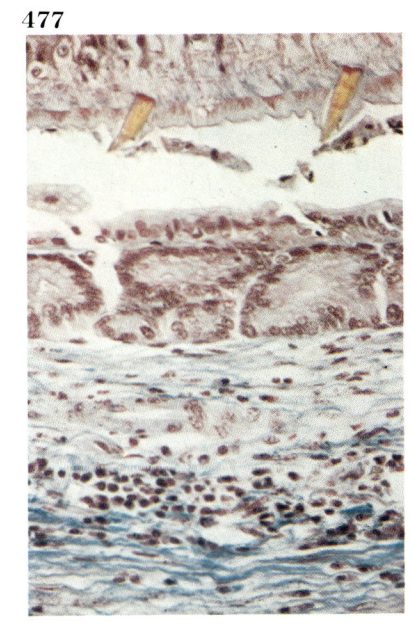

PARAGONIMIASIS

479 Distribution of lung flukes At least four species of *Paragonimus* have been found in man. *Paragonimus westermani* commonly causes human infection in the Far East where it is widely distributed among other mammals. Several other species are probably involved there. Human infections with *P. africanus* and *P. uterobilateralis* have been recognised in West Africa and *P. heterotremus* in Thailand. Unidentified species occasionally produce infection in man in parts of Central and South America.

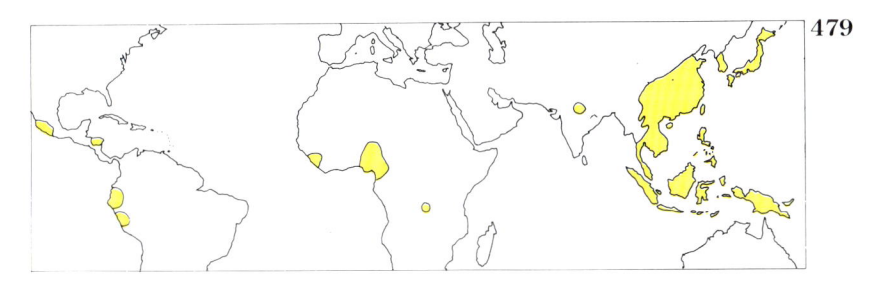

Paragonimus westermani

480 Reservoir host of *Paragonimus* The palm civet, *Paradoxurus hermaphroditus* (Viverridae), is a reservoir host for these trematodes in Thailand.

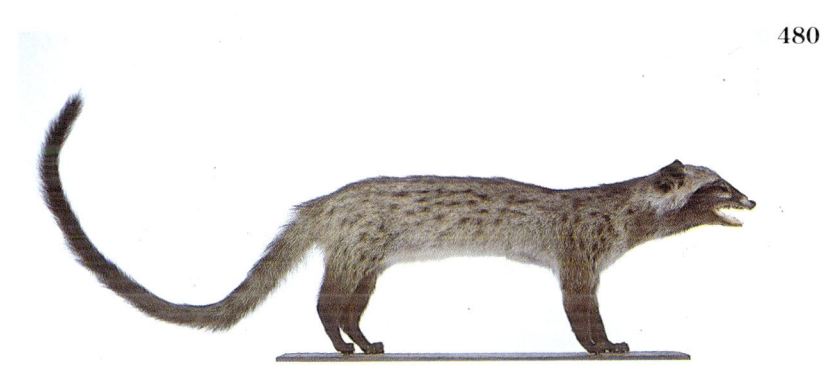

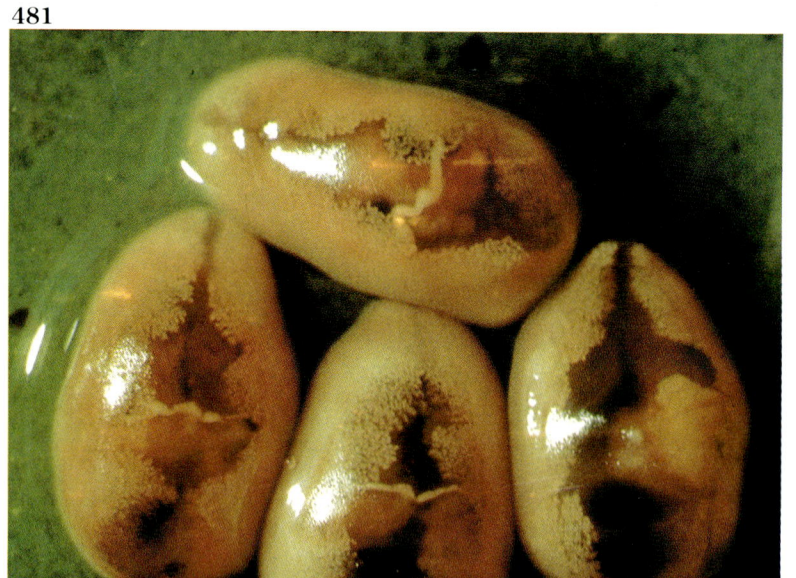

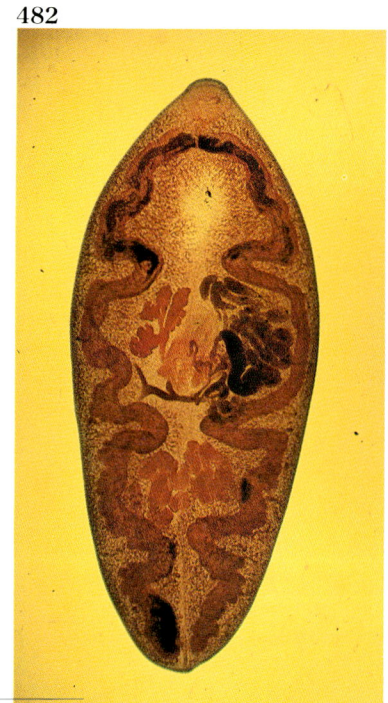

481 & 482 Adult *P. westermani* The adult fluke normally lives in the lungs. It is rather lemon-shaped and about 1 cm long when alive (**481**). Preserved specimens (**482**) become flattened and distorted during preparation. (× 6)

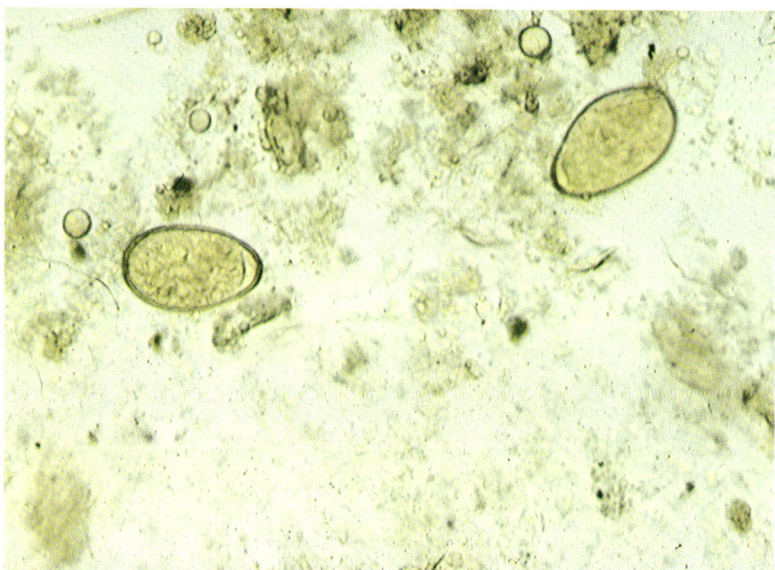

483 Eggs in human sputum Eggs (*see* **319**) are passed in the sputum or swallowed to be passed later in the faeces. The miracidia hatching from the eggs penetrate snails of various genera including *Semisulcospira* and *Thiara* (*see* **Table XII**). After the usual cycle of development in the snail, microcercous cercariae emerge and encyst inside freshwater crayfish and crabs. Various crab-eating carnivores thus become the natural reservoirs of *Paragonimus* species. (× *180*)

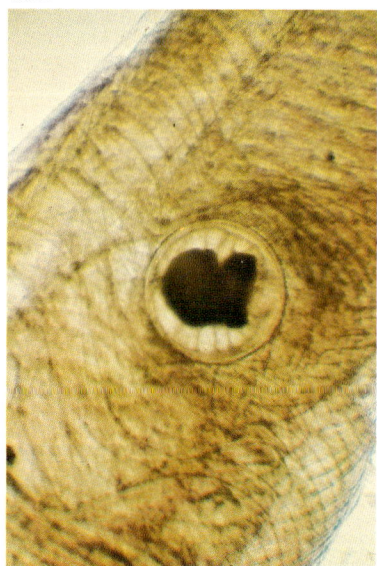

484 Metacercaria in crab gills Compare with the smaller metacercaria of *C. sinensis* (**457**). (× *10*)

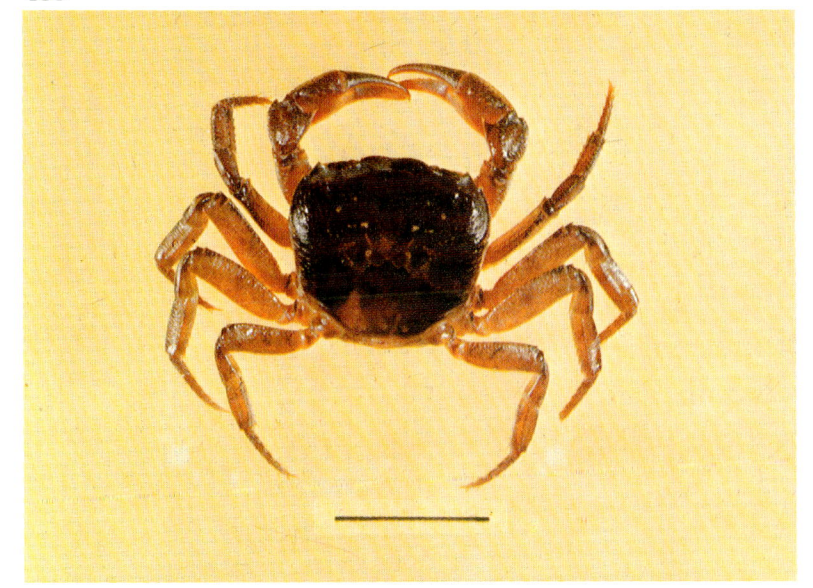

485 *Potamon rathbuni*, a host of lung fluke Crabs are commonly eaten raw, or in the form of an uncooked paste with which the metacercariae are ingested.

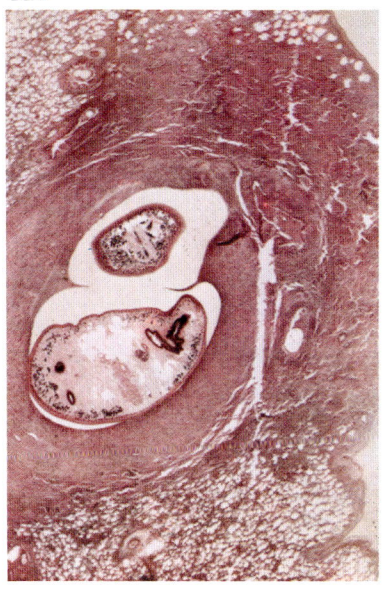

486 Section of lung The figure shows a section of lung containing encapsulated, adult *P. westermani*. (H&E × 20)

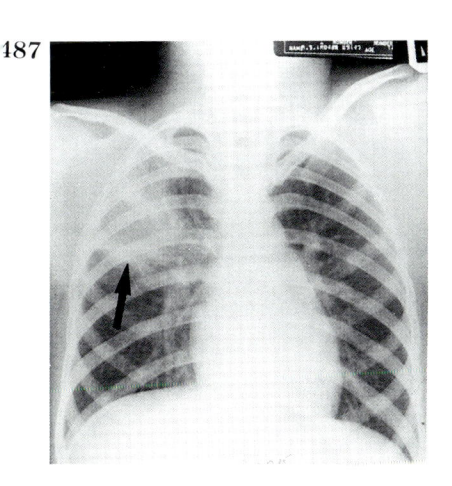

487 Chest X-ray Human infection is manifested by cough, haemoptysis, and other signs and symptoms which are commonly confused with those of tuberculosis. Typical shadows caused by the encysted adult trematodes may be seen on X-ray. This patient was infected in Thailand. *P. uterobilateralis* in Eastern Nigeria and *P. africanus* (which occurs in the nearby Cameroon Republic) have a similar life cycle and, as with *P. westermani*, man is infected by eating crabs or crayfish. The animal reservoirs are not yet known in West Africa.

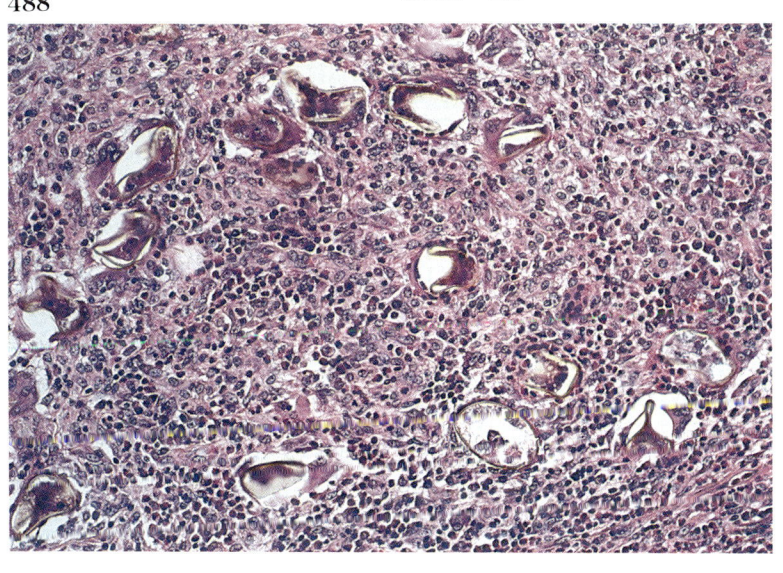

488 Eggs in mesenteric lymph node In this section several disintegrating eggs of *P. westermani* are seen in a granuloma containing numerous eosinophils in a mesenteric node. (H&E × 120)

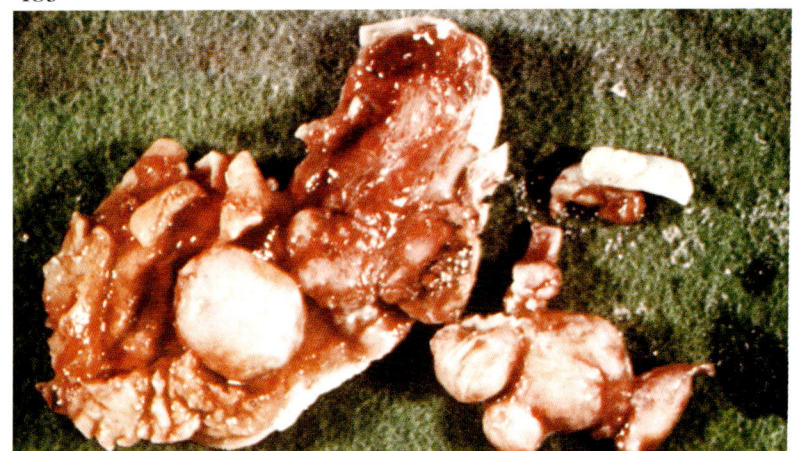

489 *Paragonimus* cyst in brain
P. westermani cyst found at post-mortem in the brain of a 21-year-old Japanese girl. Such patients usually present with epilepsy occurring for the first time in adult life.

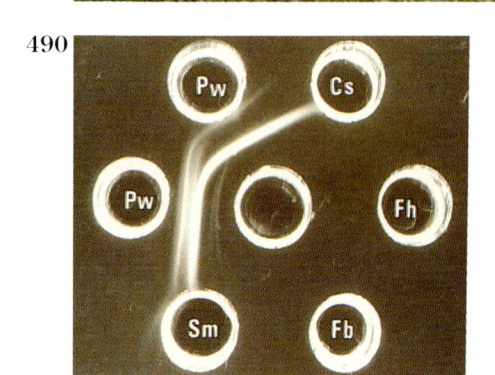

490 Gel diffusion test for paragonimiasis The reaction of antigen derived from adult worms with serum antibodies can be a useful diagnostic aid.

ANGIOSTRONGYLIASIS

The main cause of eosinophilic meningitis is infection with larvae of the rat nematode, *Angiostrongylus cantonensis*. This parasite has spread geographically in recent years with the dissemination of one of its best intermediate hosts, the giant African land snail, *Achatina fulica*, which is a popular item of food in some countries. Rats or man are infected by eating infected molluscs or food contaminated by their bodies.

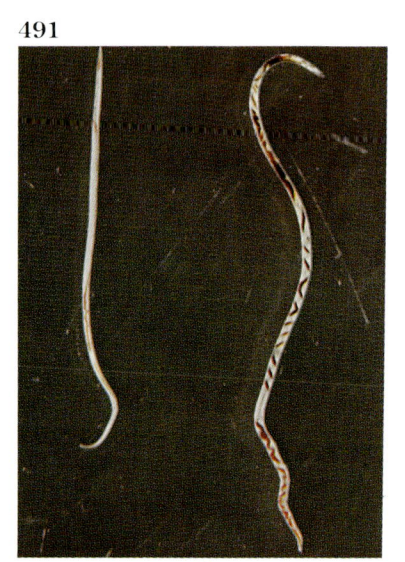

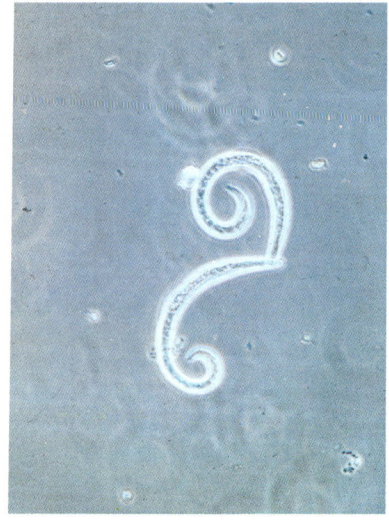

491 Adult *A. cantonensis* The adult worm, about 1 to 2 cm long, is a common parasite of rodents in the Far East and Pacific. It lives in the pulmonary arteries and arterioles. ($\times 3$)

492 First-stage larvae in rat faeces The eggs passed in the bloodstream break through the pulmonary tract, are swallowed by the rodent and are passed in the faeces in which they may hatch to first-stage larvae. ($\times 100$)

493 *Achatina fulica*, an intermediate host of *A. cantonensis* The first-stage larvae in rat faeces are eaten by snails of various genera including *Achatina*, *Cipangopaludina* and *Bradybaena*, as well as by some slugs and land planarians in which the larvae develop to the third stage. *Achatina fulica* is sometimes kept in vivaria as a 'pet' or for educational purposes in schools. It is important to ensure that such molluscs are locally bred and not imported from countries where *A. cantonensis* is enzootic. (× 1/2)

494 Third-stage larvae in *Achatina fulica* New rats become infested when they eat snails containing third-stage larvae. (× 100)

495 Larvae of *A. cantonensis* in rat brain The thread-like larvae can be seen in the subarachnoid space covering the base of this rat brain. Here they mature to young adults which migrate to the pulmonary arteries via the cerebral veins.

496 Section of larvae in meninges of human brain Man may be infested by eating freshwater prawns but how these come to contain larvae is uncertain. He may also be infected by eating molluscs which contain the larvae or food contaminated with crushed molluscs. The larvae migrate to the brain where they cause eosinophilic meningitis or meningoencephalitis. The diagnosis is aided by the examination serologically of paired specimens, using a specific antigen from adult worms. (× 60)

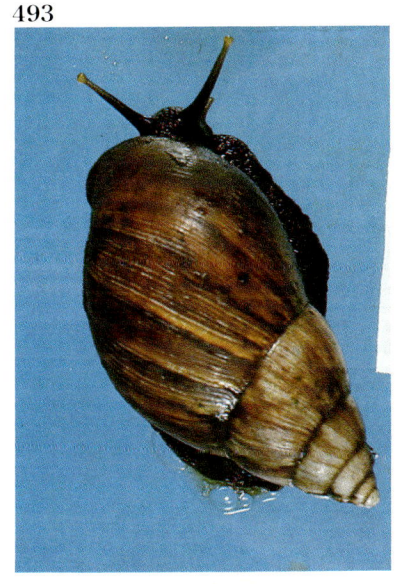

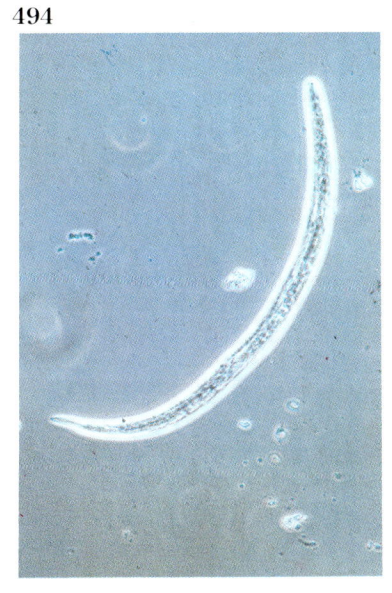

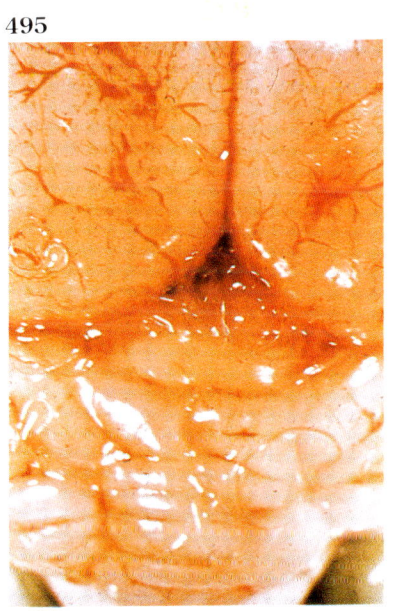

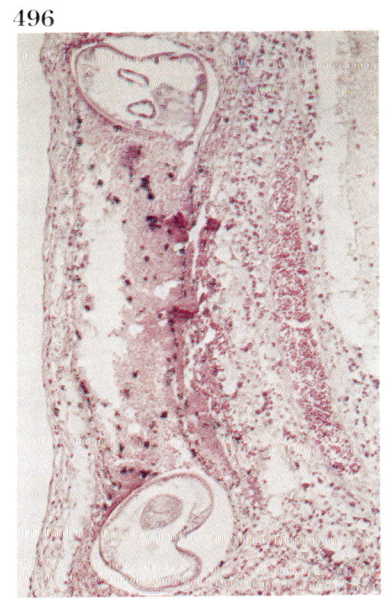

Part IV
Infections Acquired through the Gastrointestinal Tract

Many of the important pathogens that gain entry through the gastrointestinal tract are cosmopolitan in their distribution. Some cause diarrhoeal diseases (e.g. cholera, shigellosis, enteric fever) while others pass from the intestinal tract to cause disease in other organs (e.g. poliomyelitis, infective hepatitis, trichinosis). The pathogens include viruses, bacteria, protozoa, helminths and endoparasitic arthropods. The first three of these are directly infectious for man when they are passed in the faeces but, in the case of helminths, the eggs may become infectious only after maturation in the soil (e.g. *Ascaris*), or after passing through an intermediate host (e.g. *Taenia saginata*).*

The most important pattern of transmission is the passage of infective material from human faeces into the mouth of a new host, which is known as 'faeco-oral' transmission. This occurs mostly through inapparent faecal contamination of food, water, and hands—the three main points of contact with the mouth. Some of the pathogens that infect through the mouth are not excreted in the faeces: for example, guinea worm infection is acquired by drinking contaminated water, but the larvae escape through the skin. On the other hand, while the ova of hookworm are passed in the faeces, the route of human infection is by direct penetration of the skin by the larvae after a period of incubation of the egg in the soil.

A number of the infections that are acquired through the gastrointestinal tract characteristically occur in epidemic form, e.g. cholera and typhoid. The spread of El Tor cholera, for example, is facilitated by the potentiating combination of a symptomless carrier state with wide-scale local and international travel. Other infections may be more localised, affecting persons from the same household or institution, e.g. amoebiasis or enterobiasis.

[Footnote *Helminthiases acquired from the soil are included in Part II, those requiring a snail intermediate host in Part III.]

VIRAL INFECTIONS
Poliomyelitis

497 Ultrastructure of poliomyelitis virus Spherical particles measuring 25 nm in diameter. Both 'full' and 'empty' particles are shown. The virus is widely spread throughout the tropics. (× *126 000*)

498 Ethiopian boy with paralysis of left leg Thanks to the extensive use of vaccination, poliomyelitis has greatly decreased in the developed countries. Today, young indigenous children in the developing countries are predominantly affected, as well as non-immunised expatriates of all ages.

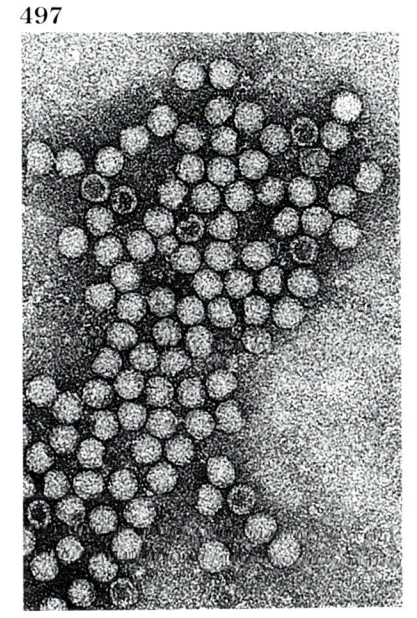

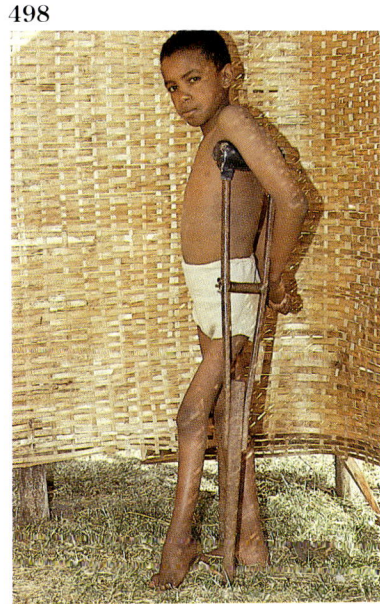

Infective Hepatitis

Infective hepatitis and its sequelae are a major problem, particularly in the tropics and subtropics, although the viruses are cosmopolitan. The four viruses responsible are hepatitis A (HAV), hepatitis B (HBV), non-A non-B (NANBV) and the recently discovered delta virus (HDV). The last virus can only exist in the presence of HBV but can cause fulminating hepatitis or lead to chronic active hepatitis. HAV is commonly acquired from contaminated food, shellfish being a notorious source of infection. HBV is usually acquired from blood or blood products by accidental inoculation, transfusion, etc. While HAV infection does not usually have serious sequelae, HBV often remains in the individual indefinitely and can induce cirrhosis and hepatic carcinoma. NANBV is usually waterborne but may also be acquired by transfusion. It is often associated with chronic liver damage.

499 Ultrastructure of 'hepatitis A virus' This electron micrograph shows virus like particles measuring 27 nm in diameter found in faecal extracts from an adult volunteer during the acute phase of HAV infection, after inoculation with MS-1 serum. The particles are heavily coated with antibody present in convalescent serum. (× *252 000*)

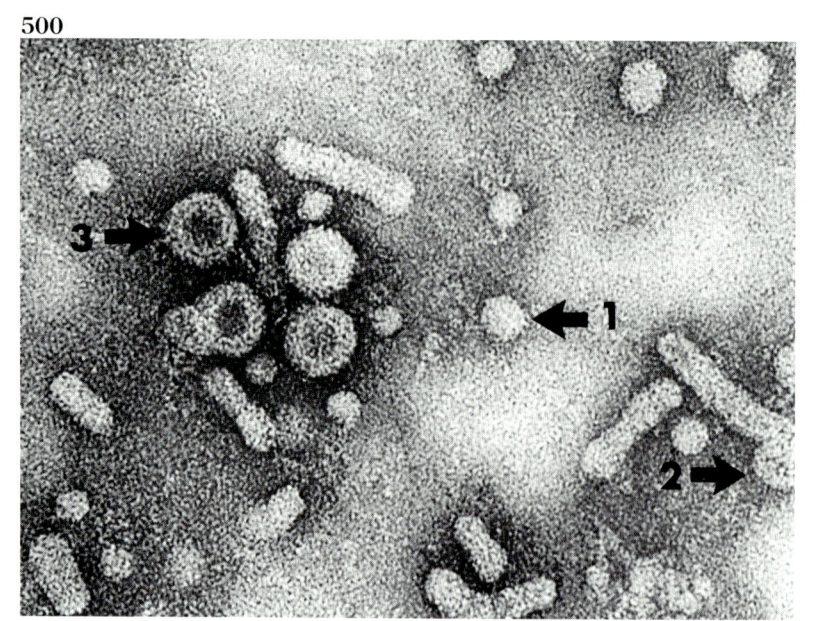

500 Hepatitis B antigen-containing serum Three distinct morphological entities are seen: Australia antigen surface coat in the form of (1) small pleomorphic spherical particles measuring 20-22 nm in diameter and (2) tubular forms of varying length with a constant diameter of 20 nm and frequently with a terminal bulbous swelling; (3) double-shelled spheroidal Dane particles of hepatitis B virus, approximately 42 nm in diameter, with a core measuring 27 nm in diameter surrounded by surface coat. ($\times 227\,000$)

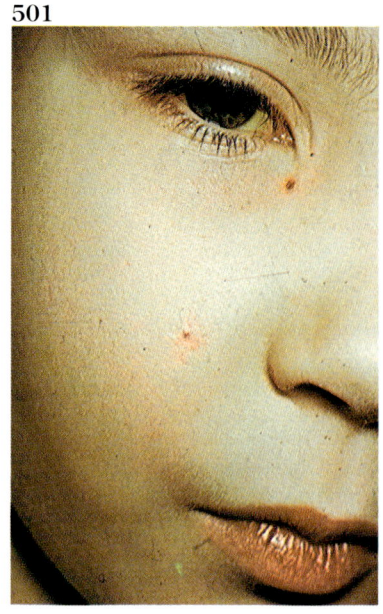

501 Jaundiced child with infective hepatitis Fever, anorexia, and later jaundice are characteristic clinical features. The disease is particularly severe in pregnancy. Note deep jaundice and spider naevus on the cheek.

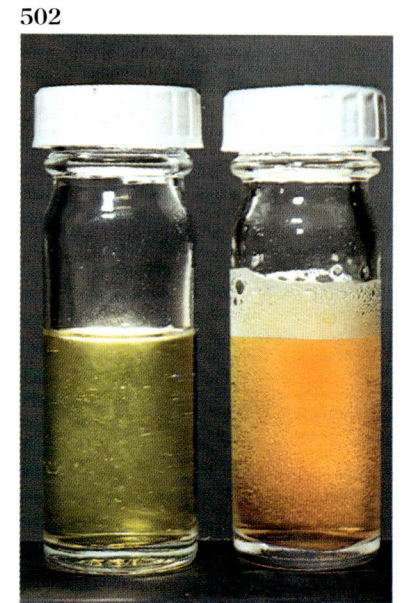

502 Urine from child with hepatitis The dark-coloured urine contains bilirubin and urobilinogen.

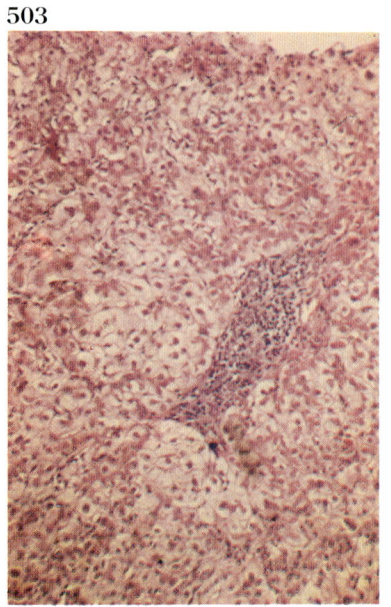

503 Biopsy of liver in hepatitis Histologically, the characteristic features are ballooning and a feathery degeneration of the liver parenchymal cells. ($\times 150$)

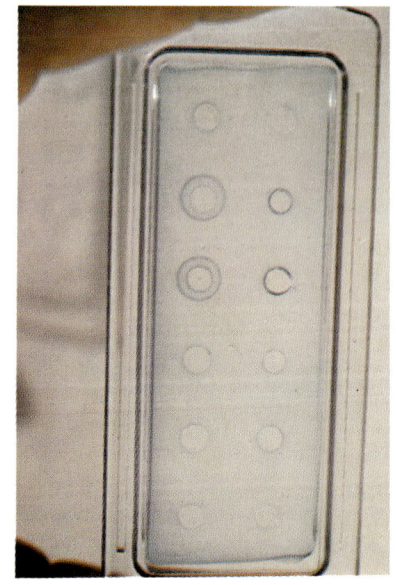

504 Single radial immunodiffusion test Hepatitis B antigen-positive serum is readily detected by this simple serological procedure.

BACTERIAL INFECTIONS
Typhoid (Enteric) Fevers

505 Rose spots The classical rose spots may appear irregularly, usually on the abdominal wall, lower thorax, and on the back of the trunk.

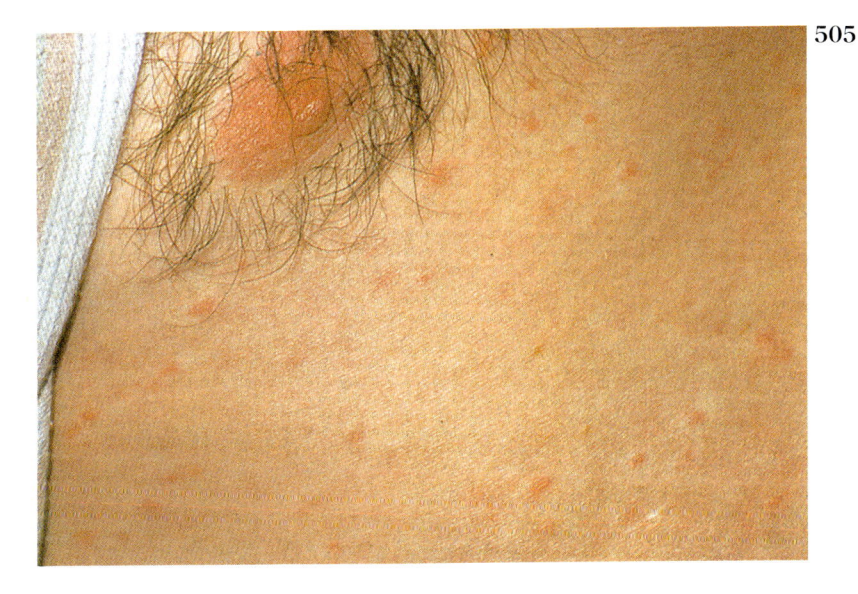

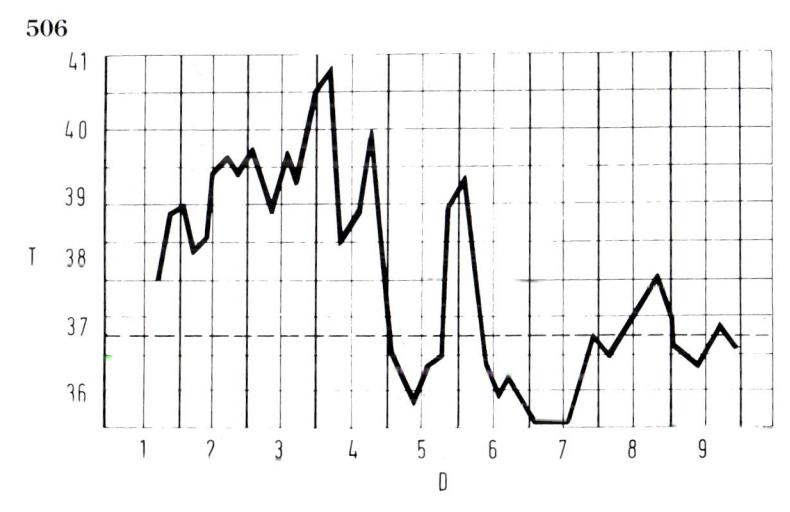

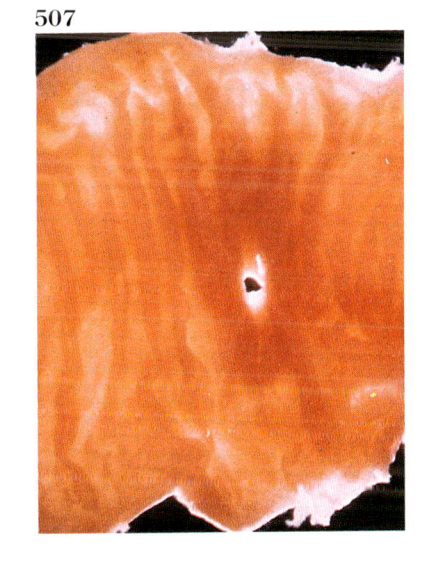

506 Temperature chart The fever is high and accompanied by confusion and severe prostration ('typhoid state'). There is often a dissociation between pulse and temperature, and an accompanying leucopenia. The tongue is frequently coated (in contrast to kala-azar when it is usually clean—*see* **183 & 184**).

507 Ulceration of Peyer's patches Intestinal haemorrhage and perforation are the two most serious complications of typhoid fever. They are due to ulceration of Peyer's patches.

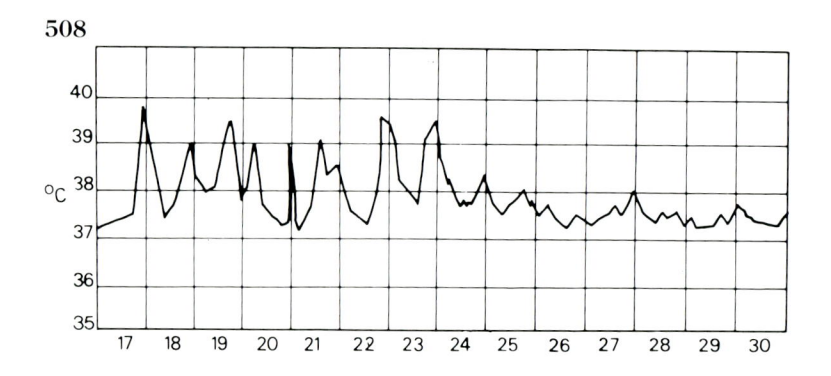

508 Salmonellosis associated with *S. mansoni* infection An association exists between fever occurring in chronic *Salmonella typhi* infection and concomitant *S. mansoni*. In such cases, clearance of the helminth infection is needed before the *Salmonella* organisms can be eliminated.

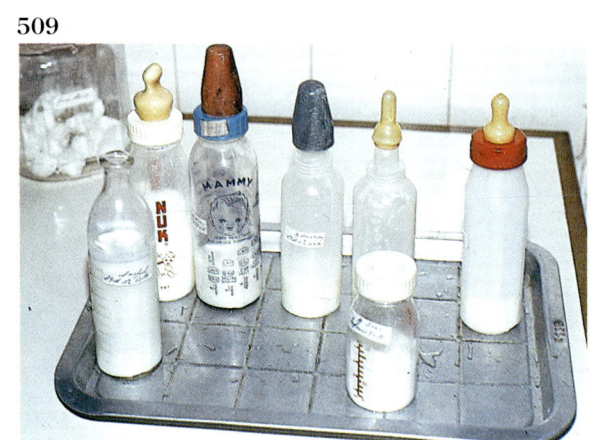

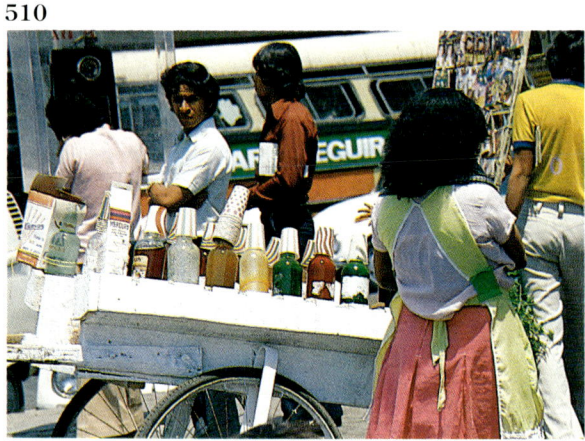

Non-specific Gastroenteritis

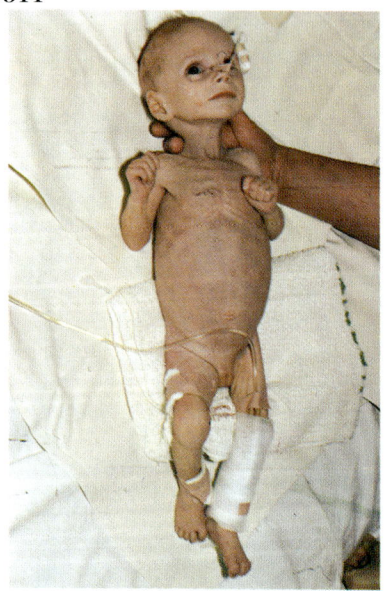

509 Sources of infantile gastroenteritis Gastroenteritis due to a variety of organisms is one of the major causes of childhood mortality in the tropics. The substitution of the milk bottle for breast feeding is increasing, rather than decreasing, the problem. Mismanagement of artificial feeding is a serious cause, due to contamination of feeds with pathogenic coliform organisms.

510 The origin of 'Turista' Dirty food containers contaminated by flies with pathogenic organisms are another common cause of non-specific gastroenteritis (often called 'Turista'), especially in travellers.

511 Dehydration due to gastroenteritis Severe dehydration due to diarrhoea and vomiting is the salient diagnostic feature. Oral rehydration with a solution containing salts and glucose or intravenous fluid replacement have revolutionised the treatment of diarrhoeal diseases.

Cholera

512

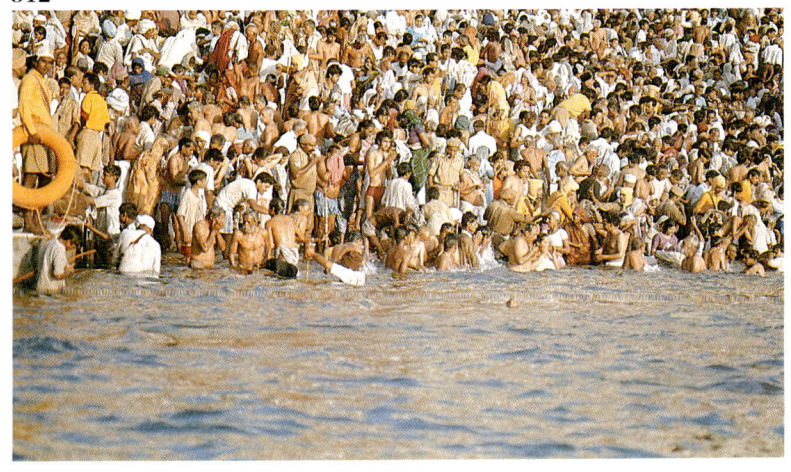

512 An ancient epicentre of cholera Mass assemblies of pilgrims for religious activities such as figured here on the river Ganges may be the source of epidemic cholera, as well as other waterborne infections. The *Vibrio cholerae* El Tor biotype was responsible for the cholera pandemic from 1961 to 1985. Symptomless carriers are very important in the epidemiology of this disease.

513

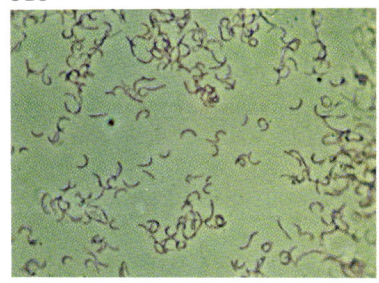

513 Cholera vibrios *Vibrio cholerae*, the classical organism, is limited to the Indian subcontinent but *V. cholerae* El Tor is almost cosmopolitan in its distribution. ($\times 600$) The organisms produce an exotoxin that causes structural and functional damage to the intestinal epithelium which can no longer reabsorb water.

514 A 'cholera cot' The disease is characterised by severe vomiting and profuse watery diarrhoea ('rice-water stools'). Nursing of patients in a 'cholera cot' facilitates the nursing and allows a rapid assessment of fluid loss to be made.

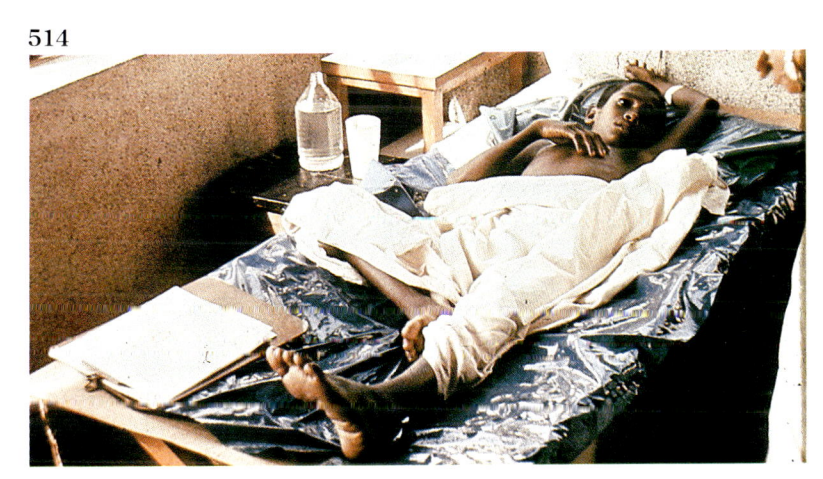

514

515 'Choleraic facies' The massive fluid loss results in severe dehydration which is the primary cause of death. Rapid rehydration with isotonic salts and glucose is life saving. This man shows the typical 'choleraic facies' with deeply sunken cheeks and eyes. With rehydration he recovered completely.

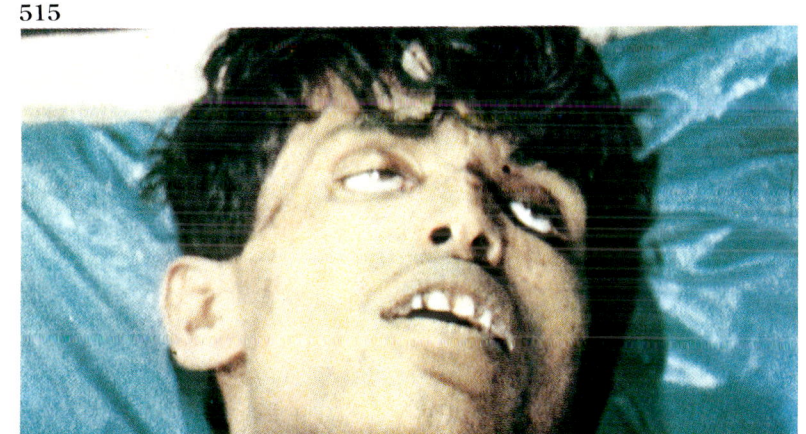

515

Brucellosis

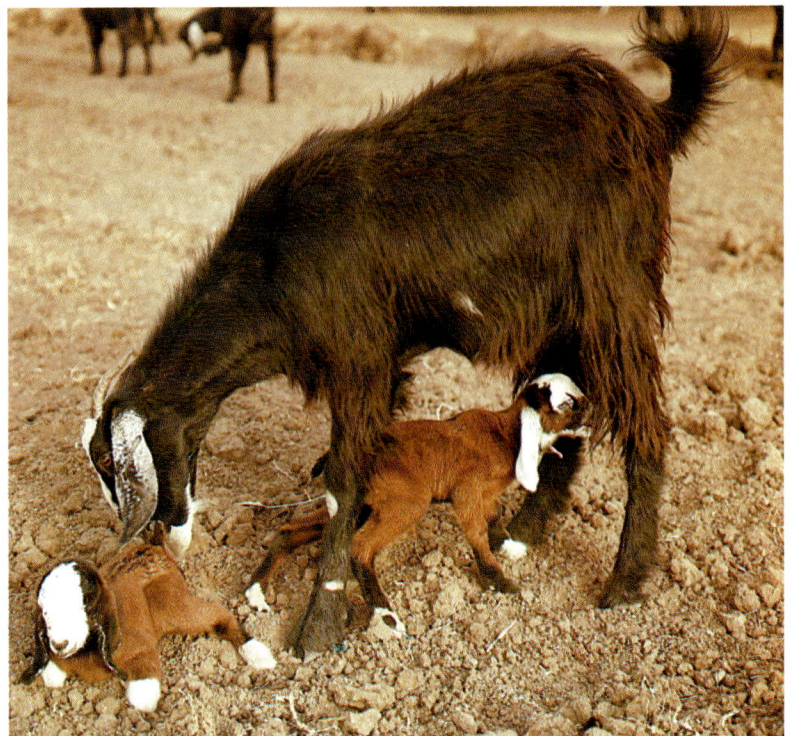

516 Reservoirs of brucellosis
Goats, cows and pigs are the most common animal reservoirs of infection with *Brucella abortus, B. melitensis* and *B. suis* respectively. Infection is acquired by drinking raw milk or milk products.

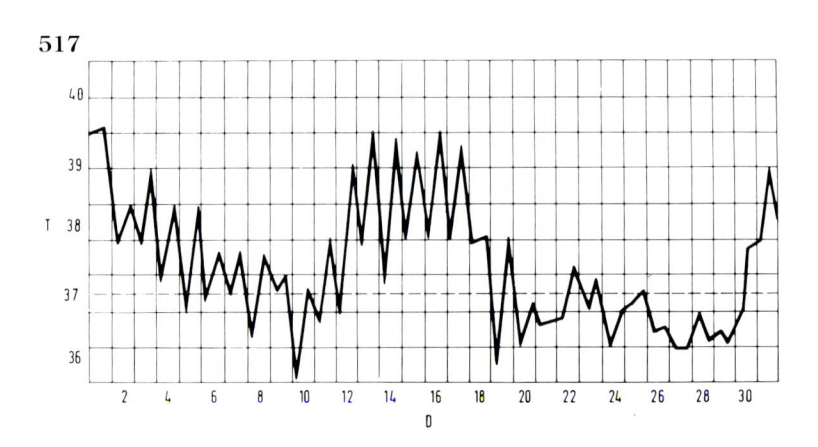

517 Temperature chart The typical fever is remittent and undulating. Moderate leucopenia and splenomegaly are usual. A sharp drop of one or more degrees somewhere in the course is common and is a useful differential feature. In some areas the fever is atypical. A persistent raised IgM is suggestive of brucellosis but a high *Brucella* agglutination titre or positive blood culture will confirm the diagnosis.

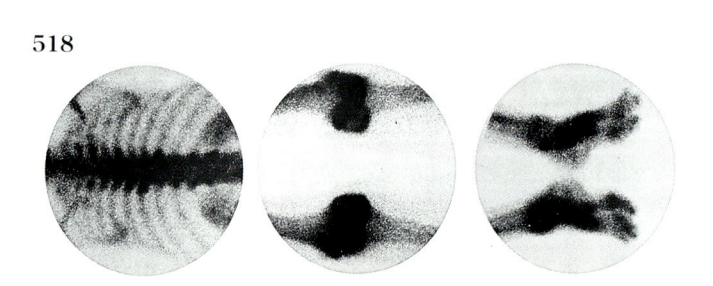

518 Degenerative osteoarthritis in brucellosis This technetium-99m MDP bone scan shows extensive osteoarthritic degenerative changes in a Bedouin shepherd who suffered from fever, painful joint swellings and backache for over a year. Brucellosis is a serious problem for many desert-dwelling pastoralists of the Middle East. While such arthritic changes are common manifestations of chronic brucellosis, the infection may also present protean neurological signs, sometimes suggestive of disseminated sclerosis.

Enteritis Necroticans (Pigbel)

519 Appearance of intestine at operation Extensive sloughing and necrosis of the large bowel occur in this condition which is endemic in the highlands of Papua New Guinea. It is associated with the β toxin of *Clostridium perfringens* type C (which can be found in the faeces of 70 per cent of highland villagers) and the intermittent consumption of inadequately cooked pork with baked sweet potatoes, especially in children whose normal diet is protein deficient. Vaccination with *C. perfringens* type C β toxoid gives protection lasting a few years.

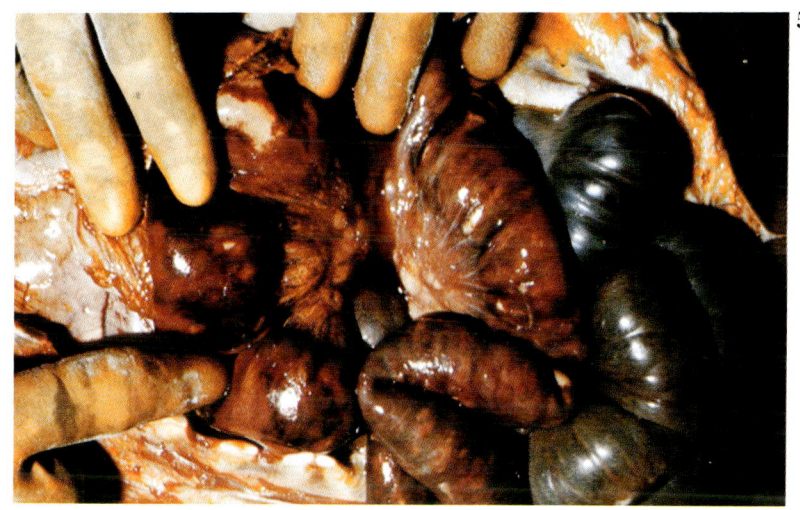

520 Necrosis of small intestine in 'Pigbel' The main lesion is patchy necrosis of the small intestine which starts in the mucosa and extends through to the serosal wall, as seen here. (*H&E × 150*)

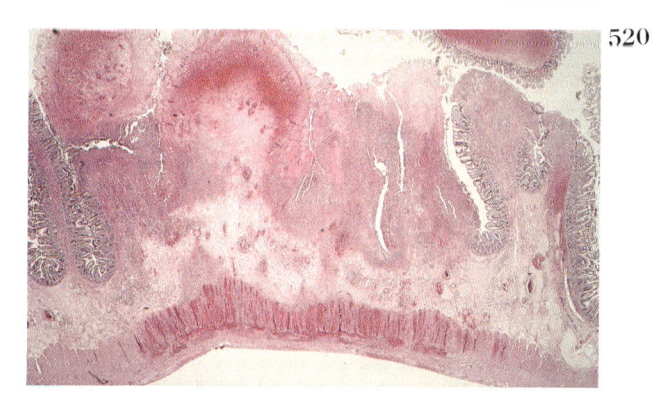

Melioidosis

521 Right upper pneumonia due to melioidosis This disease, which occurs mainly in southeast Asia, is due to infection with *Pseudomonas pseudomallei* (Whitmore's bacillus). The route of infection is uncertain but it may be waterborne or airborne, or acquired by contamination of wounds with soil. Inapparent infections are probably widespread since surveys, for example, in Thailand, have shown that 30 to 50 per cent of those examined have been seropositive but symptomless. The disease may present as acute septicaemia, followed by multiple organ abscess formation, or the disease may be subacute from the start. Chronic infections in children may present as a parotid abscess. This is an X-ray of a 14-year-old Thai boy who presented with pneumonia which failed to respond completely to antibiotic therapy. He died six months later with miliary peritoneal deposits containing *P. pseudomallei*. The diagnosis is indicated by a positive haemagglutination test and confirmed by culturing the organism from different body fluids on Ashdown's medium.

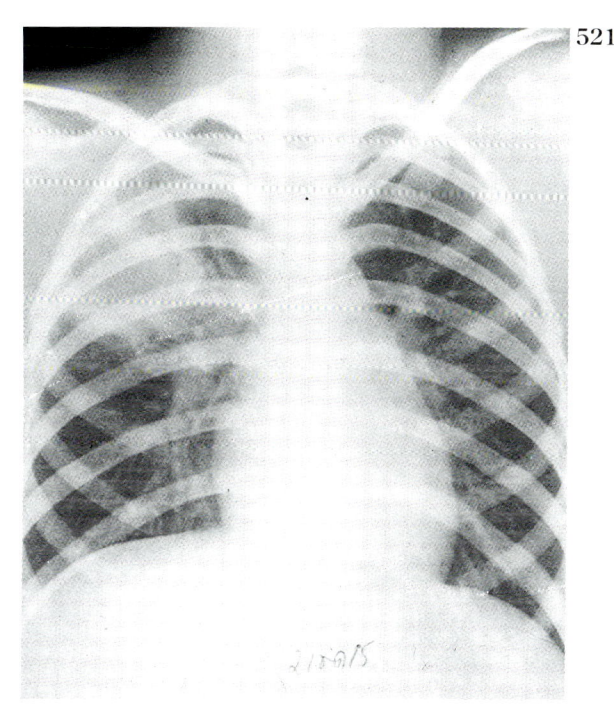

Leptospirosis (*See* **Table IV**)

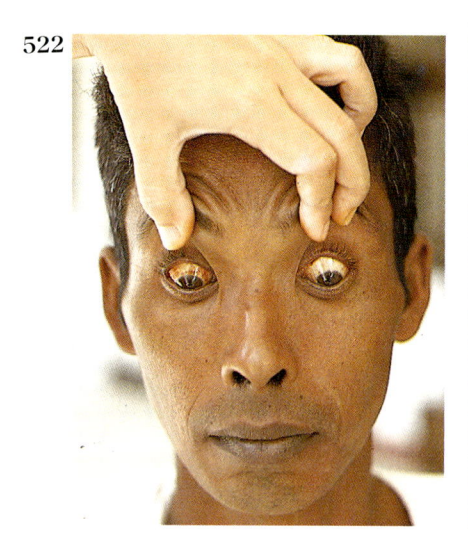

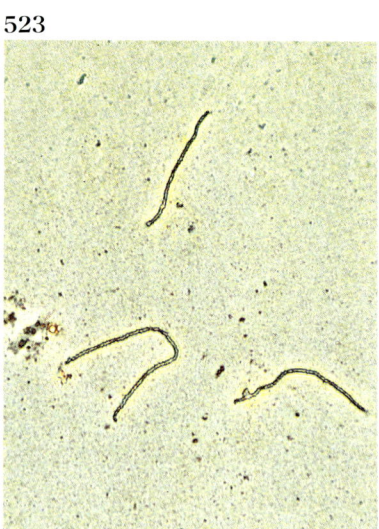

522 Injection of conjunctivae
Infection with one of a variety of organisms of the genus *Leptospira* causes illness ranging from a mild, transient fever to severe hepatitis and liver failure. Injection and small haemorrhages of the conjunctiva are not uncommon. The disease is a zoonosis usually acquired from contact with water contaminated with animal urine, especially of rodents. It is global in distribution but commoner in tropical areas.

523 *Leptospira icterohaemorrhagiae* The organisms are readily seen in silver-stained preparations, especially with a phase-contrast microscope. ($\times$ 1 350)

PROTOZOAL INFECTIONS (*See* **Table XIII**)

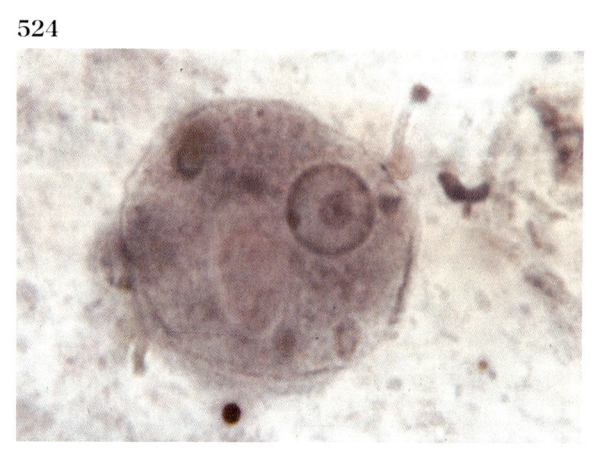

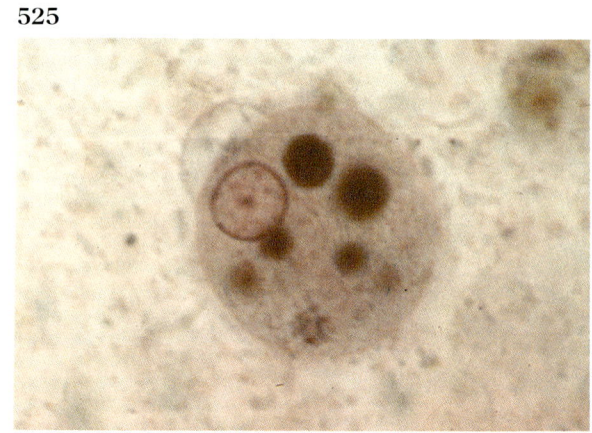

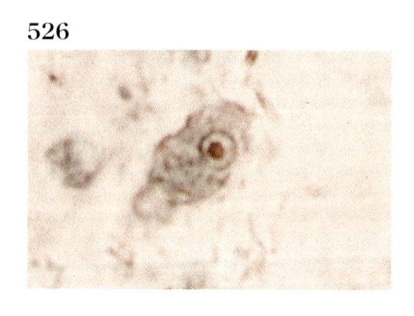

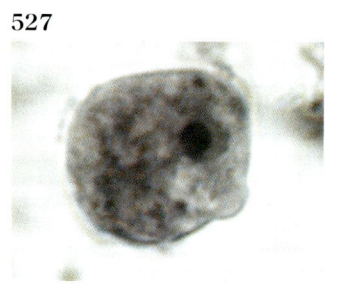

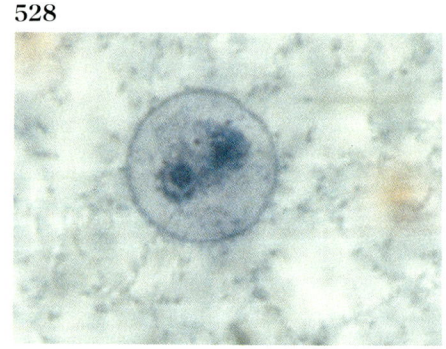

524-528 Trophozoites of intestinal protozoa *Entamoeba coli* (**524**), *E. histolytica* (**525**), *E. nana* (**526**), *Iodamoeba butschlii* (**527**), *Dientamoeba fragilis* (**528**). (**524 & 525** *trichrome stain;* **526-528** *haematoxylin*.) ($\times$ 1 800)

529-532 Cysts of intestinal protozoa
E. coli (**529**),
E. histolytica (**530**),
E. nana (**531**),
I. butschlii (**532**)
(*Iodine* × *1 800*).

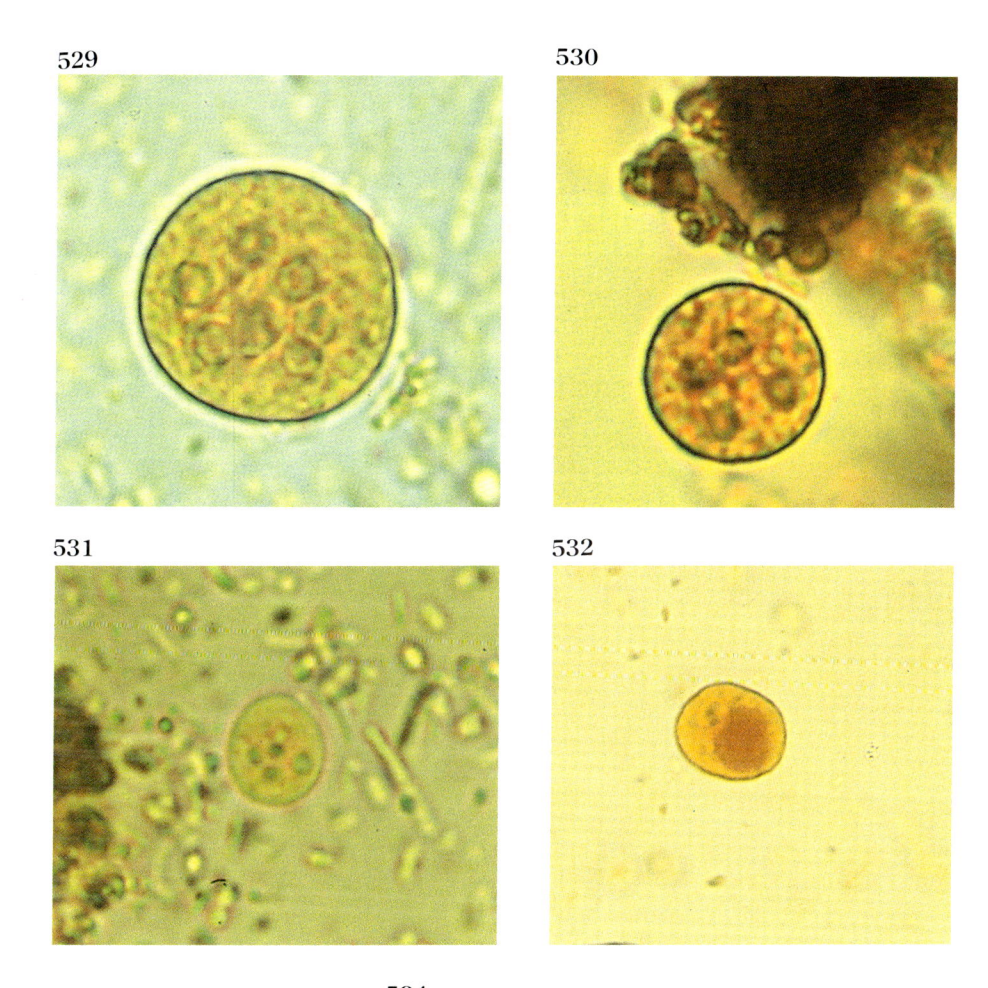

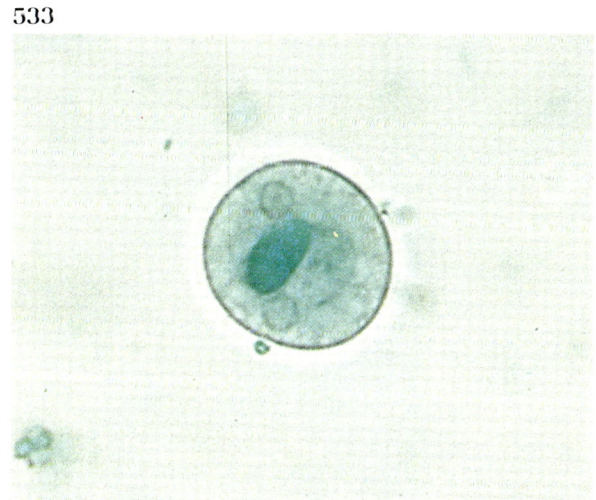

533 Chromatoid bodies in *E. histolytica* These characteristic structures are readily demonstrated with Sargeaunt's stain. (× *1 800*)

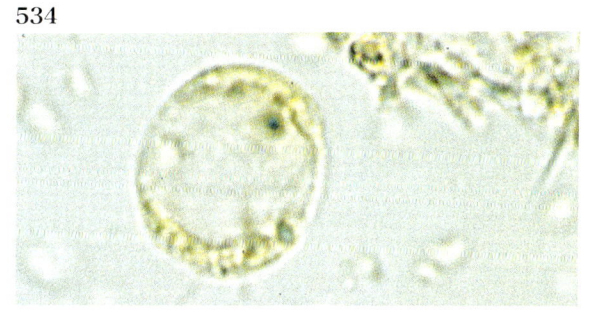

534 *Blastocystis hominis* This common faecal organism, which was formerly believed to be a commensal fungus, has recently been shown to be an anaerobic protozoon. It may be associated with acute enteritis in some immunocompromised individuals. (*Iodine* × *1 800*)

Amoebiasis

535 *E. histolytica* zymodemes By enzyme electrophoresis a number of zymodemes of this parasite can be distinguished in trophozoites cultured from cysts in human faeces. Only a few zymodemes are associated with pathogenicity, the remainder appearing to be harmless commensals.

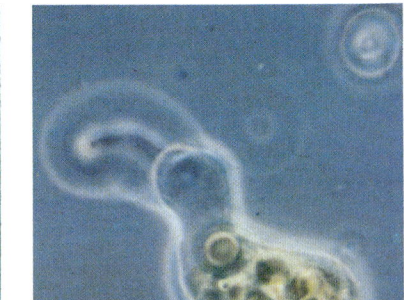

536 Living *E. histolytica* Rather rapidly moving trophozoites of *E. histolytica* containing ingested erythrocytes may be found in a freshly passed specimen. They are, unlike cysts when only those are present, clear evidence of infection with a tissue invasive (i.e. pathogenic) strain. (*Phase-contrast* × *900*).

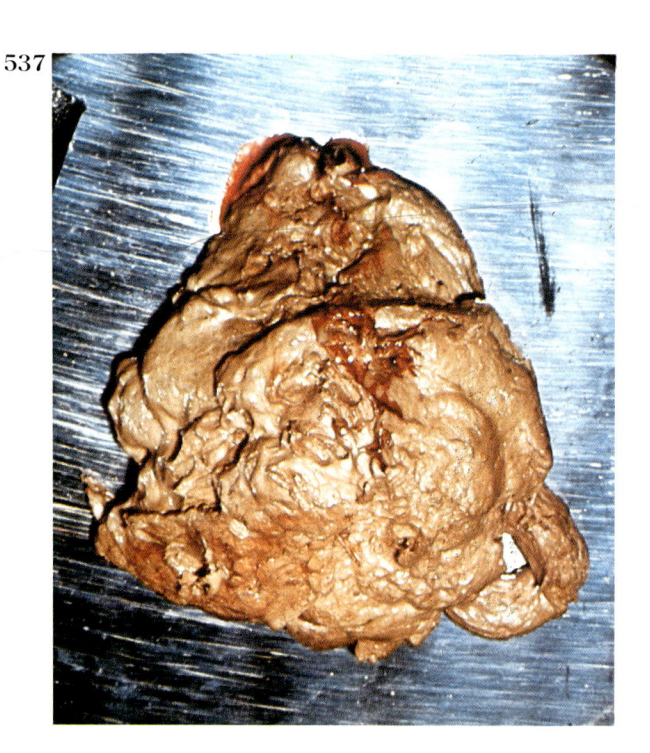

537 Macroscopic appearance of stool In amoebic dysentery the stool is loose, containing mucus and blood mixed with faecal material. As distinct from bacterial dysentery there is no cellular exudate.

538 Sites of predilection The commonest sites for localisation of *E. histolytica* in the intestine are the caecum and descending colon. Secondary sites included in the figure are liver, lung and skin.

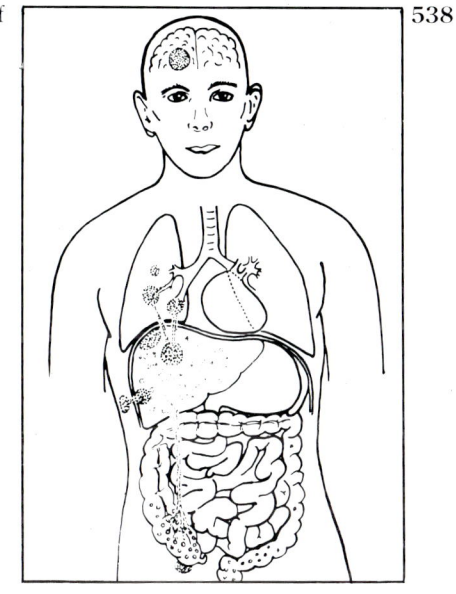

539 Gross appearance of amoebic ulceration of caecum In fulminating infections, the destruction of all layers of the intestinal wall is extensive, and ulceration may be confluent. Such lesions are frequently seen in pregnancy and the puerperium.

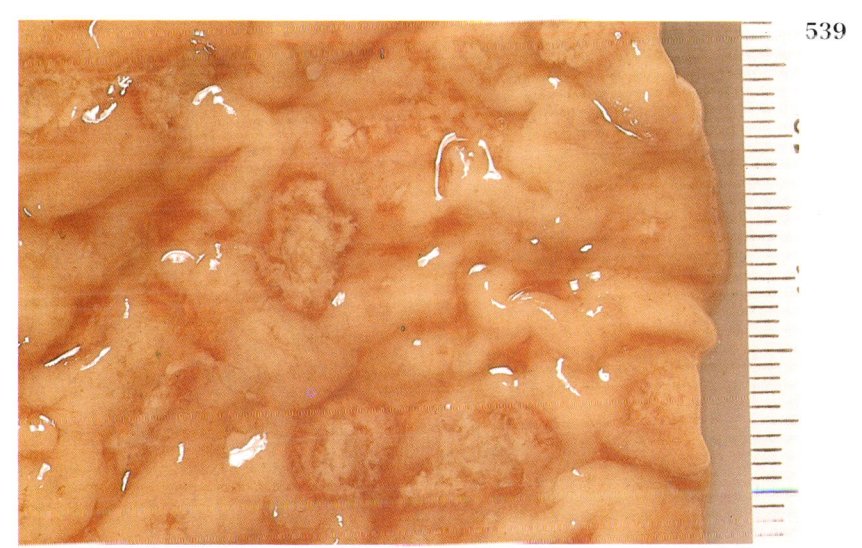

540 Section of colon wall as seen in biopsy Typical 'flask-shaped' ulcers are seen in the intestinal wall which is invaded by *E. histolytica* trophozoites. The intervening mucosa is usually normal. In this low power view, large numbers of trophozoites can be seen on the surface of and invading the mucosa. (*PAS × 40*)

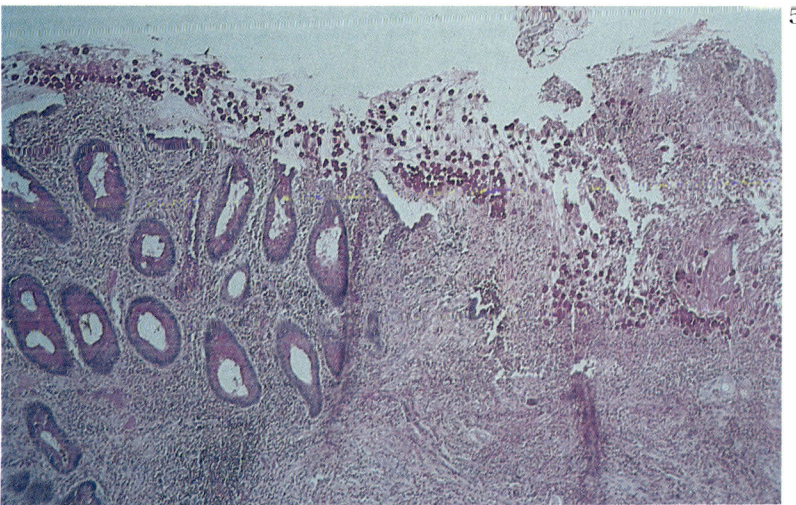

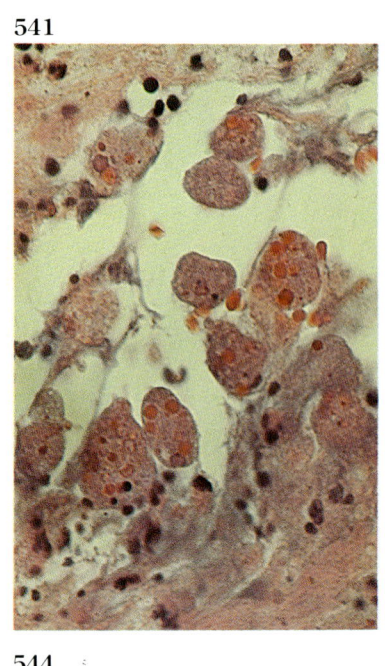

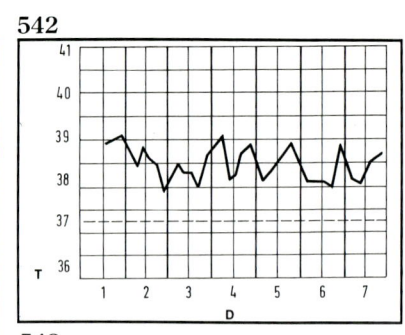

541 *E. histolytica* in mucosa
Numerous trophozoites with ingested erythrocytes are visible in this high power view. (PAS × 180)

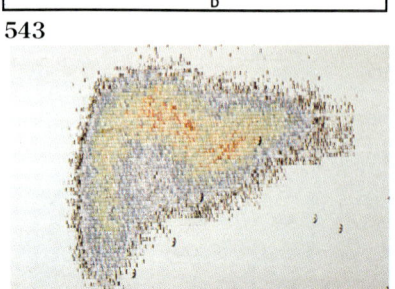

542 Temperature chart of patient with amoebic liver abscess The triad of swinging temperature, profuse sweats and leucocytosis is indicative of liver abscess, especially when associated with pain in the right hypochondrium.

543 Scintiscan of patient with amoebic liver abscess The liver is often enlarged and tender, sometimes bulging in the abscess area.

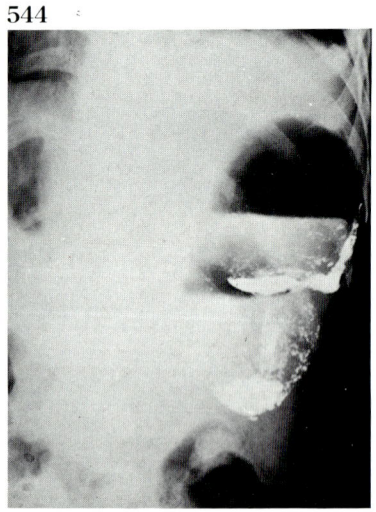

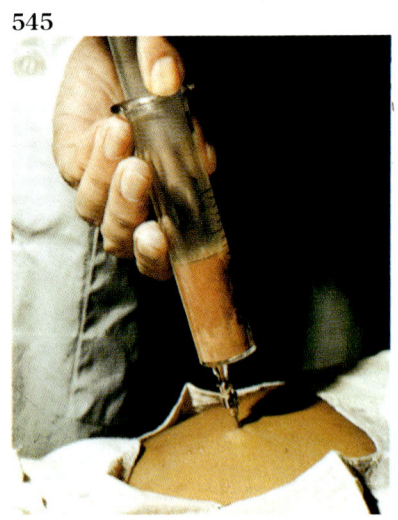

544 X-ray of liver abscess An amoebic abscess of the liver is usually single. The volume of the contents of the lesion may vary from 500 to 1 500 ml.

545 Aspiration of liver abscess Aspiration of large abscesses is usually needed as an adjunct to specific chemotherapy for successful treatment. The pus is chocolate-coloured.

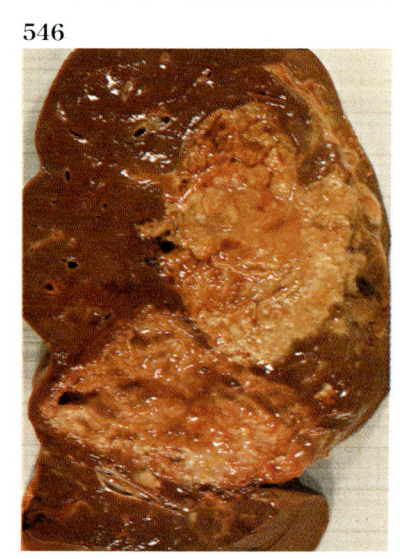

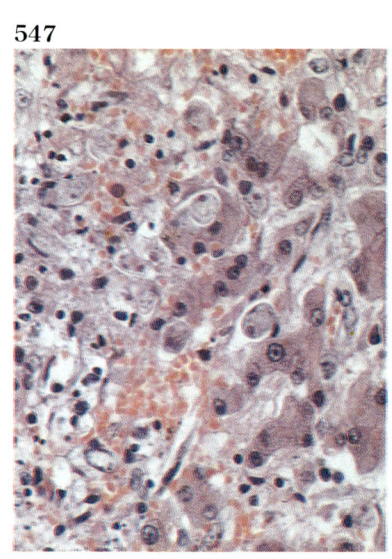

546 Macroscopic appearance of liver abscess The shaggy, irregular periphery consists of stroma and layers of compressed liver parenchyma.

547 Section of amoebic liver abscess Trophozoites, some containing ingested red blood cells, are seen in the tissues at the edge of the abscess and may be found in the pus if it is examined immediately after aspiration. (H&E × 150)

548 Amoebic abscess of lung
Extra-intestinal infections occur commonly in the liver, but any site of the body may be affected. The lung is sometimes affected by rupture of a hepatic abscess through the diaphragm. Typical amoebic pus may be coughed up with the sputum.

549 Amoebiasis of the skin
Amoebic infection of the skin may arise by direct spread from a primary abscess. This patient was erroneously operated on for a perforated duodenal ulcer and no anti-amoebic drugs were given. Sloughing of the skin occurred and amoebae were recovered from the skin lesion.

550 Amoebic balanitis Amoebic infection of the genital organs can result from normal or abnormal sexual intercourse.

551 Fluorescent antibody staining of *E. histolytica* The FAT is the most sensitive immunodiagnostic test available for invasive forms of amoebiasis. It has proved a valuable adjunct to direct microscopical diagnosis of amoebiasis. Fluorescence of cultured *E. histolytica* exposed to serum from a patient with hepatic involvement is seen in this figure. ($\times 900$)

Giardiasis

552 & 553 *Giardia lamblia* trophozoites and cysts The flagellated trophozoites (552) attach by their suckers to the surface of the duodenal or jejunal mucosa. The ovoid cysts in faeces (553) have a very distinctive structure. Contaminated drinking water appears to be a common source of infection. (552 *Giemsa* $\times 1\,000$; 553 *trichrome* $\times 1\,000$)

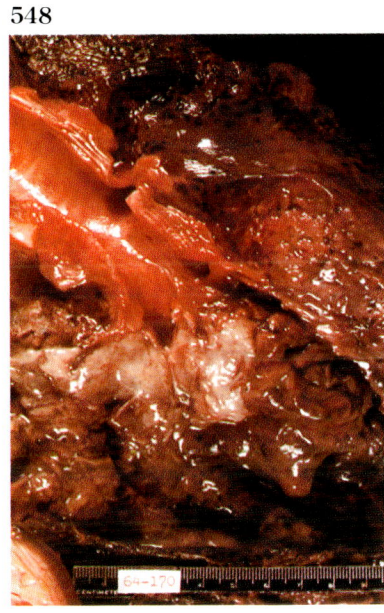

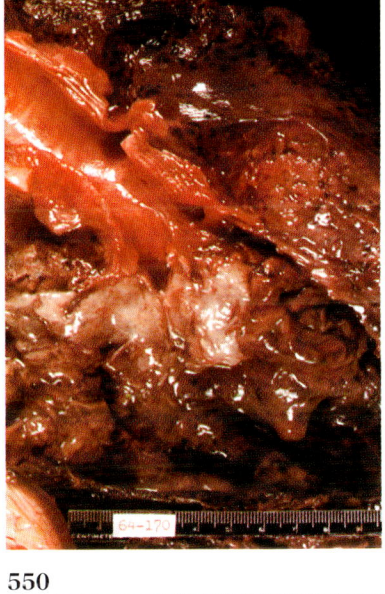

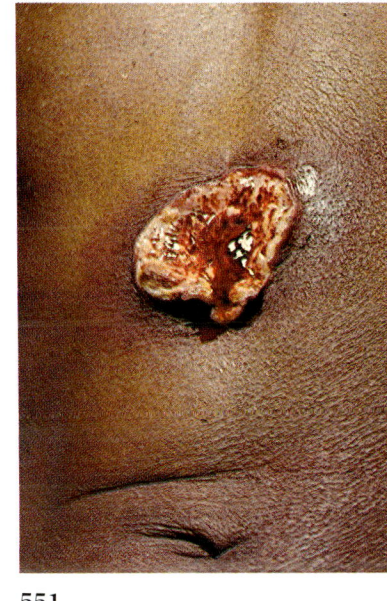

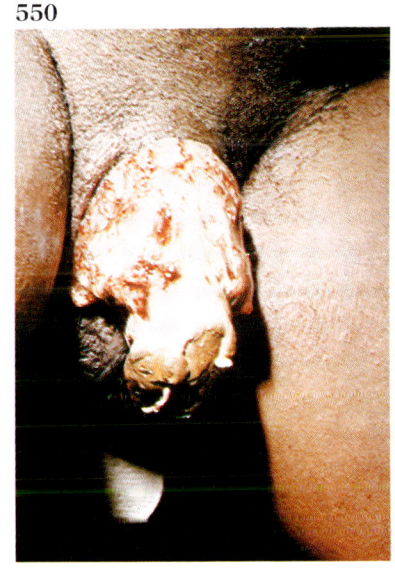

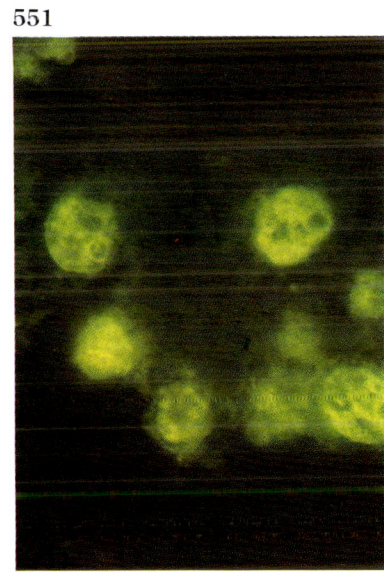

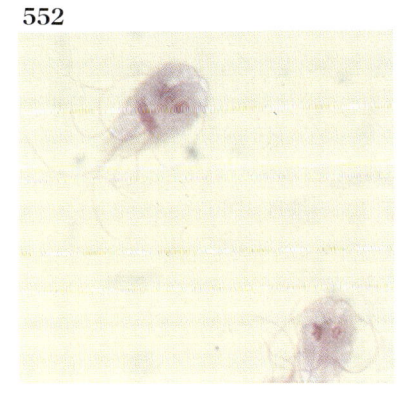

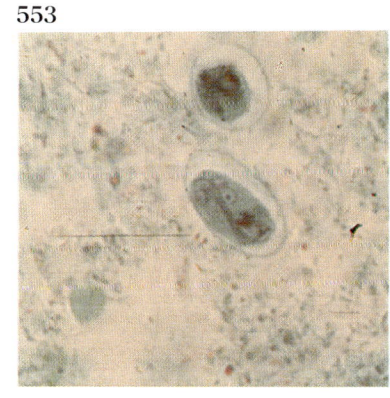

554 Scanning electron-micrograph of *Giardia lamblia* in jejunal biopsy (× 1 000)

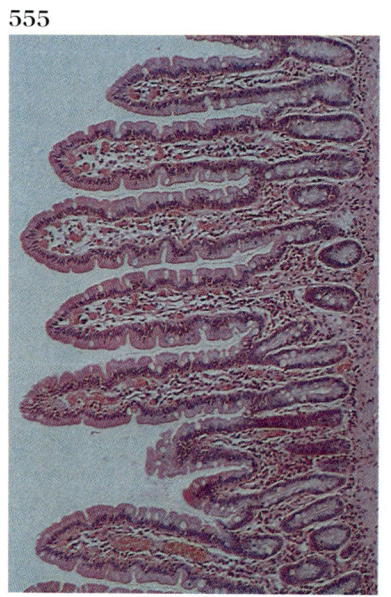

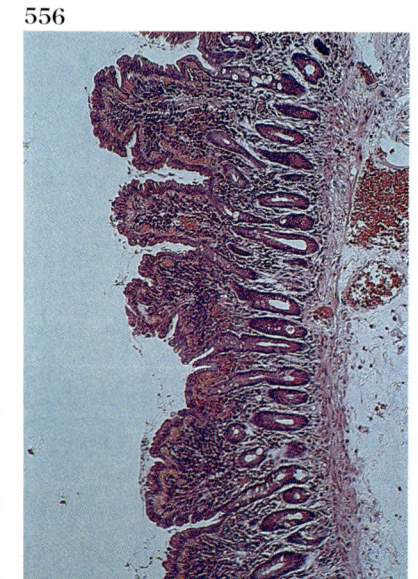

555 & 556 Jejunal epithelium
Severe infection with *G. lamblia* can result in partial villous atrophy of the duodenum or jejunum, with resulting flattening of the villi (**556**) compared with the normal pattern (**555**). Although the organism is commensal in many individuals, it is considered particularly pathogenic in children in the New World, and is a common cause of diarrhoea and a malabsorption syndrome characterised by steatorrhoea in travellers.
(*H&E* × 40)

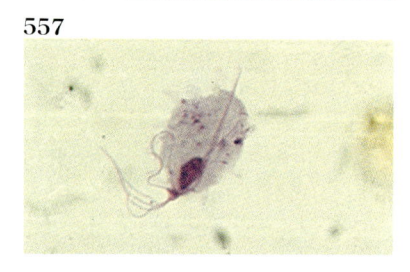

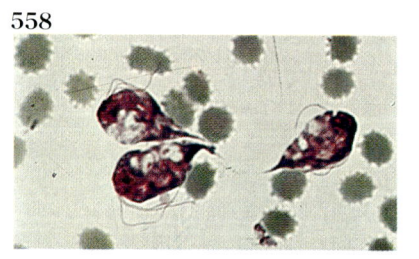

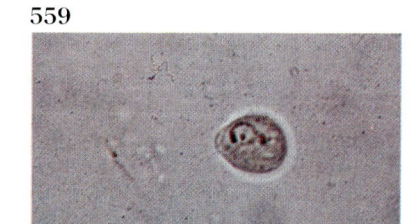

557-559 Other parasitic flagellates *Trichomonas vaginalis* trophozoite (**557**), *Cheilomastix mesnili* trophozoites (**558**) and cyst (**559**). *C. mesnili* is non-pathogenic. (Trophozoites *Giemsa*, cyst *eosin* ×900)

Coccidial Infections (See Table V)

560 Section of sarcocyst in human muscle In the muscles of the intermediate host, *Sarcocystis* forms fusiform cysts containing large numbers of bradyzoites. Although it is rarely diagnosed in life, this condition may be common in man, who harbours the sarcocysts of a number of different species, none of which has so far been identified. *'Sarcocystis lindemanni'* is no longer considered to be a valid species. (*H&E × 500*).

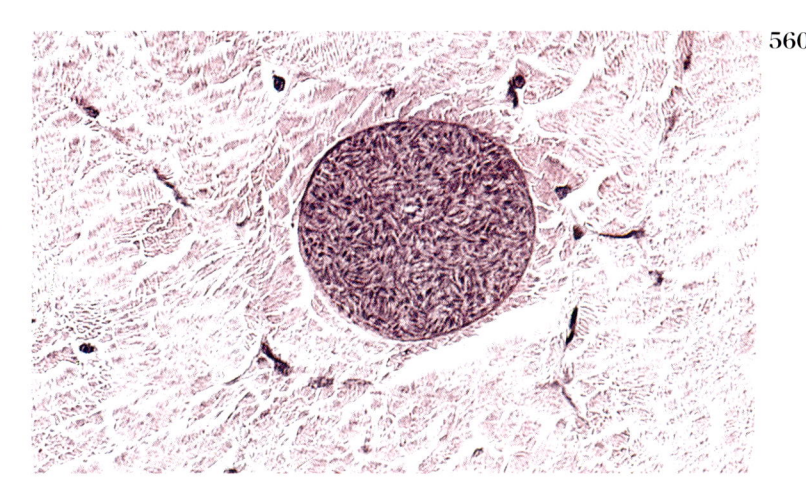

561 *Sarcocystis hominis*-like oöcysts in intestinal epithelium This coccidian parasite is common in man and is acquired from the consumption of raw or inadequately cooked beef in which the sarcocyst stage occurs. In this case man is the definitive host. Sporulated oöcysts or single sporocysts are passed in the faeces. *S. suihominis* is acquired from pork. (*Phase-contrast × 400*)

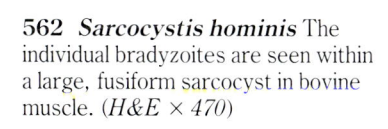

562 *Sarcocystis hominis* The individual bradyzoites are seen within a large, fusiform sarcocyst in bovine muscle. (*H&E × 470*)

563 *Isospora belli* oöcysts Unsporulated oöcysts of this species are passed in the faeces but they sporulate on storage to form eight sporozoites (of which five can be seen in this figure). The infection may be associated with diarrhoea, due to development of the parasite in the intestinal epithelium, or symptomless. Coccidian oöcysts stain dark red with Ziehl-Neelsen stain. (*Nomarksi optics × 450*)

564 *Isospora belli* in intestinal mucosa The intracellular position of two immature oöcysts is clearly seen in this section. (*H&E × 300*)

141

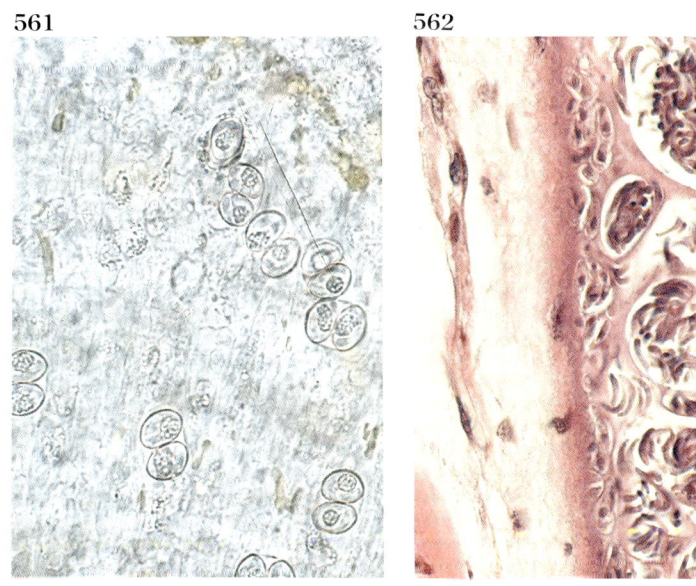

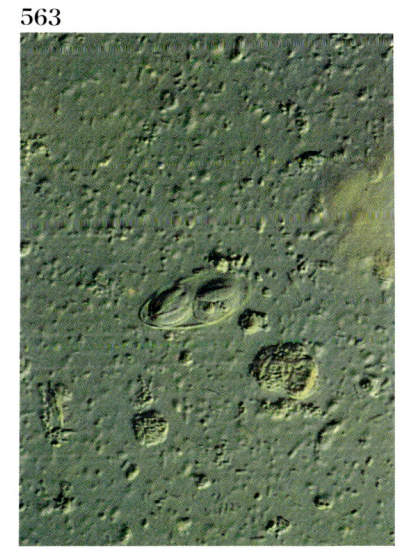

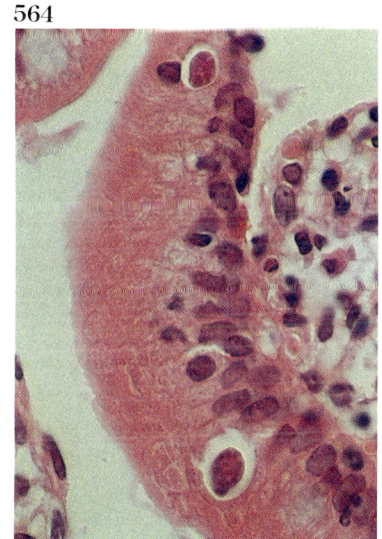

Cryptosporidiosis

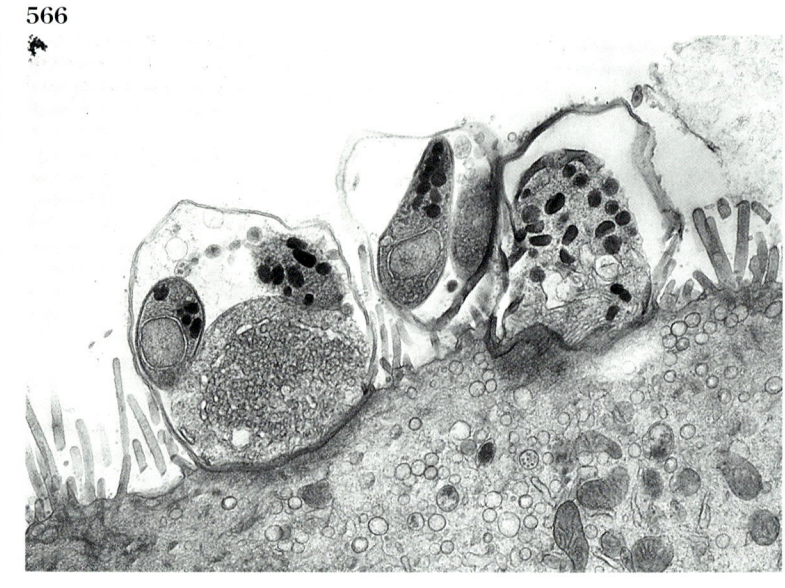

565 *Cryptosporidium* on surface of human jejunum This coccidian parasite causes intractable, profuse, watery diarrhoea in immunologically compromised subjects and is a major contributor to death in about 7 per cent of AIDS sufferers in Western countries. (*H&E* × *750*)

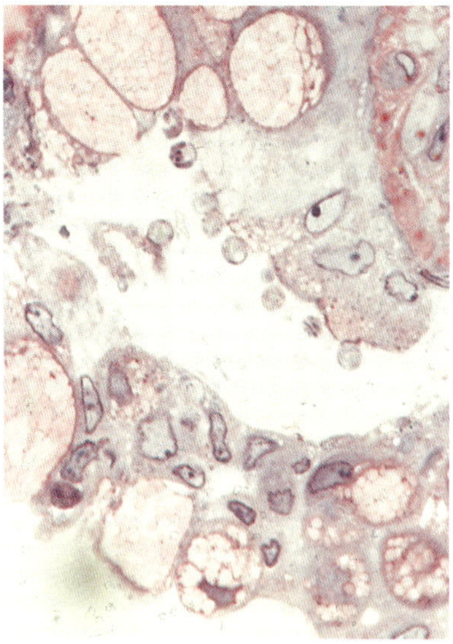

566 Ultrastructure of *Cryptosporidium* The organisms in different stages of schizogony are seen surrounded by a membrane of host cell origin, giving the parasites the false appearance of being extracellular. This section is from a biopsy of rectal mucosa from one of the earliest known victims of AIDS, who had lived in Zaïre. The parasites can colonise any part of the intestine from the pharynx to the rectum. The source of infection and the species of *Cryptosporidium* responsible for human infection are still unknown. (× *9 800*)

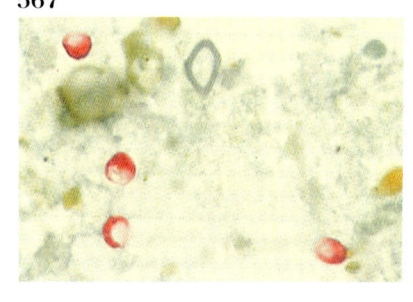

567 Oöcysts of *Cryptosporidium* in faeces The diagnosis can be made by finding oöcysts in the faeces by sugar flotation, followed by Ziehl-Neelsen or auramine staining of the concentrate. The tiny, round oöcysts (<5 μm diameter) may be present in the faeces of about 5 per cent of young children with diarrhoea, but they do not persist provided that the subject is immunologically normal. (*Ziehl-Neelsen* × *2 000*)

Toxoplasmosis

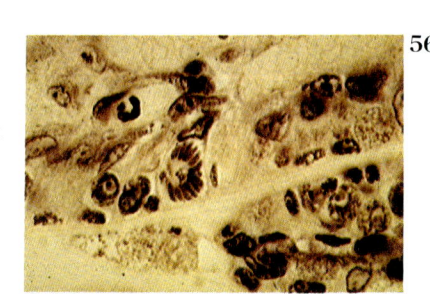

568 *Toxoplasma gondii* schizont in epithelial gut cell of a cat The definitive host of *T. gondii* is the cat, which passes infective oöcysts in its faeces. These will develop in a wide variety of mammalian hosts, including man. Infection, very often passing unrecognised, is acquired either from ingesting cystic stages containing bradyzoites from raw meat or other contaminated food, or through accidental contact with oöcysts from cat faeces. In most countries about 60 per cent of adults are seropositive. (*Giemsa* × *600*).

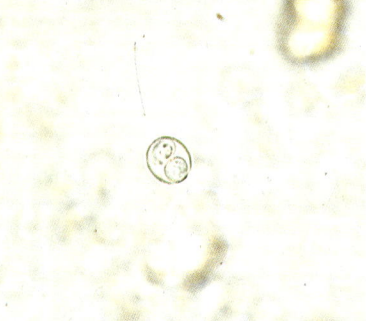

569 Sporulated oöcysts of *T. gondii* The tiny oöcysts (10 μm diameter) are passed unsporulated. (*Phase-contrast* × *440*)

570 Tachyzoites of *T. gondii* in a leucocyte Asexual and sexual reproduction occur in the epithelium of the cat's intestine. In non-feline hosts, including man, acute infection may result from ingestion of any stage, with the formation of tachyzoites which enter extra-intestinal tissues such as lymph nodes. Subsequently, following a proliferative phase of endodyogeny in many tissues, including the brain, a resting, cystic stage containing bradyzoites is produced. Tachyzoites or bradyzoites, e.g. in rodents, are infective to cats, the cycle then recommencing in the feline intestine. (*Giemsa × 900*)

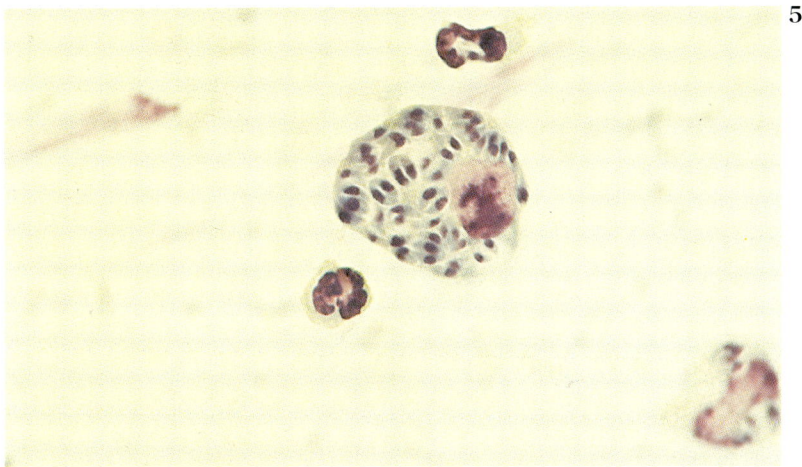

571 Post-mortem appearance of brain Acute toxoplasmosis in pregnancy seriously endangers the fetus. Transplacental infection, especially in the fourth month of pregnancy, produces congenital toxoplasmosis with typical calcification of the sub-ependymal tissues, and sometimes dilation of the ventricles due to rapid proliferation of the parasites. Irregular areas of calcification in the lateral ventricles are seen in this brain of a seven-week-old child who died of toxoplasmosis. Mental disorders and blindness are common in children who survive.

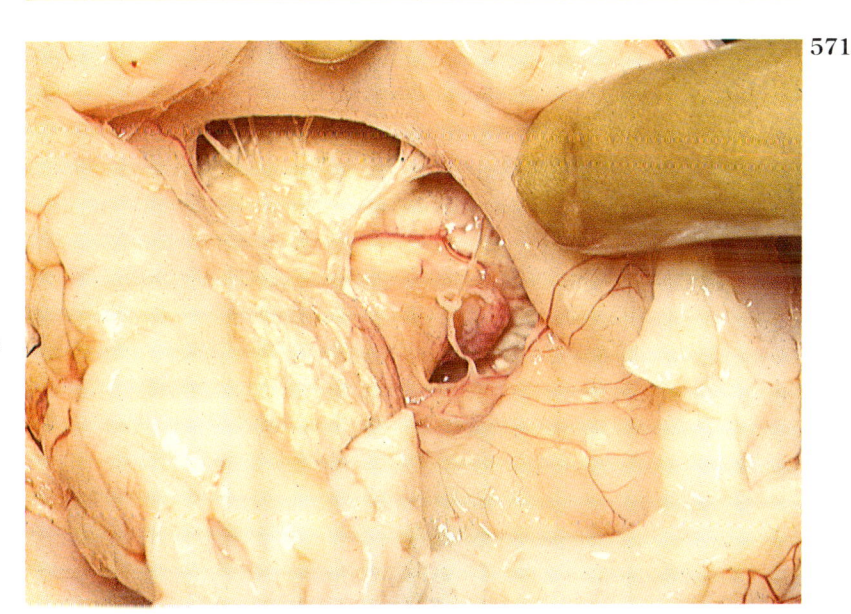

572 Brain X-ray in toxoplasmosis Calcification is seen in the ventricles and subependymal tissues.

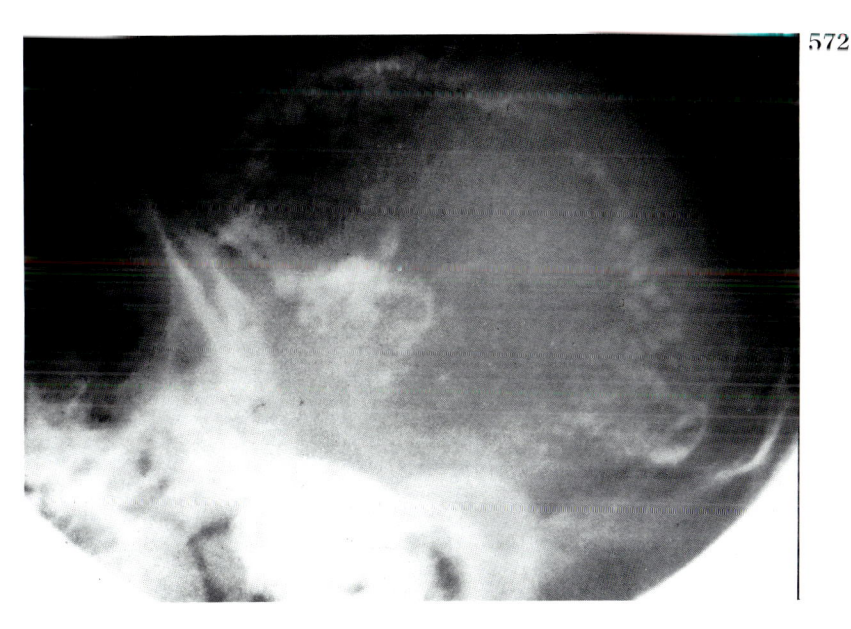

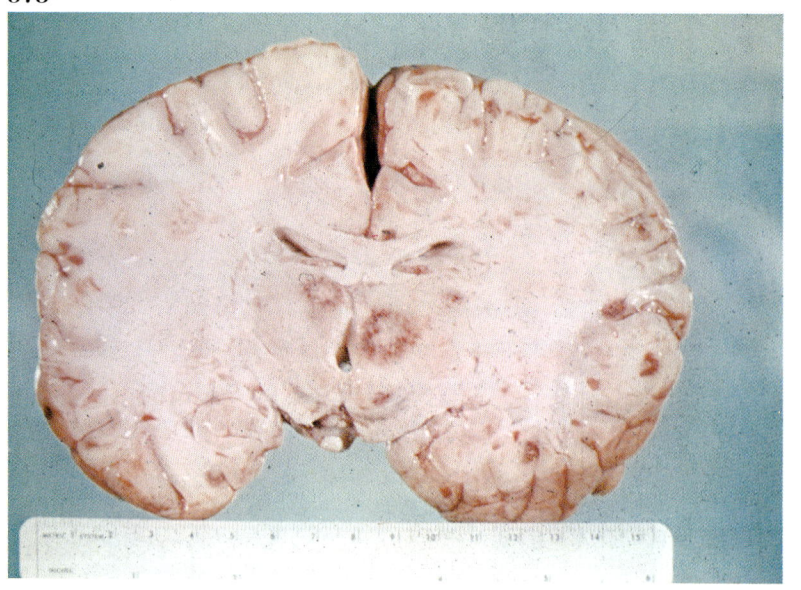

573 Fatal toxoplasmosis relapse
Brain from a 64-year-old woman who received immunosuppressive therapy for multiple myelomatosis (Case 3 of Frenkel *et al*, *Human Path* 1975, **6**, 97).

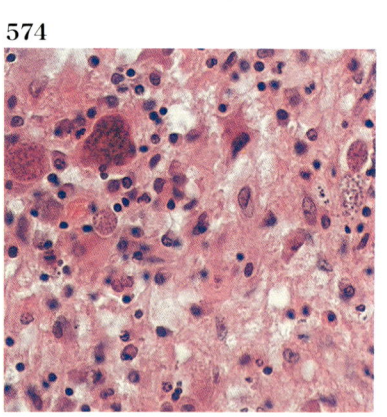

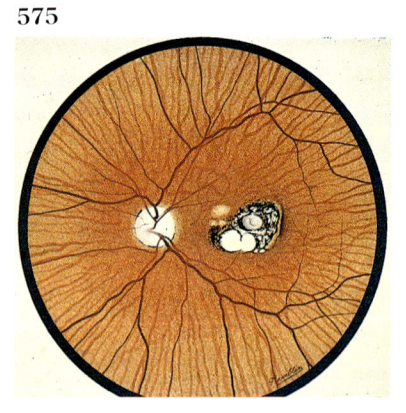

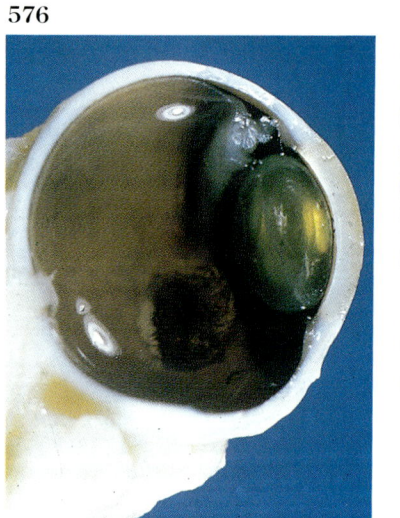

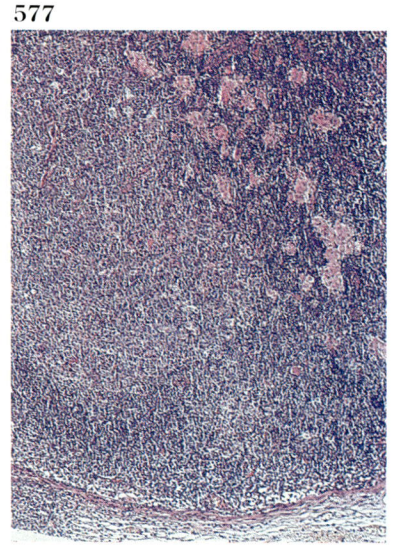

574 Toxoplasmal encephalitis
Several cysts are seen in this section of brain from an AIDS victim who died with acute encephalitis due to toxoplasmosis. The coccidian infection contributes to death in 15 per cent or more of HIV-infected individuals. (*H&E × 250*)

575 Fundal changes in congenital toxoplasmosis
Congenital toxoplasmosis may produce choroidoretinitis in later years. This painting is of a macular lesion showing ectopic choroidal pigmentation. Defective vision and squint may result.

576 Eye in congenital toxoplasmosis Severe degeneration of the eye from a one-year-old child who died from congenital toxoplasmosis.

577 Histology of lymph glands
Acute infection of older individuals may be cryptic, or it may produce a prolonged low fever with lymphadenopathy. Lymph node biopsy shows follicular hyperplasia, with active germinal centres containing large, pale histiocytes. These contain ingested plasma cells, not parasites, but *T. gondii* may be isolated from such biopsies by inoculation into mice. (*H&E × 20*)

578 Serological tests for toxoplasmosis (Negative control *left*; positive *right*). The Sabin Feldmann dye test was formerly widely employed. Methylene blue stains *T. gondii* tachyzoites obtained from mouse peritoneal exudate but, in the presence of antibody-containing serum, the uptake of dye is inhibited by 50 per cent or more. High titres occur in acute infections but a low positive titre remains indefinitely (*see comment* 568). Other useful serological tests are the CFT, direct agglutination, and toxoplasmin skin test. The most direct test is the FAT, shown here, in which antigen consists of cultured tachyzoites. ($\times 600$)

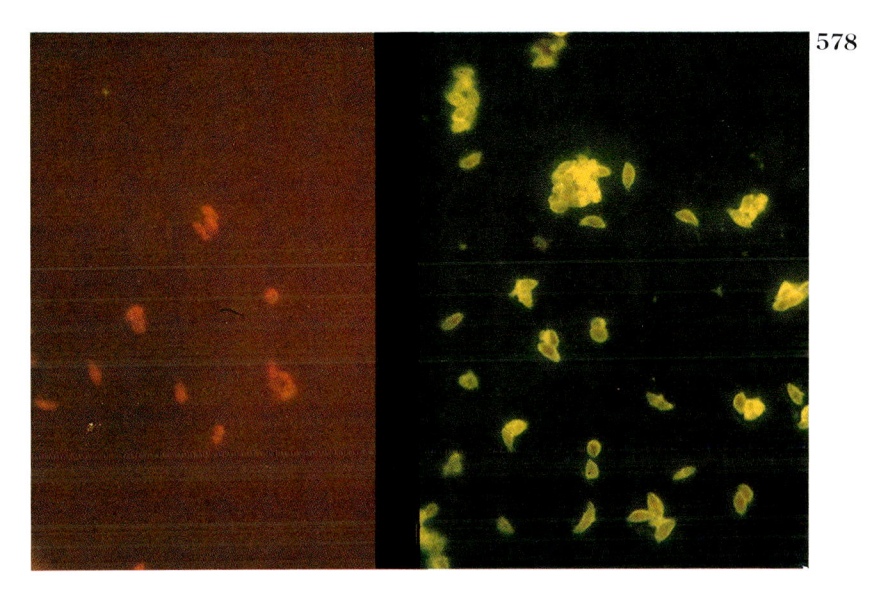

Microsporidiosis

579 Microsporidia in enterocytes Three groups of encapsulated spores of microsporidia (probably *Enterocytozoon bienusei*) in smear of cells from duodenal biopsy. The patient was a 35-year-old male suffering from chronic diarrhoea which was associated with AIDS. He subsequently developed generalised Kaposi's sarcoma and died. The presence of microsporidia in the intestinal tract is being increasingly widely recognised in such immuno-compromised individuals, although the role they play in pathogenesis is not yet clearly defined. (*Giemsa* $\times 1\,800$)

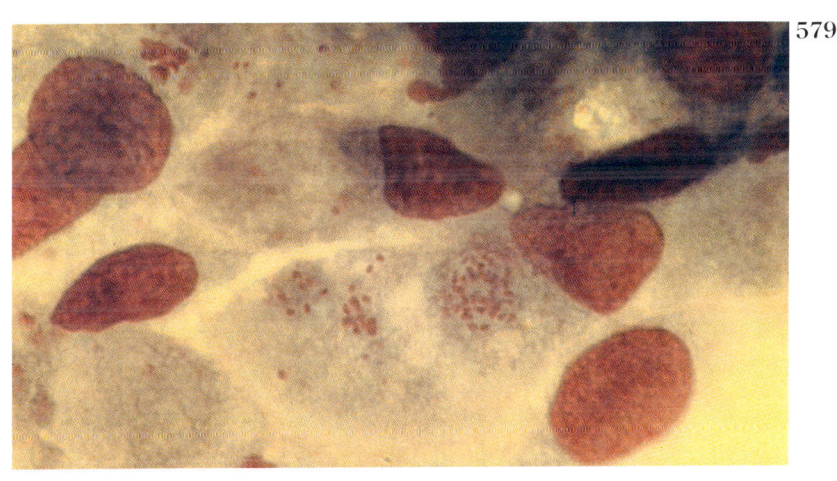

580 Electron micrograph of *Enterocytozoon bienusei* This rectal biopsy specimen from a patient with AIDS showed numerous microsporidia at different stages of development, that shown here being sporogonic plasmodium ($\times 12\,000$). (Reproduced with permission from W. O. Dobbins & W. M. Weinstein *Gastroenterology* 1985, **88**, 738-749). Microsporidia are also suspected as a cause of ill defined neurological manifestations.

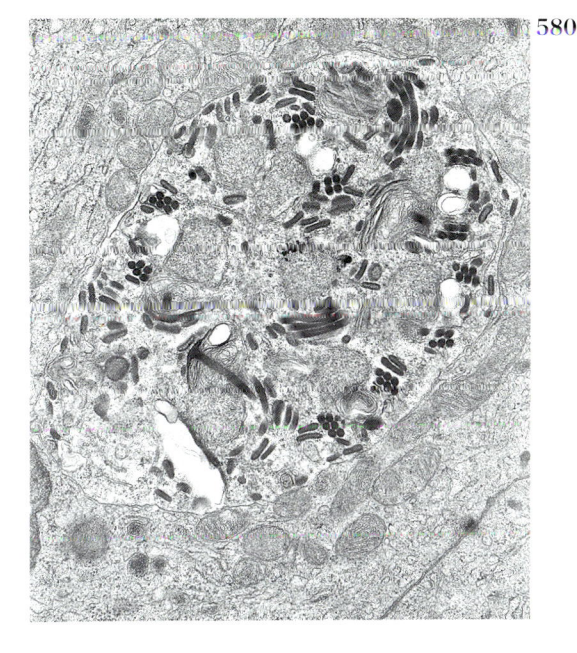

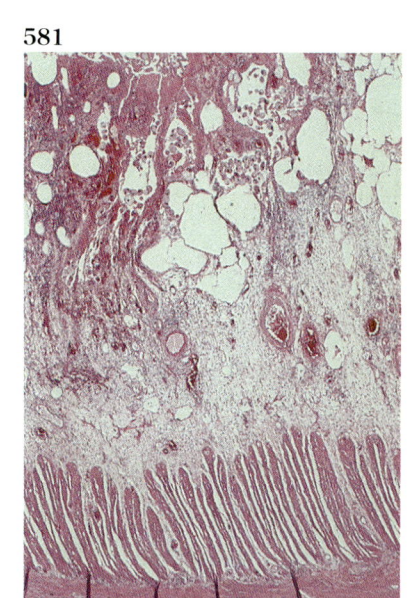

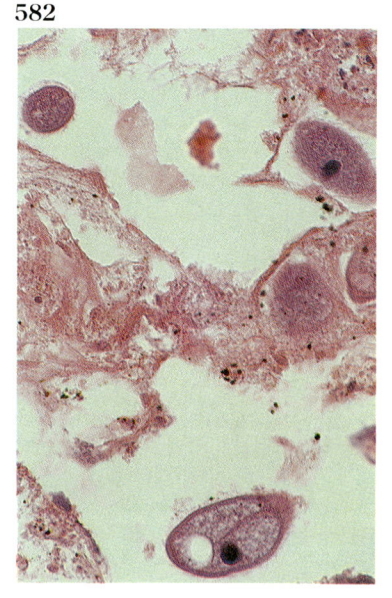

Balantidiasis

581 Balantidial ileitis
Balantidium coli is a common commensal of the large intestine of wild and domestic pigs, but is pathogenic to man and other primates in which it causes severe diarrhoea. Active, flagellated trophozoites and cysts are readily found in fresh faecal specimens. Numerous trophozoites are seen invading the submucosa in this section of human ileum. (H&E × 10)

582 Trophozoites of *Balantidium coli* Extensive ulceration of the ileum, colon and rectum may occur in severe cases. The characteristic morphology of *B. coli* trophozoites with their macro- and micronuclei is seen in this section. (H&E × 160)

HELMINTHIASES—NEMATODES
(See **Table IX** *for classification and* **313—327** *for eggs*)

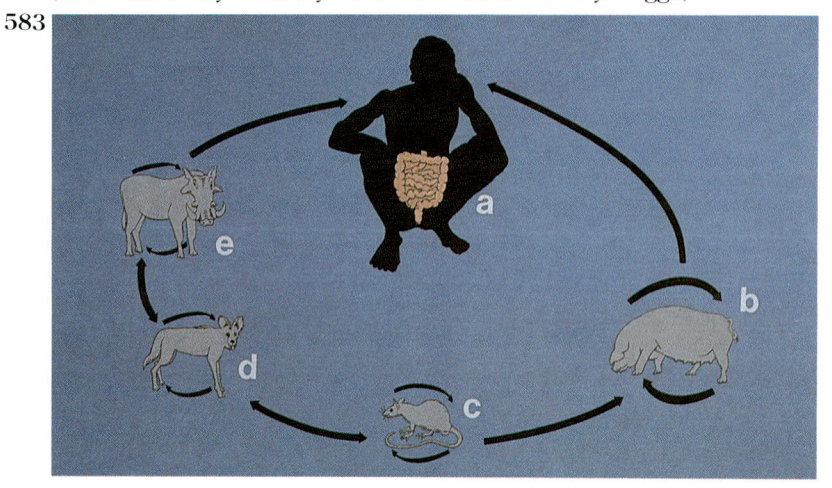

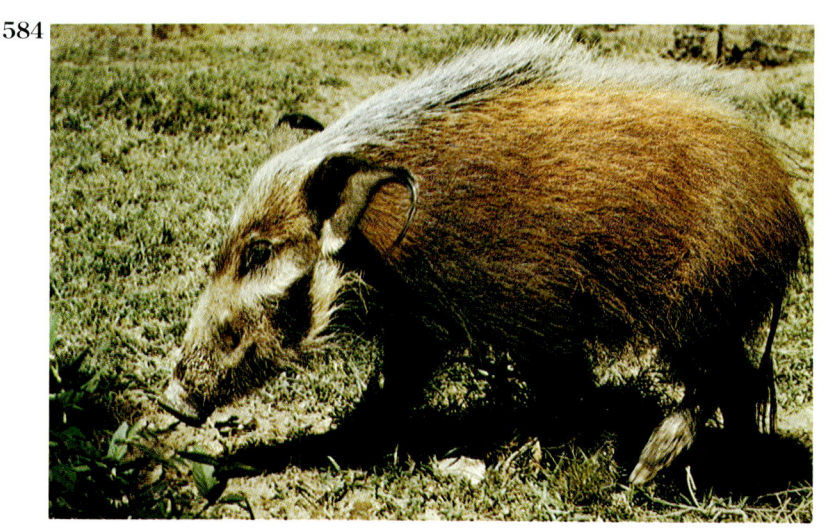

Trichinosis

583 Life cycle of *Trichinella spiralis* This nematode is a zoonotic infection that circulates between rats (c) and various carnivores. Trichinosis in man (a) commonly results from eating raw or inadequately cooked pork or pork products such as sausages. Pigs (b & e) usually acquire the infection by eating infected rats (c). Cycles of infection also exist in wild Canidae (d) that eat rodents. Infection is acquired by eating muscle containing the encysted larvae. These excyst in the small intestine and develop into minute adults in the mucosa. About five days after infection, the females, now mature, deposit larvae which migrate through the tissues to reach skeletal muscles in which they again encyst. Larviposition may continue for a week or more. Finally the larvae become calcified.

584 Wild reservoir of trichinosis
A common reservoir of infection is the wild pig such as the African bush pig, seen here. The flesh of other carnivores, such as the bear, has also served to initiate isolated outbreaks of human infection following, for example, hunting parties.

585 *Trichinella spiralis* larvae in crush preparation The larvae are easily seen in muscle by crushing the tissue between two glass plates and inspecting it through a 'trichinoscope' (a simple magnifying system). ($\times 550$)

586 Larva free in gastric juice ($\times 550$)

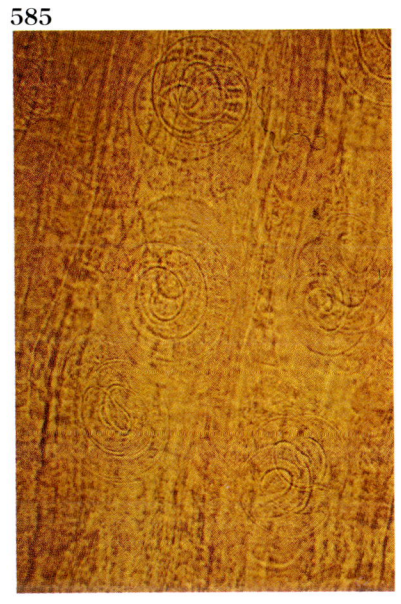

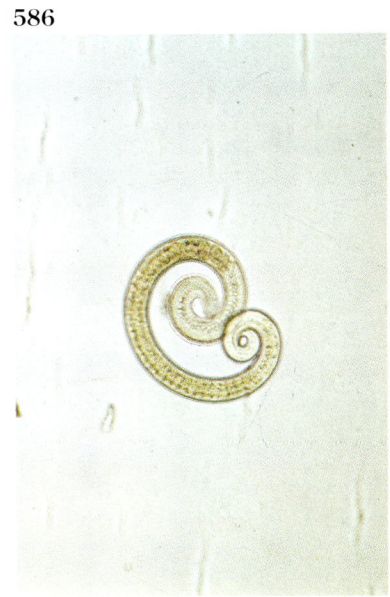

587 Parasitic female *T. spiralis* ($\times 60$)

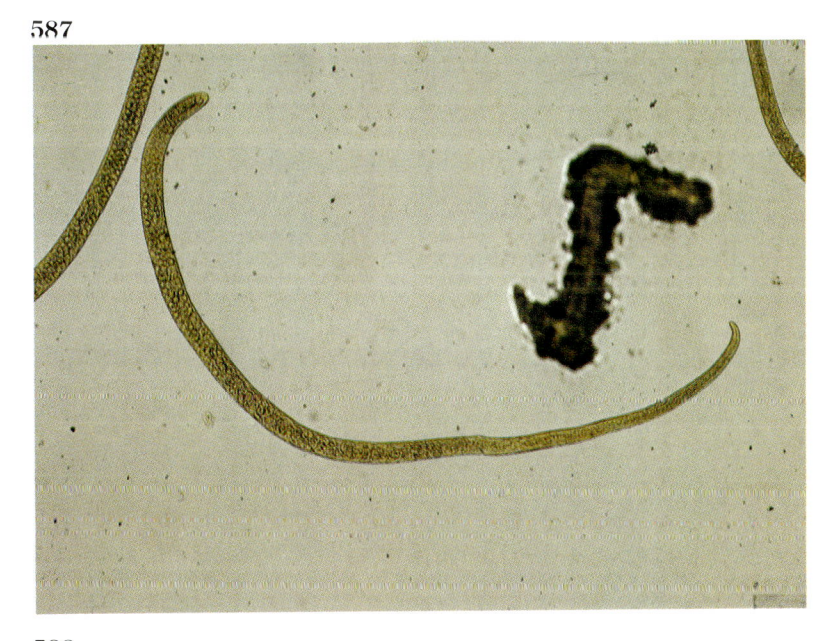

588 Larvae in muscle of fatal human case Encysted larvae are found in the muscles at biopsy (or post-mortem). Calcification of the encysted larvae occurs in about 18 months and may be detected on X-ray, but the encysted larvae remain alive for years. (*H&E* $\times 20$)

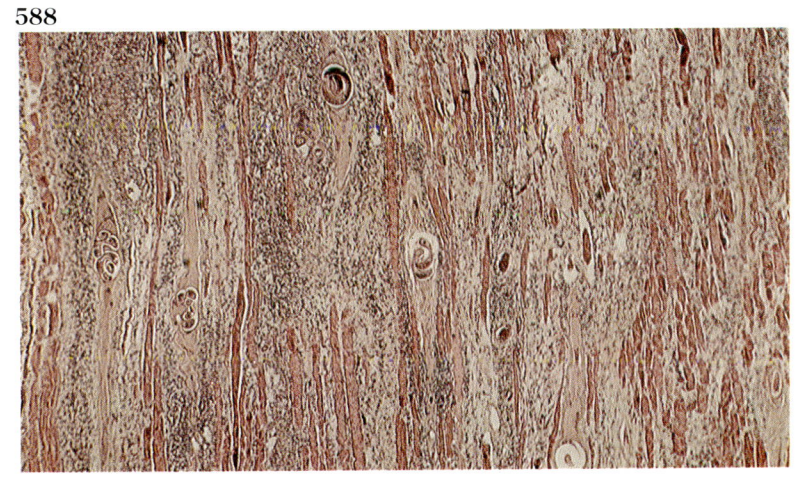

147

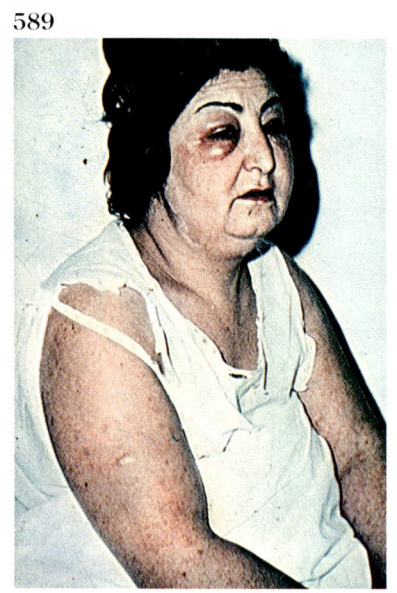

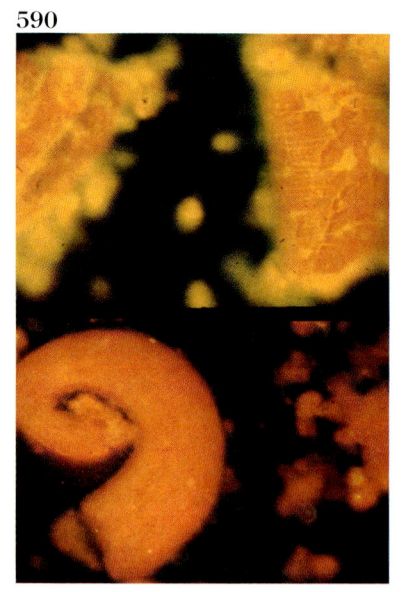

589 Patient with acute trichinosis The four cardinal features of the disease are fever, orbital oedema, myalgia, and eosinophilia.

590 Fluorescent antibody test The gel-diffusion test has also proved a useful diagnostic procedure. Other serological tests are available for the detection of humoral antibodies which reach high titres in the acute stage, but are not protective. (Immunity is largely cell-mediated.)
(*Bottom*: negative control)

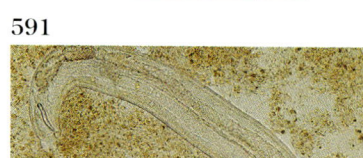

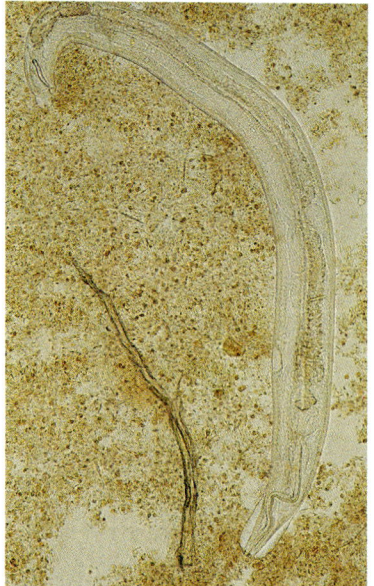

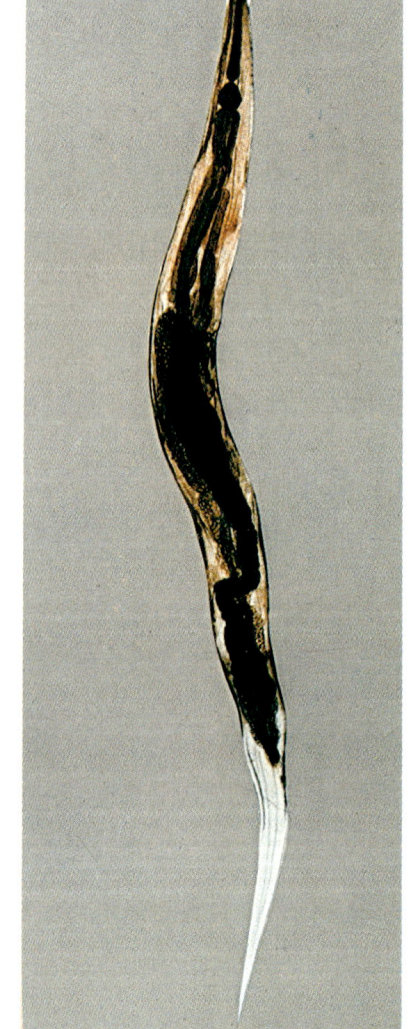

Enterobiasis

591 & 592 Adult *Enterobius vermicularis* These 'pinworms' are small, white, and threadlike. The males (**591**) have coiled tails and measure 2.5 mm. The females (**592**), which are about 10 mm long, emerge to the perianal region where they lay some 10 to 15 000 eggs, then die. In the process they cause severe pruritus. The embryonated eggs which are directly infectious on ingestion, hatch in the duodenum and the larvae pass to the caecum where they mature. (♂ × *30*; ♀ × *15*)

593 Adult pinworms in appendix The worms are occasionally found in the appendix but their role as a cause of acute appendicitis is uncertain. (*H&E* × *6*)

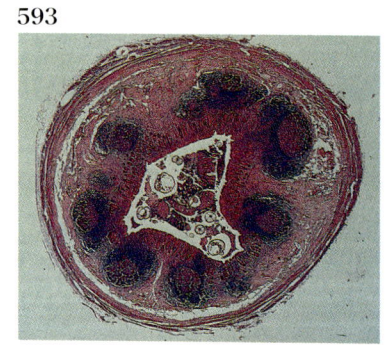

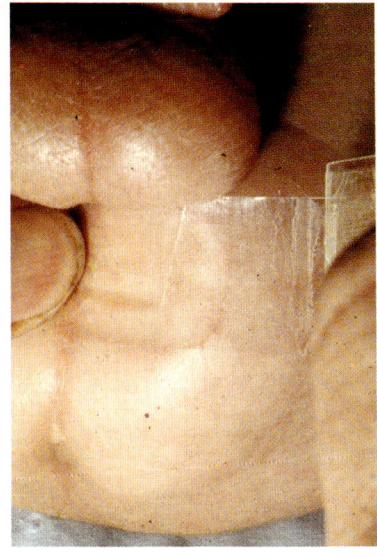

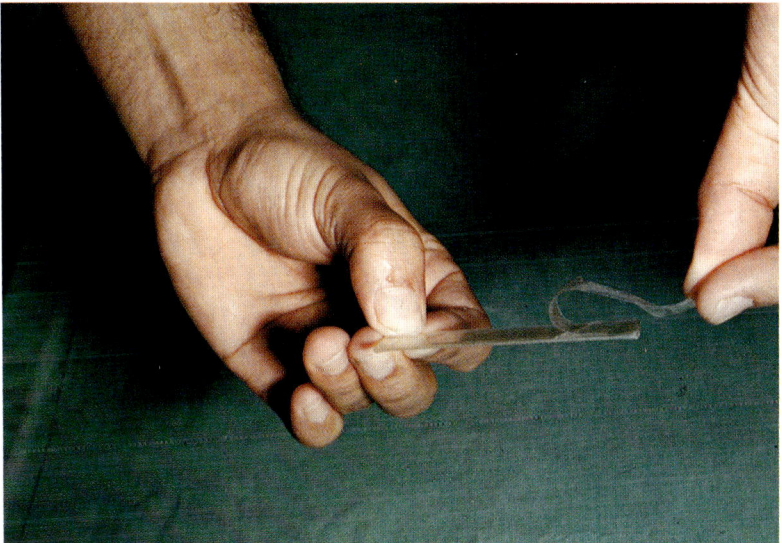

594 & 595 Scotch tape swab to demonstrate perianal eggs The eggs (**323**) are found on the perianal skin. They adhere to the Scotch tape, which can then be placed on a slide and examined directly under a microscope. Because of severe pruritus ani, children frequently reinfect themselves from eggs under their fingernails. Bedding is also a source of infection which tends to persist in households and institutions such as orphanages.

Capillariasis

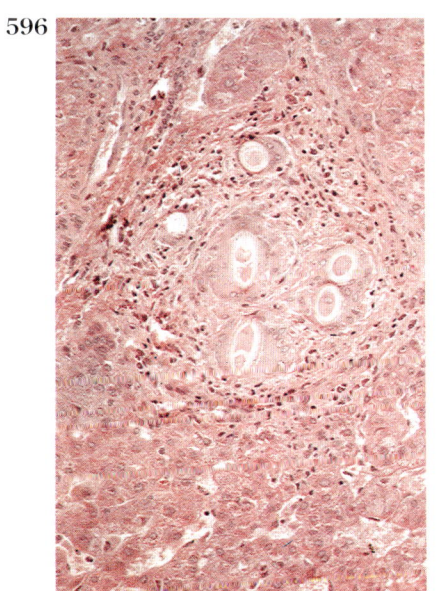

596 *Capillaria hepatica* in liver section Human infection with this rodent nematode is very rare. The adult worms live in the portal tracts. Eggs, resembling those of *Trichuris* (see **322**), are infective only after undergoing maturation in the soil. Adult worms in the liver cause hepatic enlargement and severe parenchymal damage. Note the giant cell reaction around the eggs. (*H&E × 150*)

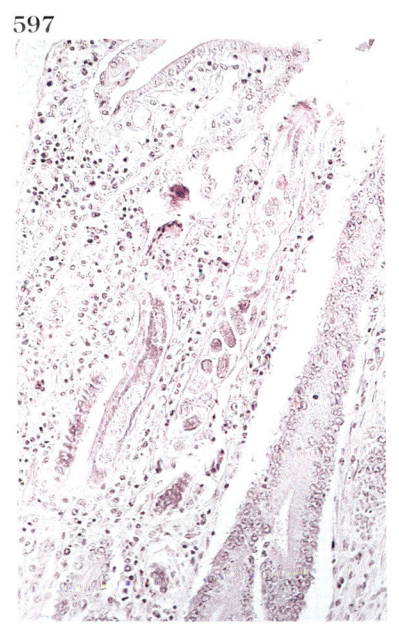

597 *C. philippensis* invading small intestine This species, of which the adults live in the upper small intestine, has occurred in epidemic form. A malabsorption syndrome, sometimes fatal, develops in heavy infections. The life cycle remains unknown. (*H&E × 150*)

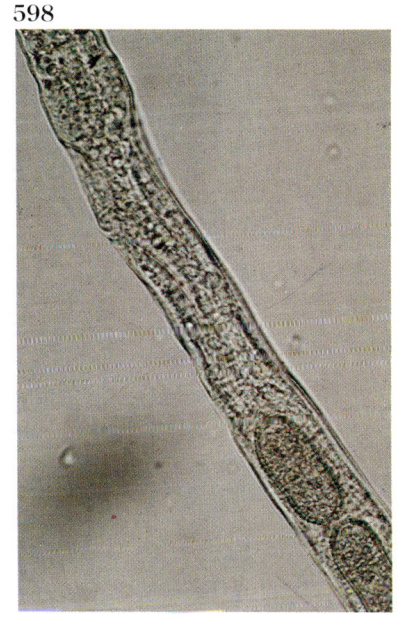

598 Female *C. philippensis* from human faeces The figure shows the vulval region of the female, in which two typical eggs can be seen. (× *300*)

Anisakiasis

This term is used for human infection with the larvae of *Pseudoterranova decipiens*, a common nematode parasite of marine mammals, cod, pollock and other sea fish, or with larvae of species of *Anisakis* which infect such fish as herring and mackerel. Infection is acquired by consuming uncooked fish, a custom that is increasing because of the popularity of Japanese-style 'sushi'.

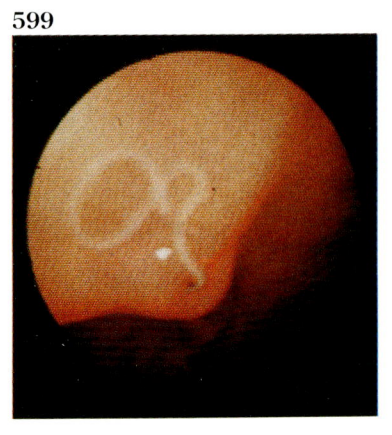

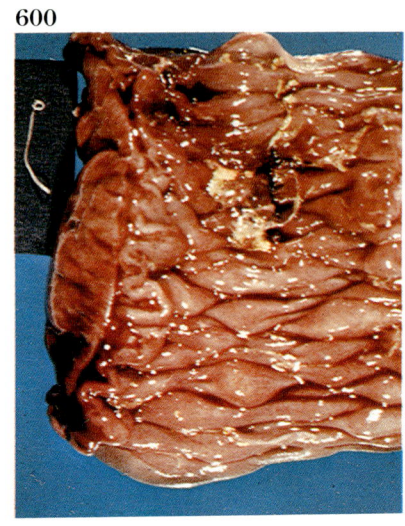

599 Larval *Pseudoterranova* The yellowish larvae, about 2 cm long, usually invade the gastric mucosa, causing acute epigastric pain within a few hours of their being ingested. Various intestinal symptoms may develop following infection with *Anisakis*, depending upon the location of the invasive larvae as they move further down the intestine. The figure shows a *Pseudoterranova* larva as seen by gastroscope in the stomach wall of a 53-year-old Japanese woman.

600 Larva removed from small intestine This larval *Anisakis* produced ulceration of the intestine in another Japanese patient.

Gnathostomiasis

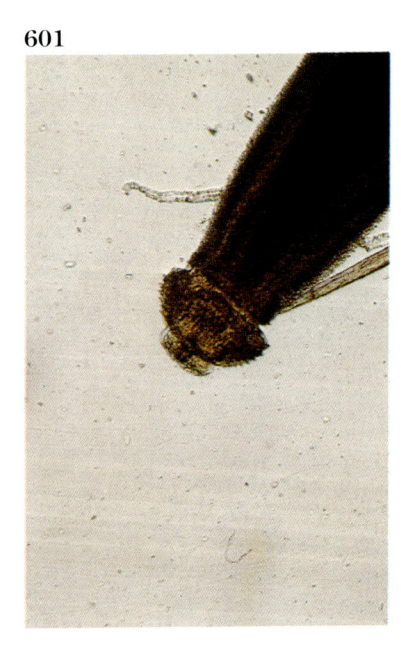

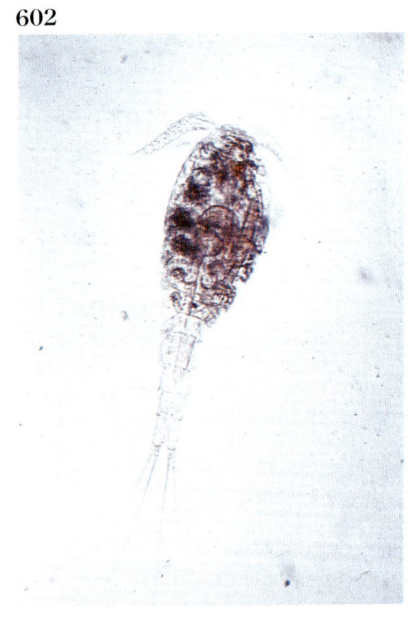

601 Head of adult *Gnathostoma spinigerum* The adult, which is about 2 to 3 cm long, usually lives in the stomach of dogs, cats and wild felines. It is found throughout SE Asia. There are two intermediate hosts. Man acquires infection by eating fermented fish, a delicacy in Thailand, or any other form of raw fish. The parasite cannot mature in man but migrates, causing cutaneous and visceral larva migrans. ($\times 30$)

602 Second-stage larva in *Cyclops* Larvae hatching from eggs passed with faeces into fresh water infect *Cyclops* water fleas and, later, fish that eat the *Cyclops*. Here the third-stage larva develops. ($\times 45$)

603 Periorbital larva migrans
One of the characteristic clinical features is a migrating, subcutaneous swelling associated with boring pain and eosinophilia. Third-stage larvae may be recovered surgically from swellings in suitable locations. Cerebral lesions with focal signs are not uncommon in Thailand.

Dracontiasis (Guinea Worm Infection)

604 Insanitary water supply being infected Note the open infective lesions on this girl's foot. Guinea worm occurs in parts of Africa, India, the Middle East and Brazil where water is drawn from shallow pools or primitive wells. Larvae are swallowed inside water fleas.

605 Contamination of surface water A papule forms where the adult female worm reaches the skin surface and ulcerates when the skin is immersed in water. A loop of the worm's uterus prolapses and ruptures, releasing large numbers of rhabditoid larvae into the water.

606 Larva of *Dracunculus medinensis* The free-swimming, first-stage larvae enter water fleas of *Cyclops* and allied genera. Here they develop and await ingestion by a new definitive host when unboiled water is drunk. The larvae emerge in the intestine from where they migrate to, and mature in, the subcutaneous tissues. ($\times 70$)

607 X-ray of calcified worms The size of an adult female *D. medinensis* can be judged from this X-ray of a calcified worm in the ankle. Females attain up to 100 cm, but males only 10 to 40 cm in length.

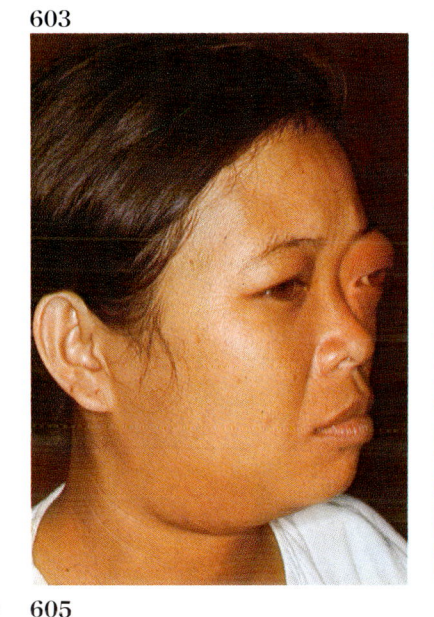

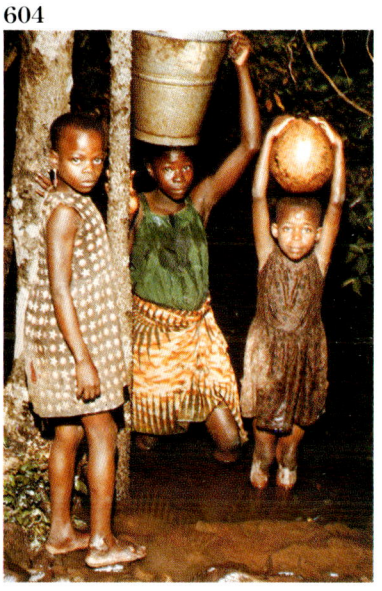

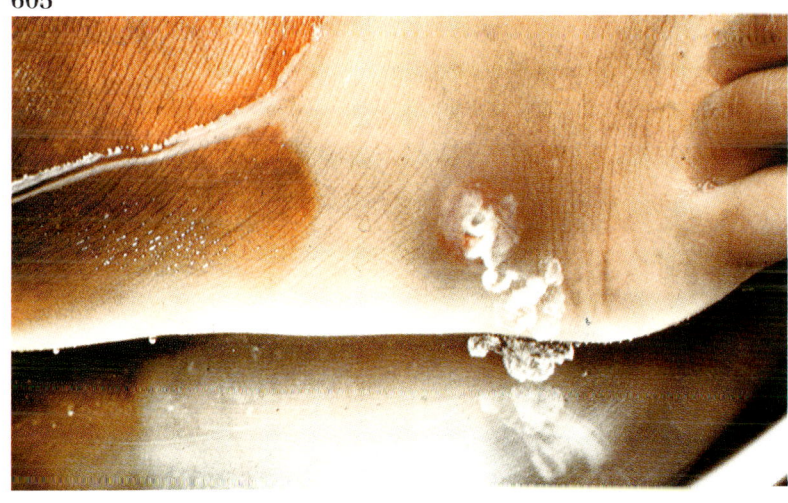

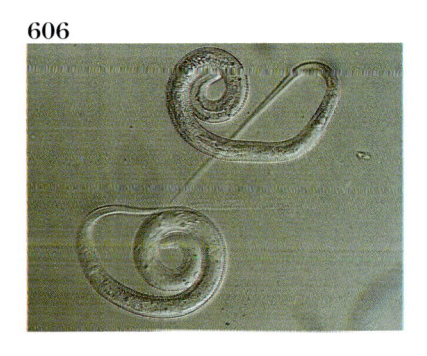

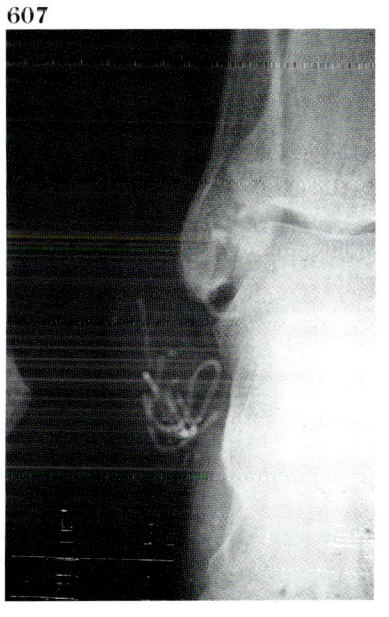

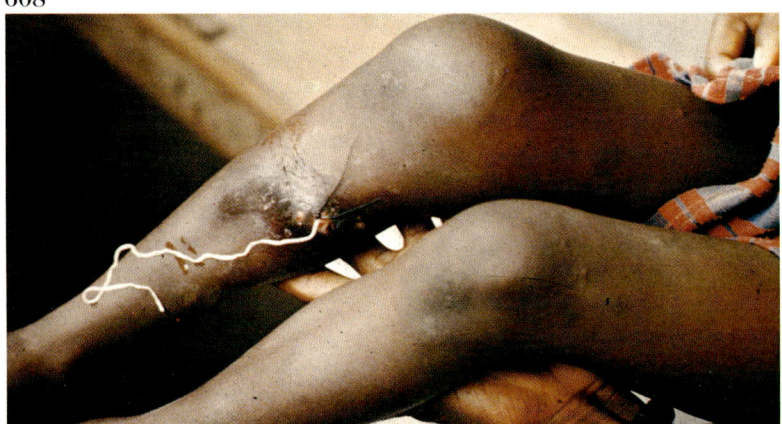

608 Adult guinea worm in knee joint Heavy infestations may cause considerable disability and arthritis may be caused by female worms in the vicinity of joints.

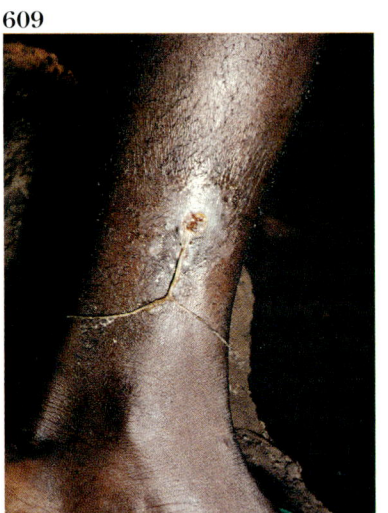

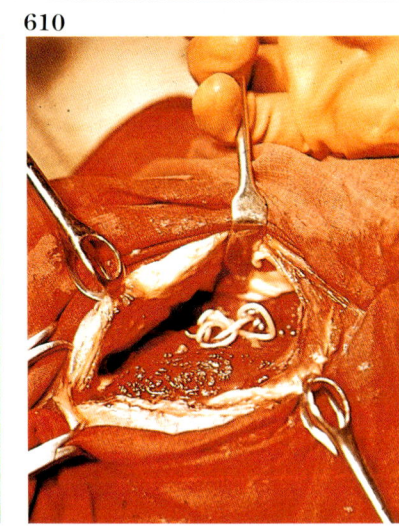

609 Extraction of female worm Adult females are commonly extracted by progressively winding them round a matchstick as they emerge from the subcutaneous tissues. Chemotherapy has made the procedure easier and less hazardous.

610 Operative removal of worm from knee A wide-scale campaign for the eradication of guinea worm infection throughout its distribution is currently in progress.

HELMINTHIASES—CESTODES (*See* Table XIV)

Diphyllobothriasis (Fish Tapeworm)

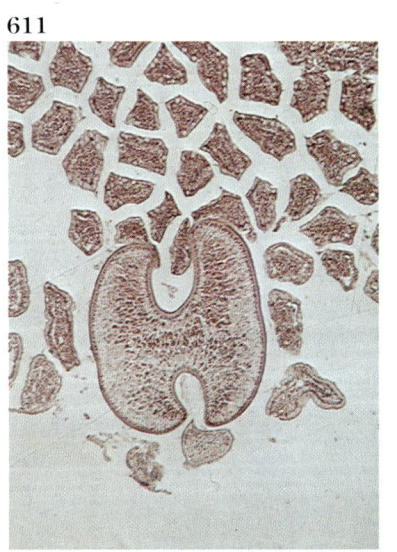

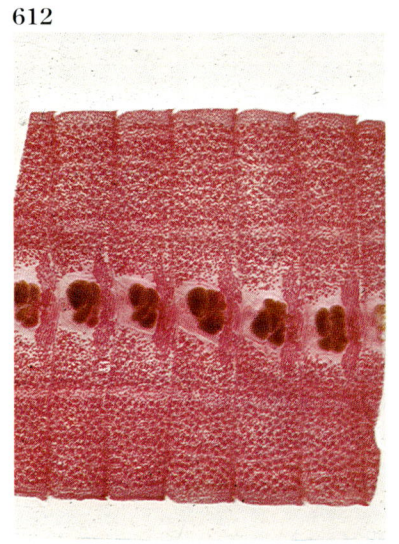

611 & 612 Cross-section of head, and segments of adult tapeworm The fish tapeworm, *Diphyllobothrium latum*, is common around large lakes in Europe, North America and elsewhere. A mature adult may reach 10 m in length. The head and mature proglottids are readily distinguished from those of *Taenia* in man (*see* **633, 643**). Mature worms may produce one million eggs daily. (× 8) (*See* **320**.)

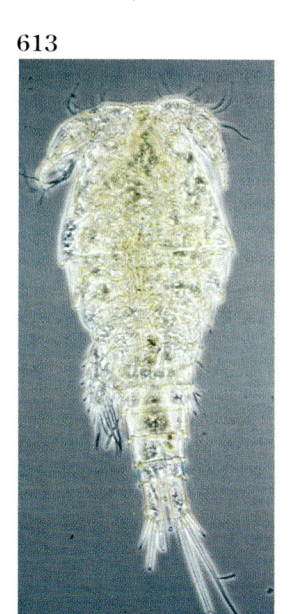

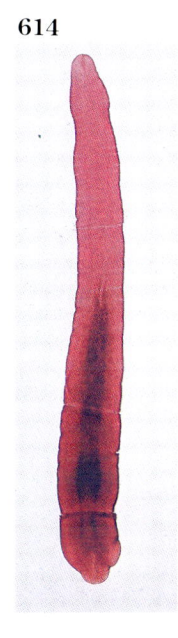

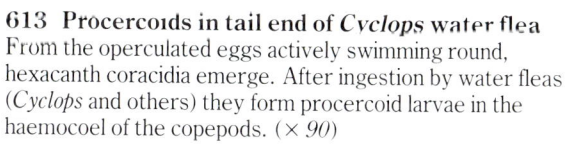

613 Procercoids in tail end of *Cyclops* water flea
From the operculated eggs actively swimming round, hexacanth coracidia emerge. After ingestion by water fleas (*Cyclops* and others) they form procercoid larvae in the haemocoel of the copepods. (× 90)

614 Plerocercoid in fish When the *Cyclops* is ingested by a fish, the larva emerges to form a migrating plerocercoid (sparganum) which comes to lie in the muscle. These develop into adults in the gut of man if the fish is consumed incompletely cooked. (× 6)

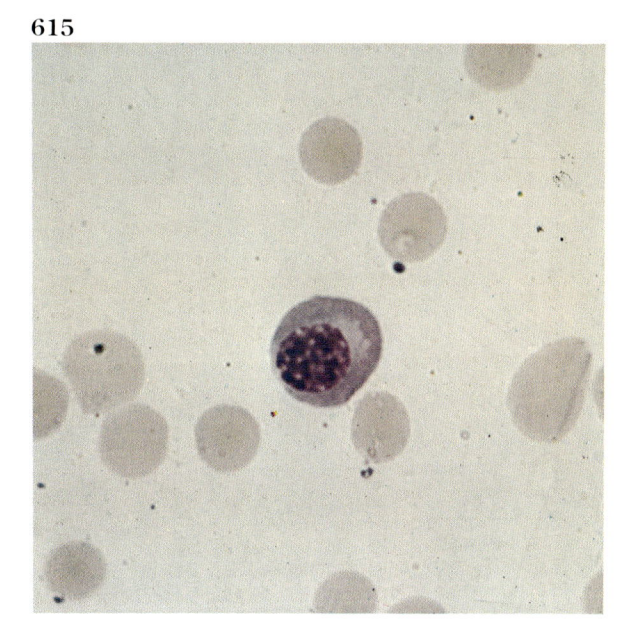

615 Macrocytic anaemia in blood film The classical clinical feature of the infection is the development of Vitamin B12 deficiency, with a resultant macrocytic anaemia. (*Giemsa* × 1 250)

Sparganosis

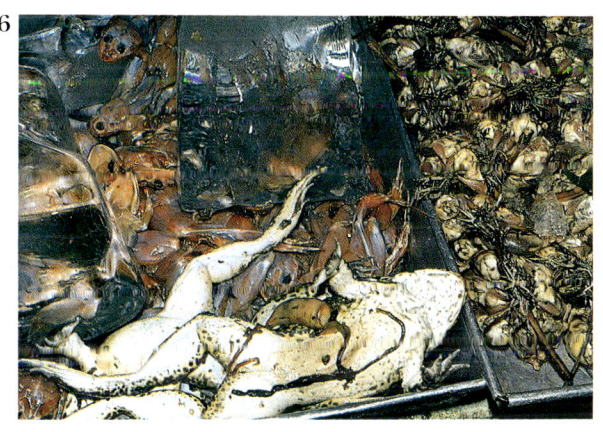

616 Edible frogs and sea food on a Thai market stall Sparganum occurs in a variety of amphibious animals including frogs, and these also may be infective to man if ingested. They are the larvae of tapeworms of the genus *Spirometra* that are common in various canines and felines. The first-stage larvae are formed as procercoids in *Cyclops*. Ingestion of these larvae produces sparganosis in man, since the larvae cannot mature in this abnormal host.

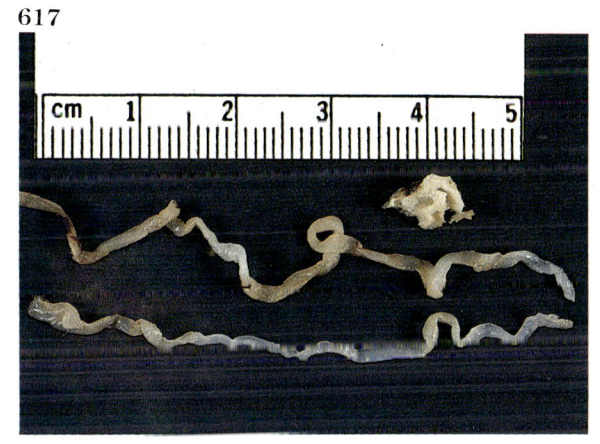

617 'Sparganum mansoni' The sparganum larvae proliferate, often in the subcutaneous tissues, where they become encysted in large nodules from which they can be removed surgically. The specimen shown here, for example, was found when a 'hernia' was opened in the groin of a Ugandan woman. When localised in the periorbital tissues or under the conjunctiva, severe oedema may result. In Vietnam and Thailand this infection may follow the application of frogs as a poultice for inflamed eyes!

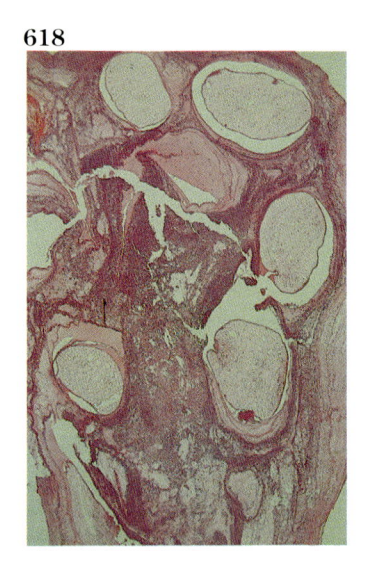

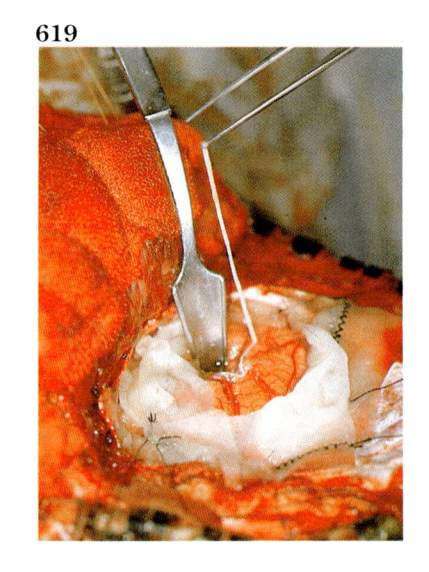

618 Section of Sparganum in a nodule The larval cestode is walled off by an intense cellular and fibrotic reaction. (H&E × 7)

619 Sparganosis of the brain A 10 cm long larva being removed from the subcortical area of the brain of a Japanese patient.

Dipylidium caninum (Dog Tapeworm)

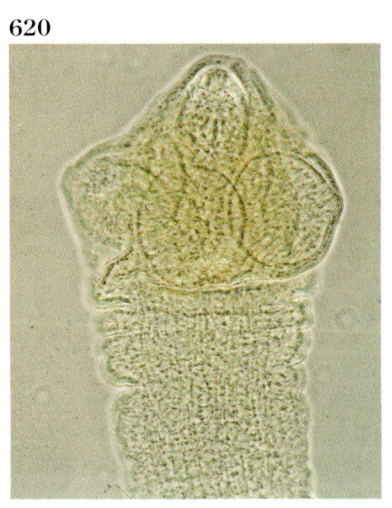

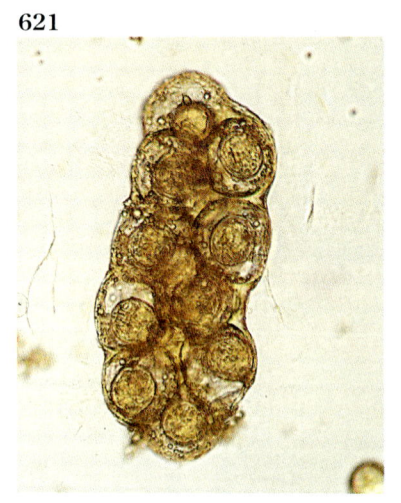

620 & 621 Scolex and egg capsule The adult *D. caninum*, which reaches a length of 10 to 70 cm, is the common tapeworm of domestic and wild canines and felines. In addition to mature segments, encapsulated clusters of eggs in which larval hooks may be seen, are passed as the mature segments disintegrate. (Scolex × 15; egg capsule × 200)

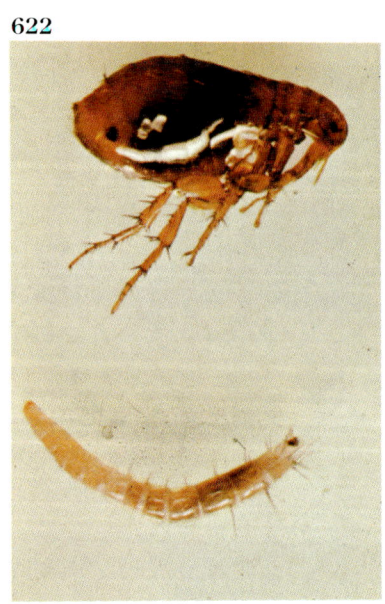

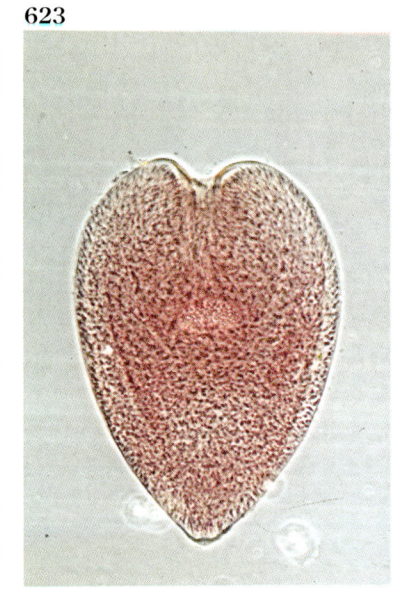

622 Dog flea larva and adult The eggs are ingested by larval dog, cat or human fleas. They develop first procercoid, then cysticercoid larvae in the haemocoel of the insects in which they remain when the fleas grow to the adult stage. Man becomes infected by accidentally swallowing infected fleas. (× 15)

623 Immature cysticercoid from dog flea (× 90)

Vampirolepsis (= *Hymenolepis*) *nana* (Dwarf Tapeworm)

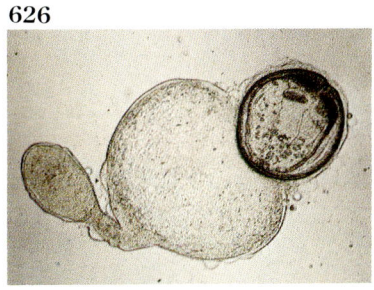

624 Hexacanth oncosphere This cosmopolitan tapeworm, which reaches only 2.5 to 4 cm in length, lives in the small intestine of man and rodents. Infection is acquired directly by ingesting eggs. After ingestion by a mammal or by certain insects the eggs (**324**) hatch into the hexacanth oncospheres. (*Phase-contrast* × 500)

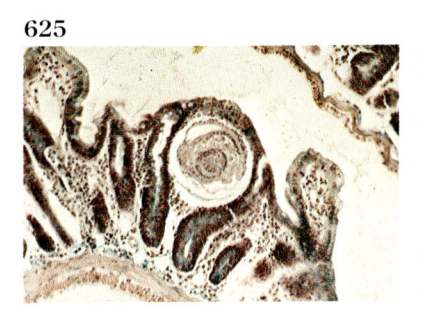

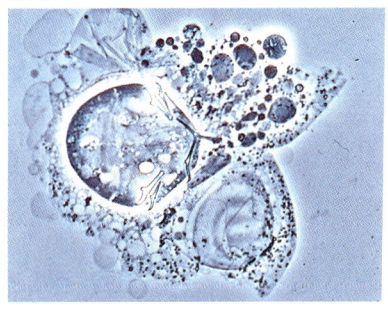

625 Cercocyst in intestinal villi In the mammal the oncospheres penetrate into the villi of the small intestine. There they mature into tailless cysticercoids (cercocysts) which leave the villi, move further down the gut and become attached to other villi where they mature to adult tapeworms. (× 100)

626 Cysticercoid in insect If the egg is eaten by an insect, the oncosphere metamorphoses to form a tailed cysticercoid in the insect's body cavity. Further development takes place if the insect is ingested by man. (× 60)

627 Mature proglottids Man is probably the only source of human infection, rodents being infected possibly by a different (non-human) strain. (× 15)

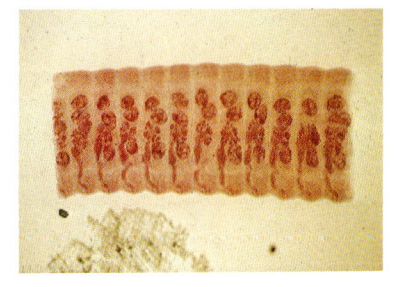

Hymenolepis diminuta (Rat Tapeworm)

628 Cysticercoid of *H. diminuta* in arthropod The adults of this, the common cestode of rodents, are 20 to 60 cm long. Their eggs (**325**) resemble those of *H. nana* but lack the polar filaments. An intermediate insect host is essential in this life cycle and a wide variety of coprophagic arthropods serve in this capacity. Occasionally man is infected by accidentally swallowing infected arthropods, e.g. rat fleas, or larvae of grain moths and beetles. (× 90)

629 *Tribolium confusum* These grain pests are typical intermediate hosts of *H. diminuta*. (× 9)

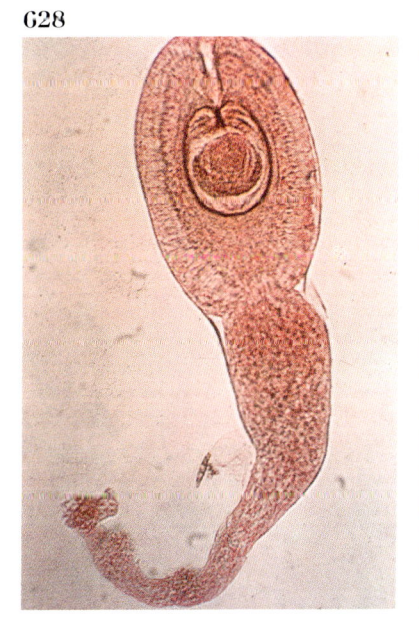

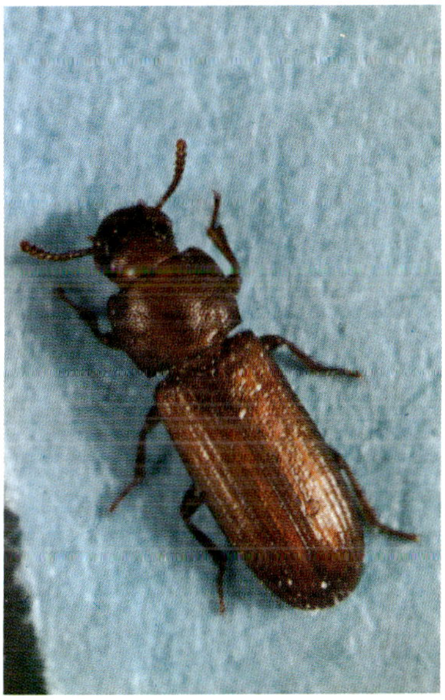

Taenia solium (Pork Tapeworm)

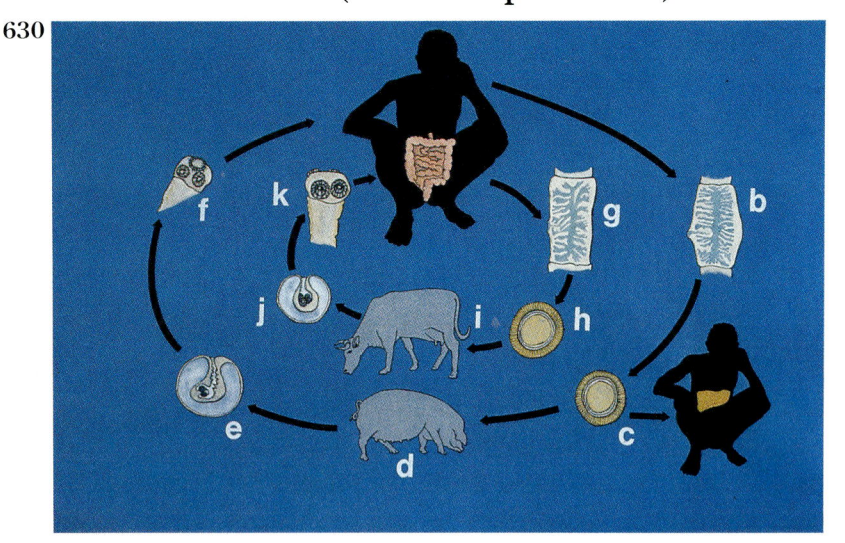

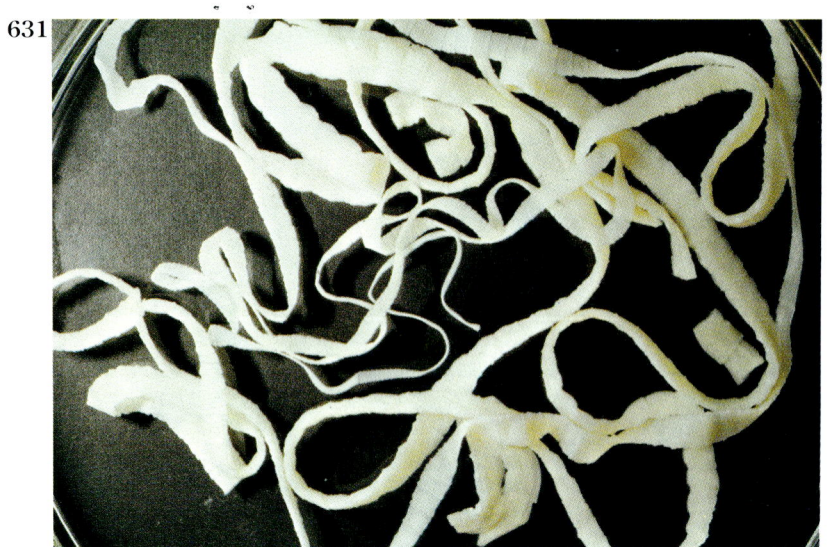

630 Life cycle of *Taenia solium* and *T. saginata* The adults of both species live in the small intestine of man, the definitive host. The gravid segments (b & g) are very active and escape through the anus, releasing large numbers of eggs (c & h) in the perianal region or on the ground, where they can survive for long periods. Faecal egg loads are, therefore, relatively light. When ingested by pigs (d) (*T. solium*) or cattle (i) (*T. saginata*), the eggs hatch, each releasing an oncosphere which migrates through the intestinal wall and blood vessels to reach striated muscle within which it encysts, forming cysticerci (e & j). When inadequately cooked meat containing the cysts is eaten by man, the oncospheres excyst (f & k), settle in the small intestine and develop there into adult cestodes over the next three months or so. The segments of *T. solium* are somewhat less active than those of the beef tapeworm but its eggs, if released in the upper intestine, can invade the host (autoinfection), setting up the potentially dangerous larval infection known as cysticercosis in muscle or any other site.

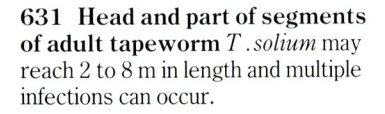

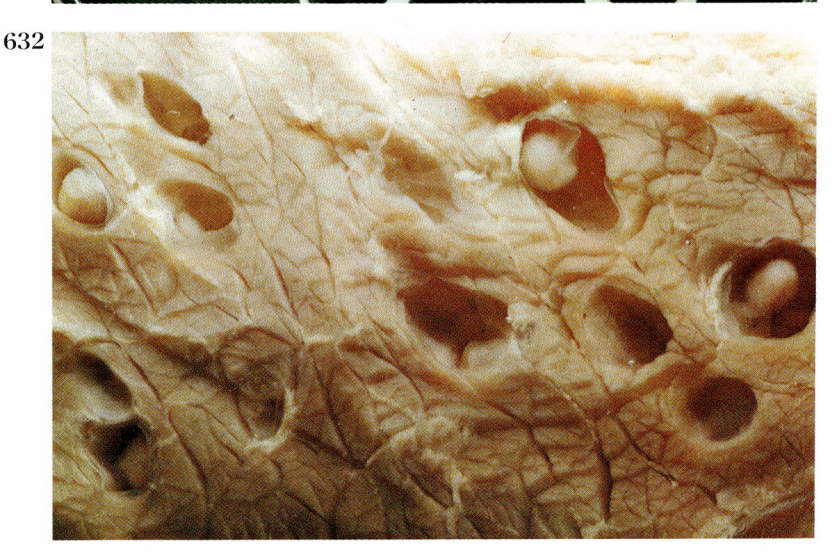

631 Head and part of segments of adult tapeworm *T. solium* may reach 2 to 8 m in length and multiple infections can occur.

632 Cysticercus in pork The larval cysticercoid stage occurs in the pig, giving rise to 'measly pork'. Man is infected by ingesting the meat inadequately cooked. ($\times 3$)

633 & 634 Scolex of *T. solium* and *T. saginata* The head of *T. solium* (**633**) is armoured with hooks, in addition to four suckers. *T. saginata* has no hooks. (× 40)

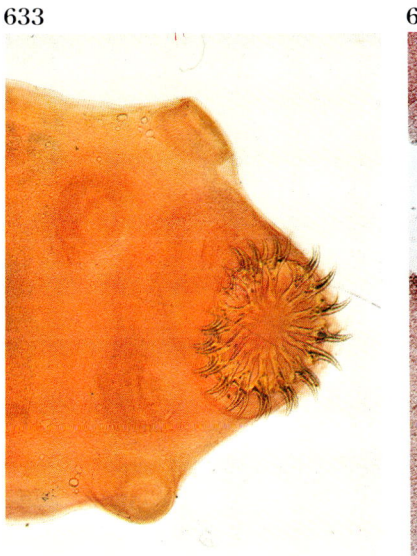

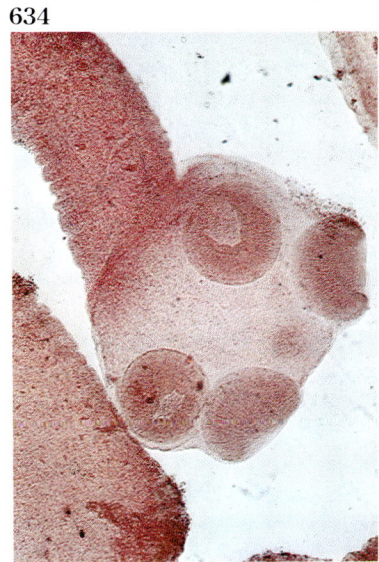

635 ***T. solium* cysticerci in chest wall** Auto infection due to the release of eggs may follow the incorrect use of taeniacidal drugs. The cysts (Cysticerci cellulosae) may be formed in any tissue. This agricultural student was infected in Thailand.

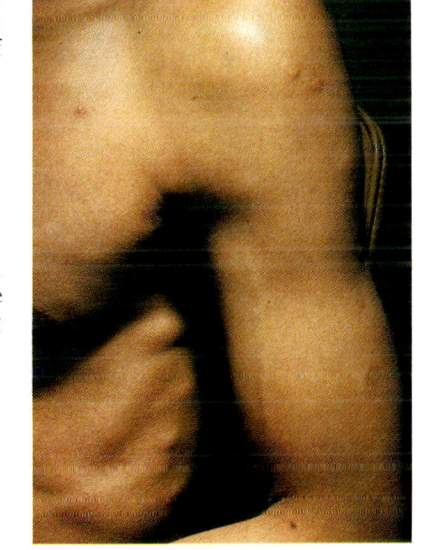

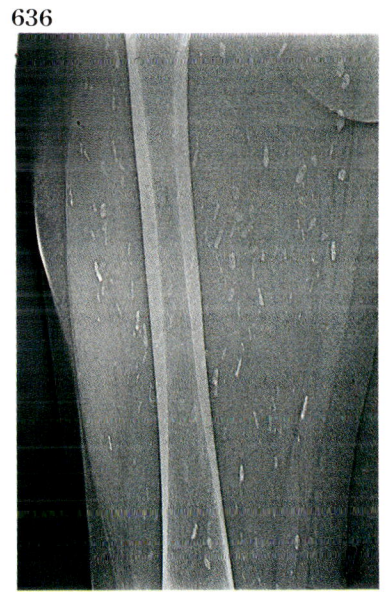

636 X-ray of cysticercosis of soft tissues When calcification occurs, the cysticerci are readily seen by X-raying the soft tissues.

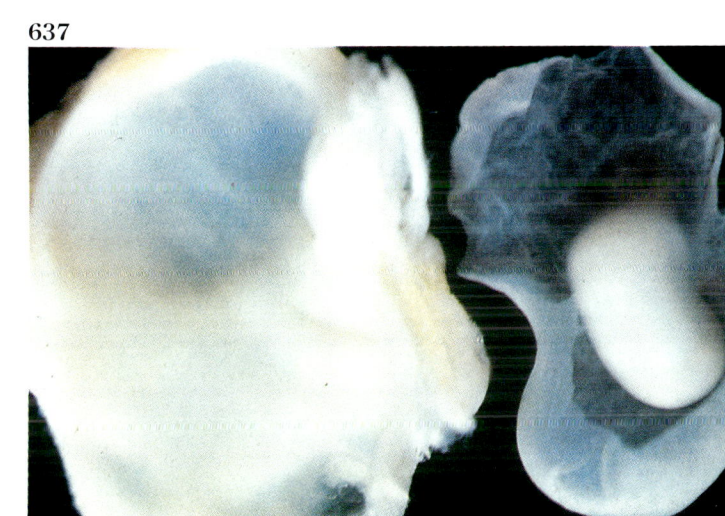

637 Cysticercus removed from subcutaneous tissues This fibrous nodule containing a cyst was from the patient shown in **635**. (× 10)

157

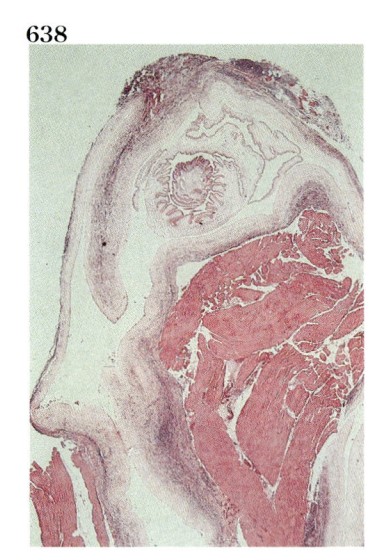

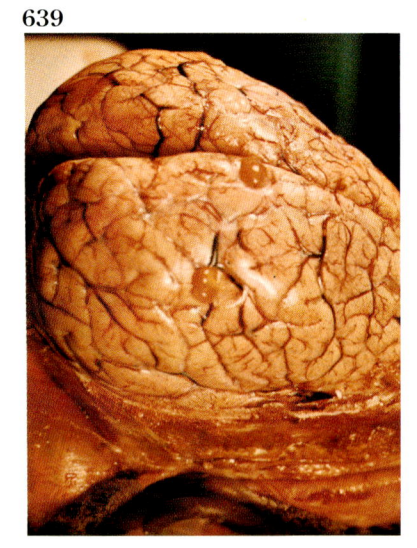

638 Section of cyst in human muscle The figure shows a section of a typical Cysticercus cellulosae removed from a chest wall. (× 6)

639 Cysticercosis of brain When cysticerci lodge in the brain calcification can occur, but usually much later than in tissues such as muscle and often after epilepsy has manifested itself.

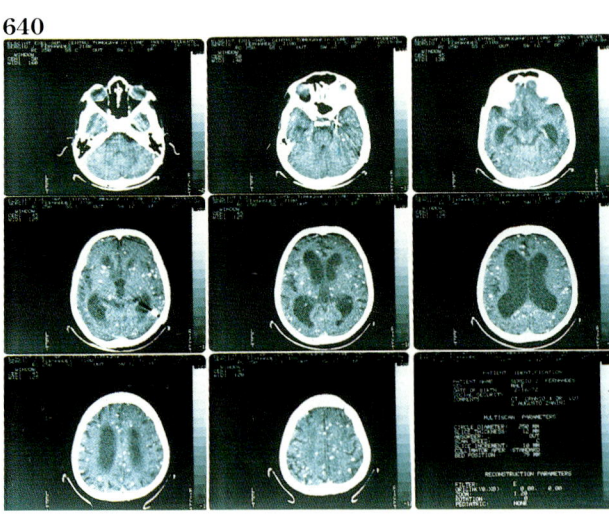

640 CAT scan in cerebral cysticercosis A large number of pea-sized nodules is seen in this scan of a Brazilian patient who later died with severe neurological lesions.

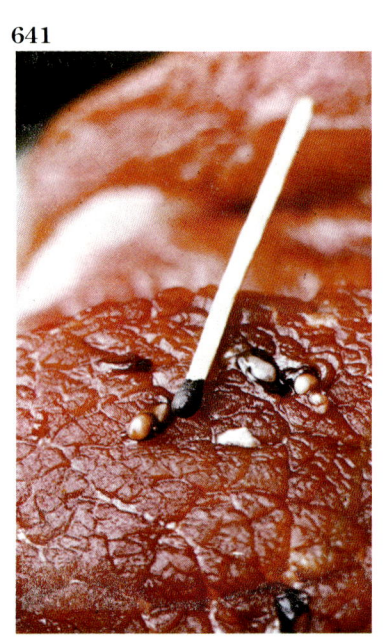

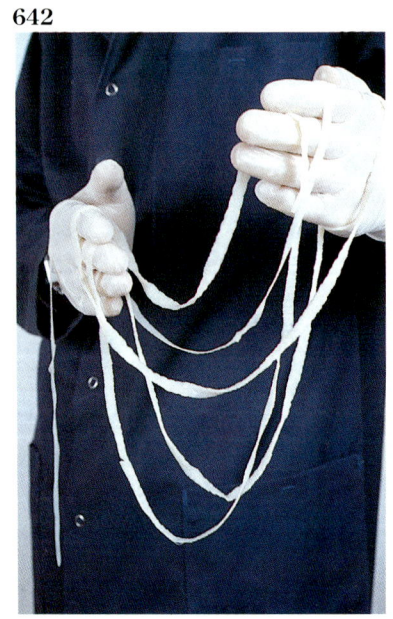

Taenia saginata (Beef Tapeworm)

641 Cysticercus in beef The cysticercal stage occurs only in cattle, man becoming infected when he eats raw or partially cooked beef.

642 Adult *T. saginata* The figure gives an impression of the size of this cestode, which can attain 10 m in length. This was only part of a worm passed after treatment with a taeniacide.

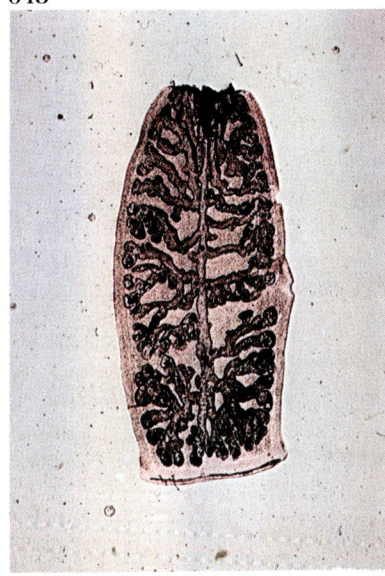

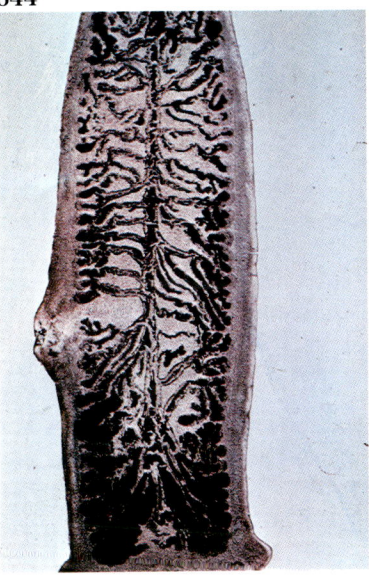

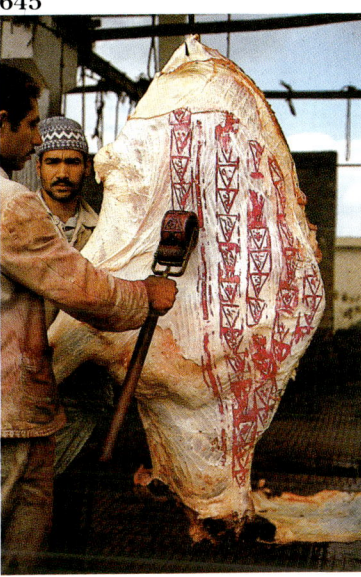

643 & 644 Mature proglottids of *T. solium* and *T. saginata* The gravid segments of *T. solium* (**643**) contain a central uterus with less than a dozen lateral branches. The eggs (**326**) are similar to those of other *Taenia* species. The gravid segments of *T. saginata* (**644**) contain a central uterus with 15 to 20 lateral branches. (× 6)

645 Meat inspection—certificate of health Taeniasis is prevented by strict abattoir supervision, including adequate inspection of carcasses and condemnation of 'measly' meat.

Hydatidosis

646 Life cycle of *Echinococcus granulosus* The adult tapeworm (a) inhabits the small intestine of dogs in the faeces of which typical taeniid eggs (b) (**326**) are passed. Eggs ingested by herbivorous animals hatch in the duodenum, the hooked embryos entering the circulation where they are carried to various sites to develop into cysts (d). The liver is most commonly infected. Man (e) is infected when he accidentally ingests eggs.

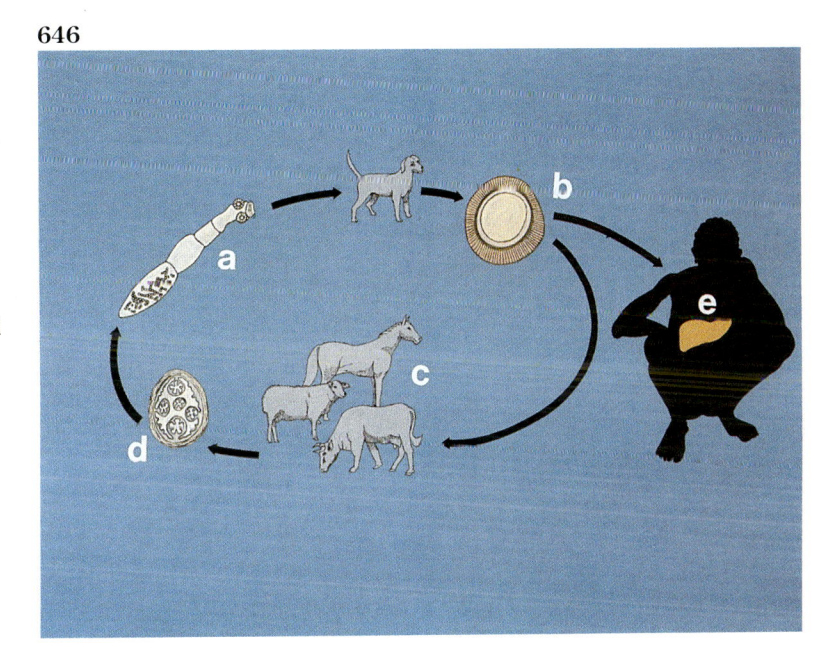

159

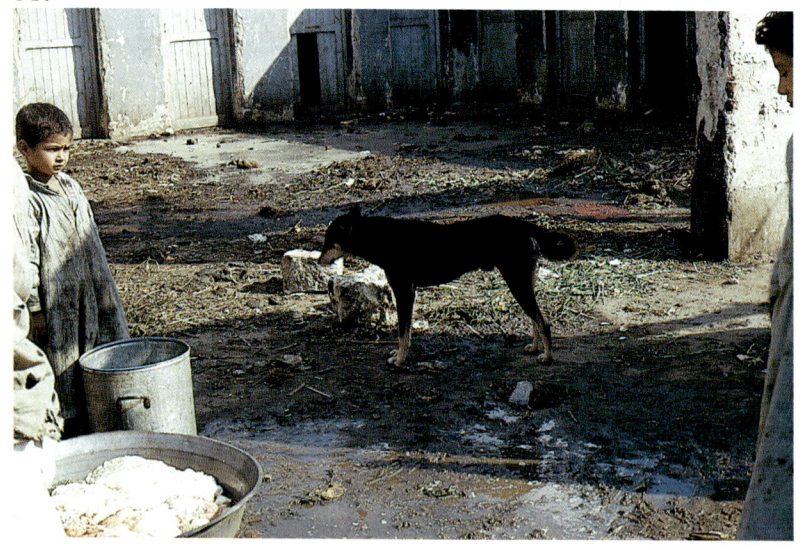

647 Dog in an insanitary abattoir Hydatidosis can be largely prevented by strict control of abattoirs and disposal of infected offal. In some primitive rural communities which slaughter animals for food in an entirely uncontrolled and *ad hoc* fashion, hydatid disease is very common.

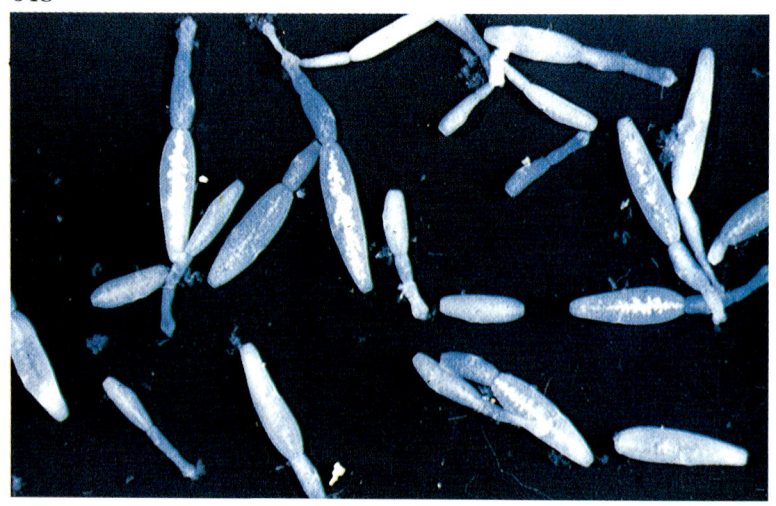

648 Adult *Echinococcus granulosus* This tapeworm is about 5 mm long. Large numbers may be found in the small intestine of dogs which are infected by eating offal of sheep, cattle or other animals containing hydatid cysts. The scolices in the cysts evaginate in the animal's intestine and mature into the adult worms. ($\times 9$)

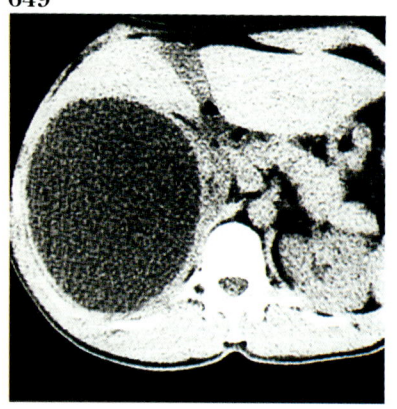

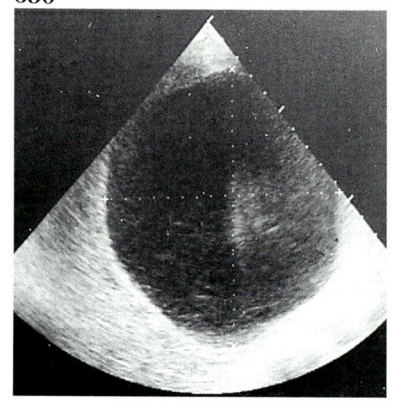

649 CAT scan of hydatid cyst in liver If man accidentally ingests eggs he becomes the host of the larval (hydatid cyst) stage. The liver is most commonly affected. The hydatid cyst is usually unilocular, with a double wall comprised of an outer laminated layer and an inner nucleated germinal layer. The figure shows a massive cyst in the right lobe of the liver of a 14-year-old Kuwaiti boy.

650 Ultrasound scan of hydatid cyst (Same case as **649**) This is an invaluable diagnostic aid that is accessible in many hospitals.

651 Daughter cysts The germinal layer produces brood capsules, inside which grow scolices.

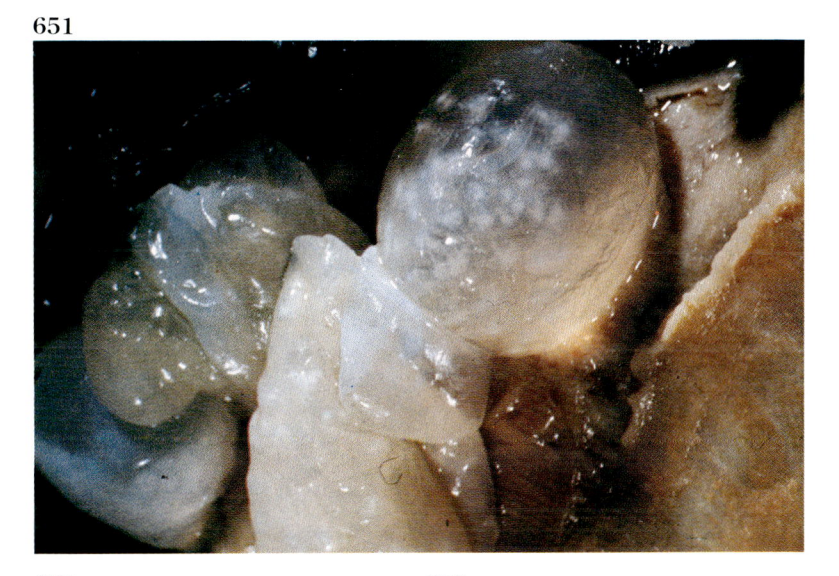

652 'Hydatid sand' The daughter cysts are attached to the parent cyst wall or may float free in its milky fluid contents as the so-called 'hydatid sand'. Rupture of a cyst into the tissues results in dissemination and further growth of the scolices. (× 250)

653 X-ray of lungs Hydatid cysts of the lung are not uncommon.

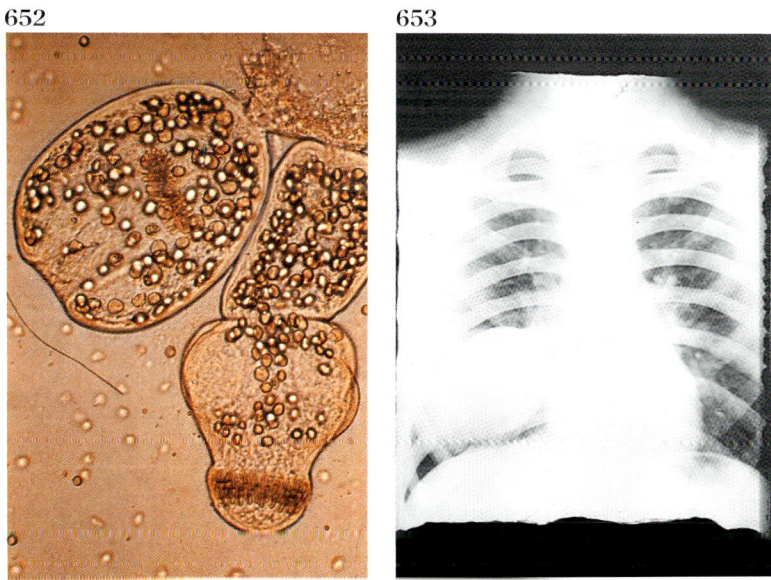

654 Hydatid cyst of lung Section of cyst removed from a lung showing the multi-layered cyst wall and numerous daughter cysts produced by the germinal layer. (H&E × 40)

655 Hydatid cyst in brain This cyst was found in the brain of a four-year-old girl.

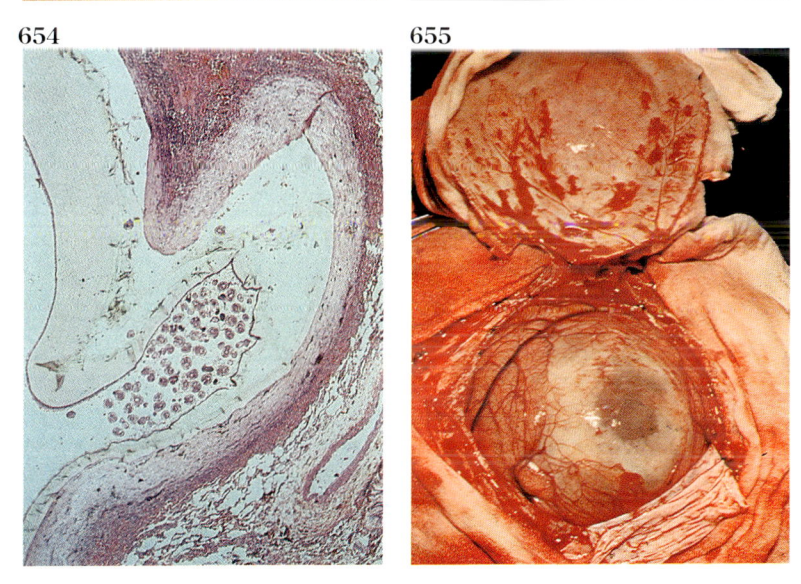

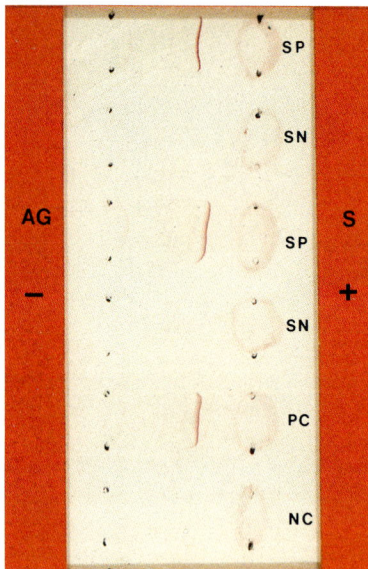

656 Immunodiagnosis of hydatidosis The Casoni skin test formerly employed used crude hydatid fluid as antigen. This has been largely replaced by purified antigens such as 'arc 5' which is employed in counter immunoelectrophoresis.
(SP = positive, SN negative sera; PC = positive, NC negative controls; AG = antigen at cathodic ends; S = serum at anodic ends.)

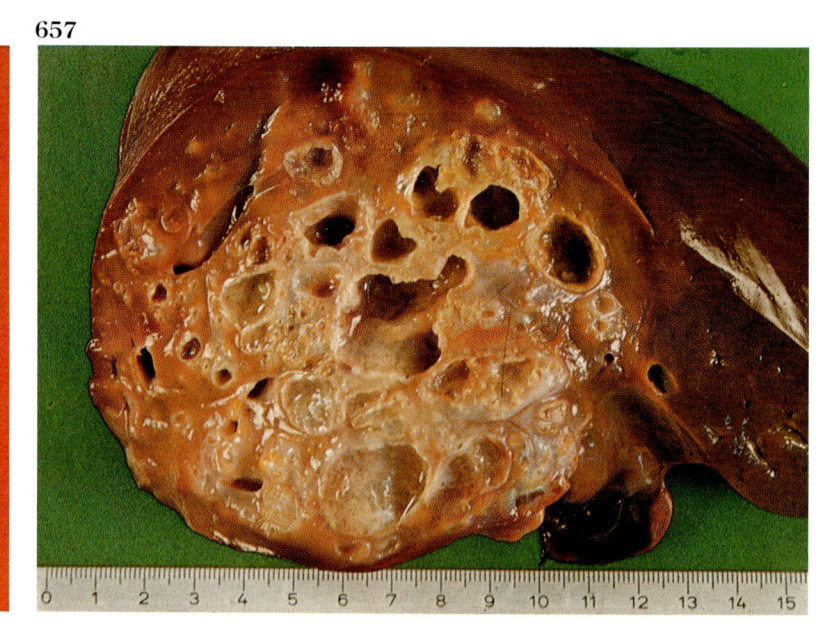

657 Multilocular hydatidosis in human liver Multilocular or alveolar cysts are caused by infection with *Echinococcus multilocularis*. The adult of this species is found in wild canines, and the usual larval hosts are rodents. The alveolar cyst in the human liver may mimic hepatic carcinoma, but it is usually only discovered at post-mortem, as in this case.

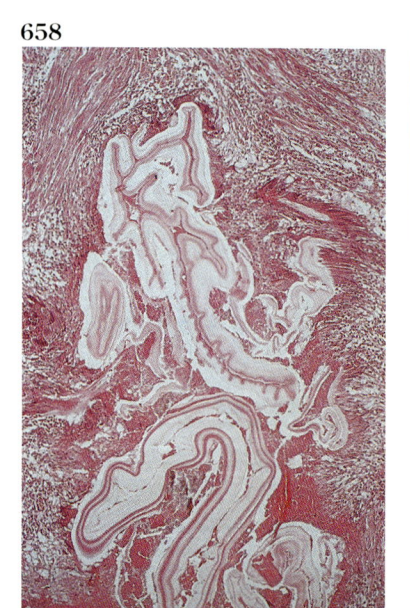

658 Section of alveolar hydatid cyst Unlike *E. granulosus*, cysts of *E. multilocularis* do not contain daughter cysts with scolices in man. (× *40*) (cf. **654**)

659 *Coenurus cerebralis* of sheep This is the larval stage of *Multiceps multiceps*. The adult lives in the intestine of the dog and the 'bladder worm' larva is usually found in the brain of sheep. Fortunately infection of man is rare.

660 *Coenurus* in human eye This infection necessitated enucleation of the eye.

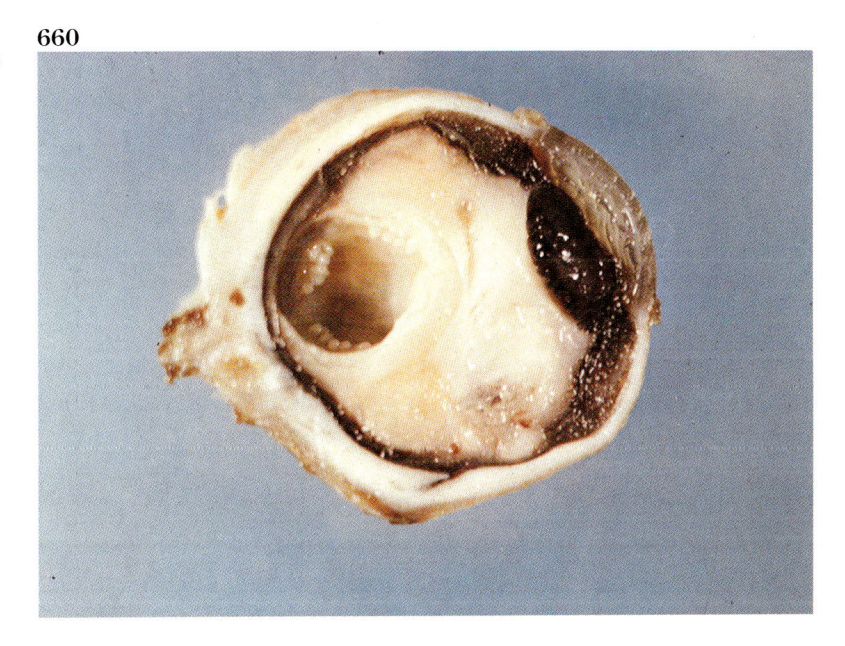

PENTASTOMIASIS
Linguatula serrata (Tongue Worm)

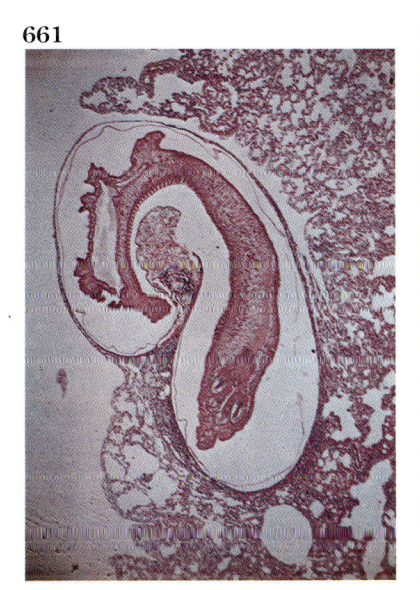

661 Third-stage larva in rabbit lung These endoparasitic and highly specialised parasites have embryonic and ultrastructural affinities to the Arthropoda. Man may be infected by eating inadequately cooked food containing third-stage larvae. Other carnivores are also infected. ($\times 20$)

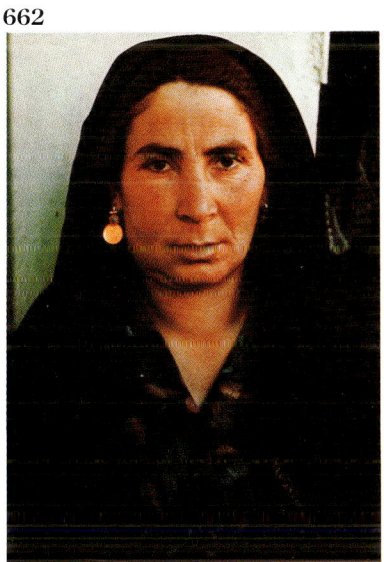

662 Halzoun syndrome The parasites migrate to the nasopharynx where they produce large adults which block the airways and cause deafness. Eggs are passed in the nasal secretions. Facial oedema is a common sign.

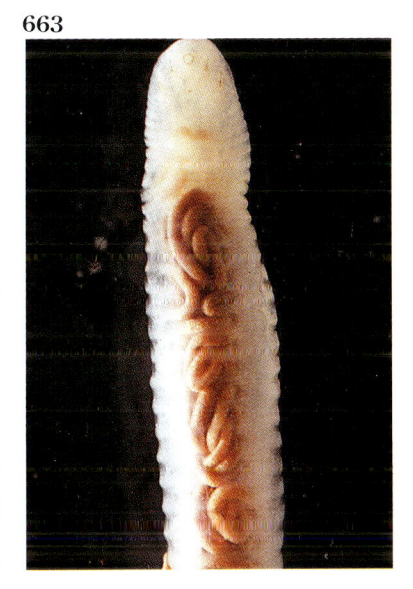

663 Adult *Linguatula serrata* Cephalic third of a typical adult tongue worm. Note the oral opening and four hooks. ($\times 3$)

Other Pentastomids

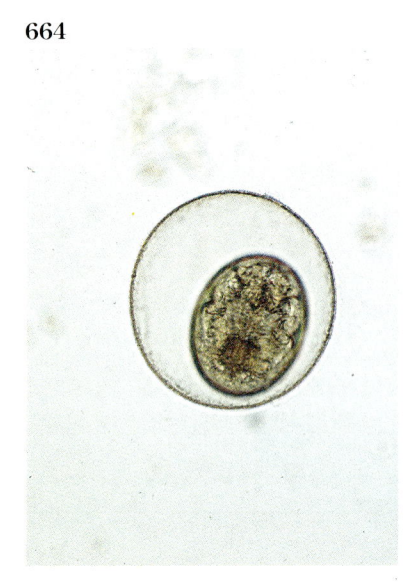

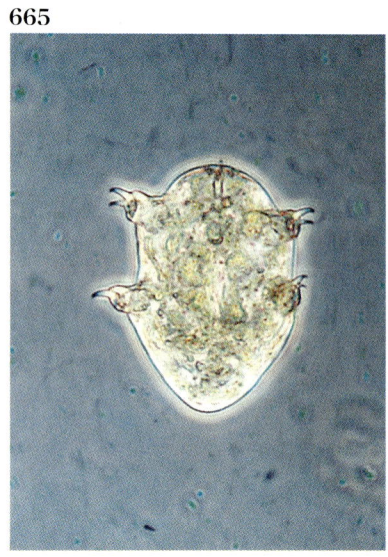

664

665

664 & 665 Eggs and first-stage larva of *Porocephalus* The eggs and primary larvae with their four bifurcate legs point to the arthropod origin of this parasite of North American snakes (*Porocephalus crotali*) (**664** × *200*; **665** × *320*)

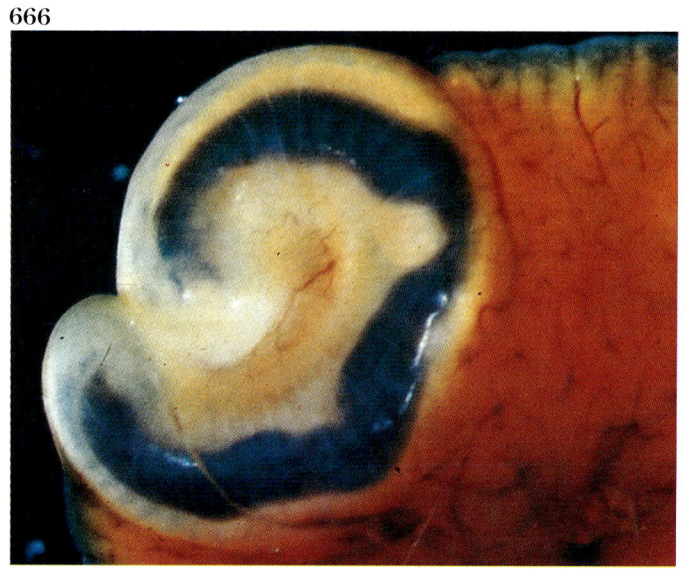

666

667

666 *P. crotali* third-stage larva After ingestion of eggs in food or water by a secondary host (usually a rodent), primary larvae emerge in the gut. They penetrate the gut wall and encyst in various tissues. This infective third-stage larva lies subperitoneally in a rodent, the normal intermediate host. (× *6*)

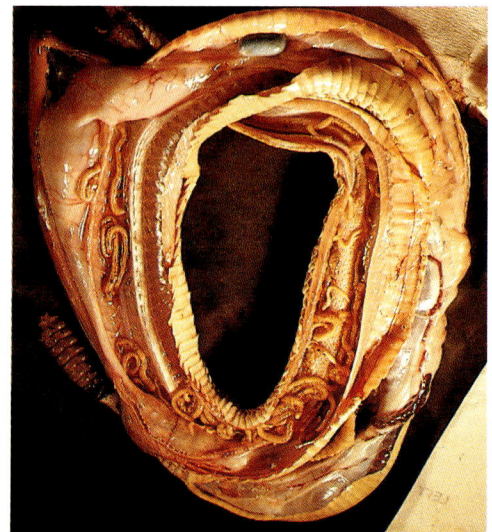

667 Adult *Porocephalus crotali* in rattlesnake lung Eggs of this 'lungworm' are passed in saliva or in faeces. The parasite is common in snakes, which acquire infection by eating rodents containing third-stage larvae. (× $1/7$)

668 Adult males and a female *Armillifer armillatus* This lungworm is a common parasite of several species of African snakes. The usual intermediate hosts are rodents, but man is quite commonly infected with the larvae.

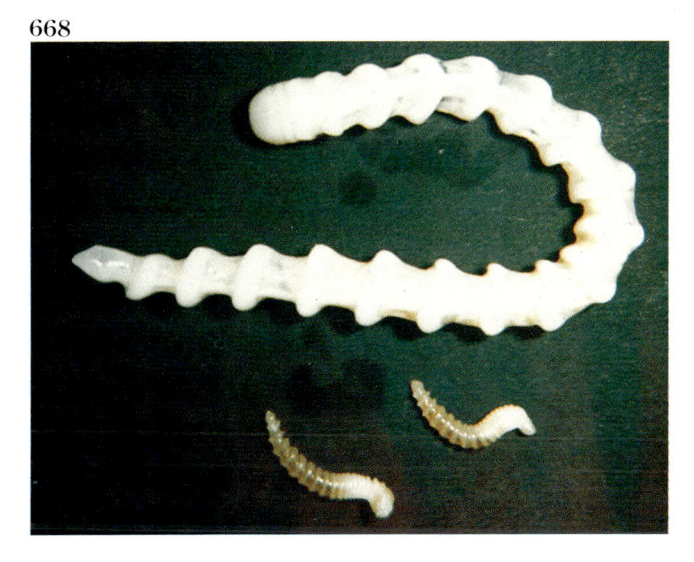

669 Larvae of *Armillifer armillatus* Third-stage larvae are seen under the capsule of the liver of a Nigerian at post-mortem.

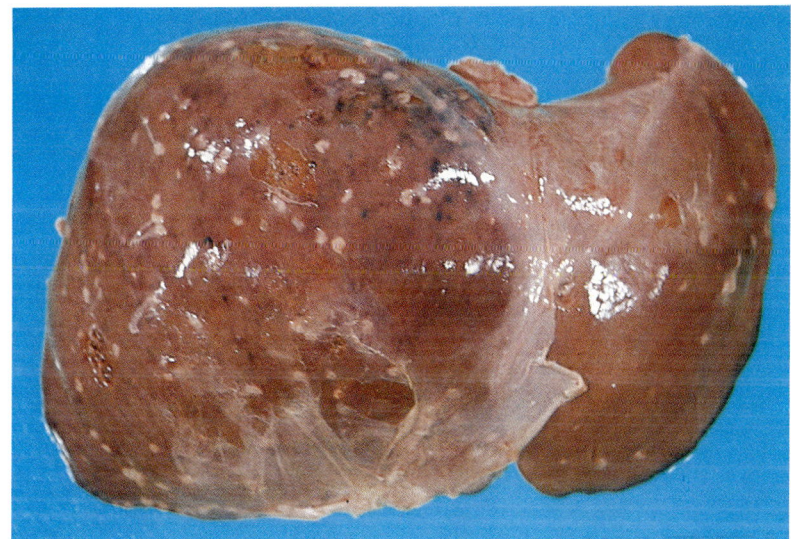

670 X-ray of pentastomid larvae in man Calcified third-stage larvae are seen in this X-ray of an African patient.

671 Pentastomid larva in eye The eye is a rare site for pentastomid larvae, the abdomen being mainly affected in man.

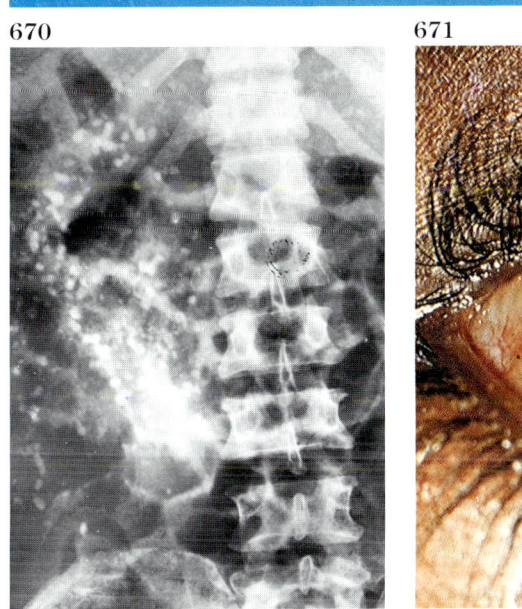

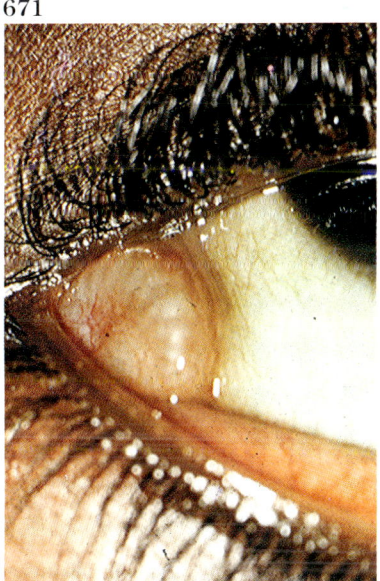

Part V
Infections Acquired through the Skin and Mucous Membranes

The infective agents include viruses, bacteria, protozoa, helminths and arthropods. In one group, transmission of infection is by contact with contaminated persons or objects. In the other group, infection may be acquired by exposure to infected soil (hookworm)*, water (schistosomiasis*, leptospirosis), by the bites of animals (rabies) or through wounds (tetanus). The mode of transmission may be by direct, or by indirect, contact.

The smallpox eradication campaign organised by the World Health Organization has resulted in the disappearance of the disease. Yaws is now almost a curiosity, although some cases do still occur. Trachoma, however, remains an important blinding disease despite the considerable progress made in its control, especially in the Middle East. The venereal diseases are more important in the tropics than has hitherto been appreciated, while the non-venereal treponematoses are widely distributed in the world.

A newly recognised and rapidly spreading disease caused by several viruses that suppress the human immune system, especially the Human Immunodeficiency Virus (HIV), which is believed to have its origins in Central Africa, has assumed pandemic proportions. It is spread both by sexual contact and by the injection of virus in blood or blood products. The fully developed 'Acquired Immune Deficiency Syndrome' (AIDS) produces death from a multiplicity of opportunistic infections: viral, bacterial, fungal or parasitic, or neoplasms.

The greatest concentration of leprosy is in the Indian sub-continent (3 million), while the highest prevalence rates are in Africa (about 100 per 1 000). One fifth of the estimated 15 million cases are under treatment. Europe has 52 000 (mainly in Southern Europe), and over 900 patients have been notified in England since 1951.

A wide variety of fungi infect skin, hair and nails without deeper penetration of the host tissues. Other fungi cause deep mycoses that can result in some of the most disfiguring lesions seen in clinical medicine.

*These conditions are dealt with in Parts II and III respectively.

VIRAL INFECTIONS
Smallpox

Twenty years ago smallpox was endemic in many countries of the tropics. Following a successful smallpox eradication campaign organised under the auspices of WHO, this disease has now been eradicated. As far as is known, the only *Variola major* virus surviving is in a very small number of top-security virology laboratories.

672 Distribution of rash The distribution of the rash was centrifugal and concentrated on the face as shown here, hands and feet. It was accompanied by marked toxicity and left severe scarring ('pockmarks') in those surviving.

673 Ultrastructure of smallpox virus *Variola major* is a large, ovoid DNA virus which could readily be identified in fluid from the cutaneous lesions. ($\times 63\,000$)

674 Primary smallpox vaccination response Vaccination immunises the individual for a period of three years. It is no longer carried out, except on military personnel in a few countries.

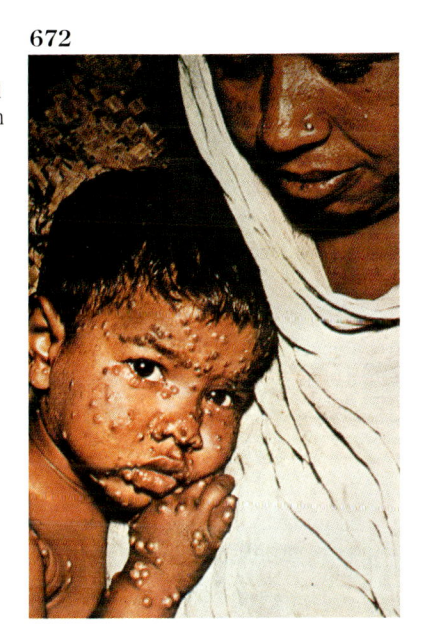

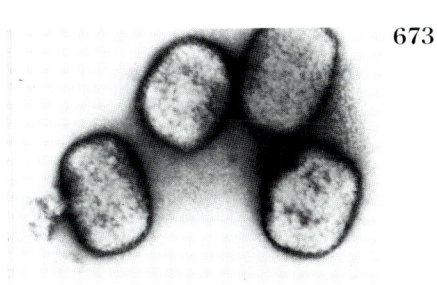

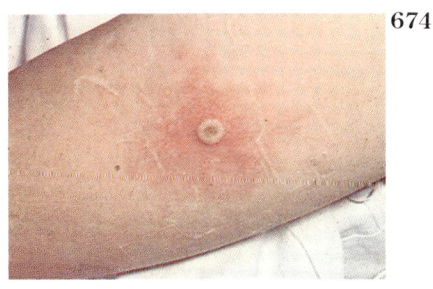

Trachoma

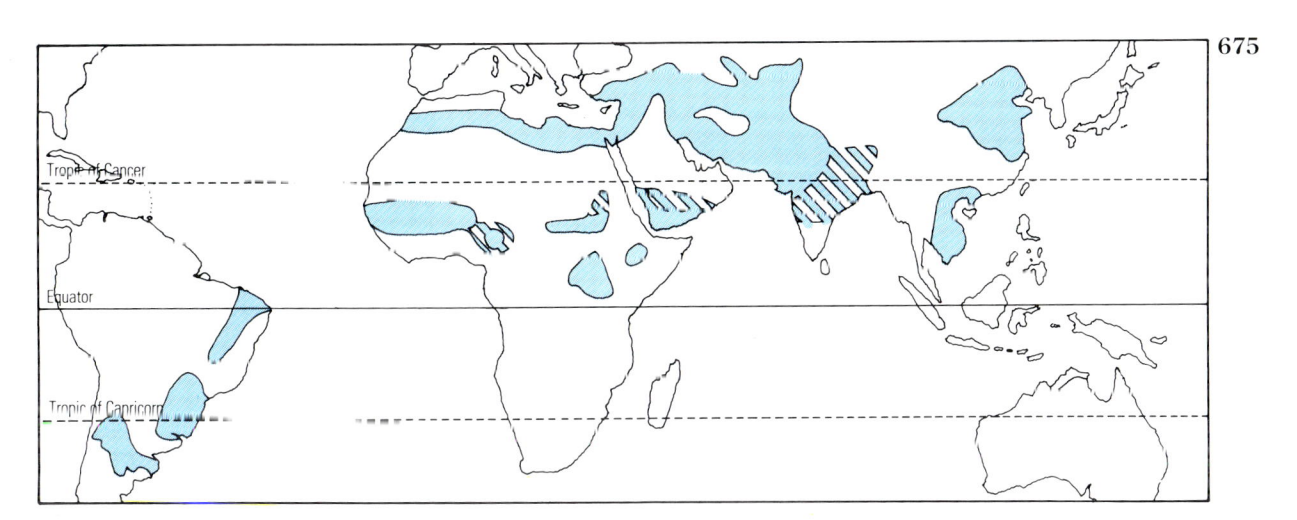

675 Trachoma distribution Trachoma is particularly common in the Middle East and Africa, as well as other parts of the tropics. It is caused by a virus of the *Chlamydia* group (also known as *Bedsonia*). (Solid colour on the figure indicates high incidence, lines indicate lower incidence.)

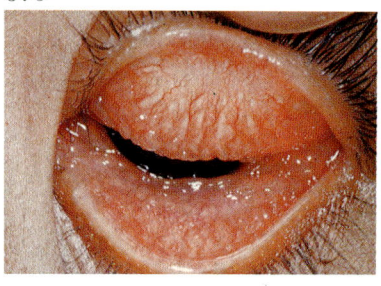

676 Early lesions Small, pinhead-sized, pale follicles beneath the epithelium over the tarsal plates, especially in the upper lid, are a characteristic feature of the disease. The so-called 'TRIC' virus may be identified at this stage and up to the time scarring commences, in epithelial scrapings.

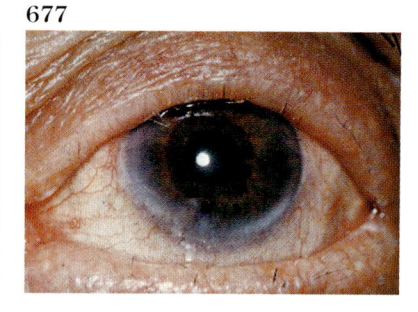

677 Entropion and trichiasis Scarring of the tarsal plates may be extensive and result in entropion of the edge of the lid. The eyelashes point inwards and rub against the cornea (trichiasis), adding to the damage already done by the virus.

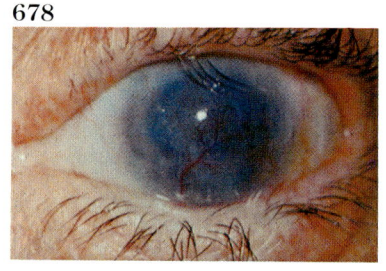

678 Late corneal scarring and trichiasis The end point of trachoma is frequently blindness due to corneal scarring and other complications.

Lymphogranuloma Venereum

679 Inguinal adenitis Inguinal lymphadenitis is a common feature, resulting in a large, sausage-shaped mass, over which the skin is shiny and purplish in colour. The disease is caused by another *Chlamydia* species which can be seen as elementary bodies in Giemsa-stained leucocytes. Serious genito-anorectal lesions can result.

680 Frei test The Frei skin test is a delayed hypersensitivity reaction of value in the diagnosis. The test is read at 48 hours and 96 hours after the injection of 0.1 ml of the antigen, which is prepared from virus cultured in chick embryos. (This disease is also called lymphogranuloma inguinale, climatic bubo or esthiomène.)

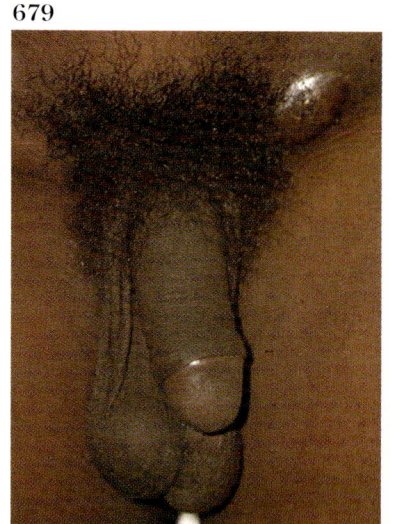

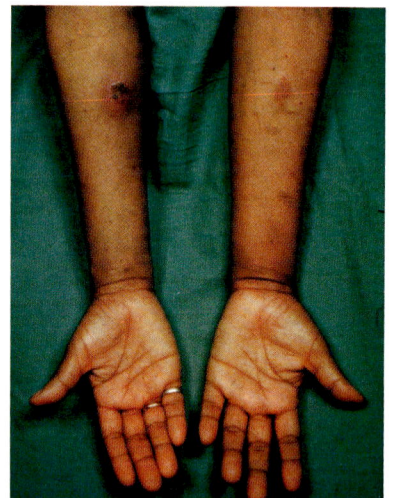

Acquired Immune Deficiency Syndrome (AIDS)

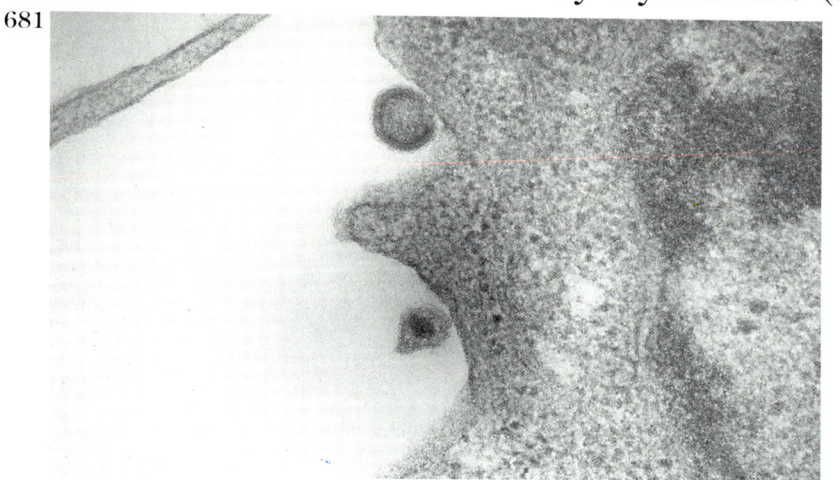

681 The Human Immunodeficiency Virus HIV is the major aetiological agent of AIDS. This type C retrovirus, also known as HTLV-III (human T-lymphotropic virus type III) or LAV (lymphadenopathy associated virus), is one of several in the genus *Lentivirus* that grow in mammalian T-cells. HIV is related to HTLV-IV and LAV-2 which are associated with AIDS in Africa, as well as to the STLV-III group of viruses of African Green monkeys (**815**) and mangabeys. The HIV particles seen here are growing in a lymphocyte cell line. (× *90 000*)

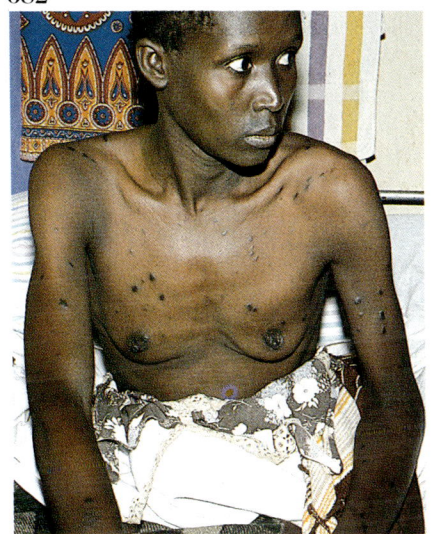

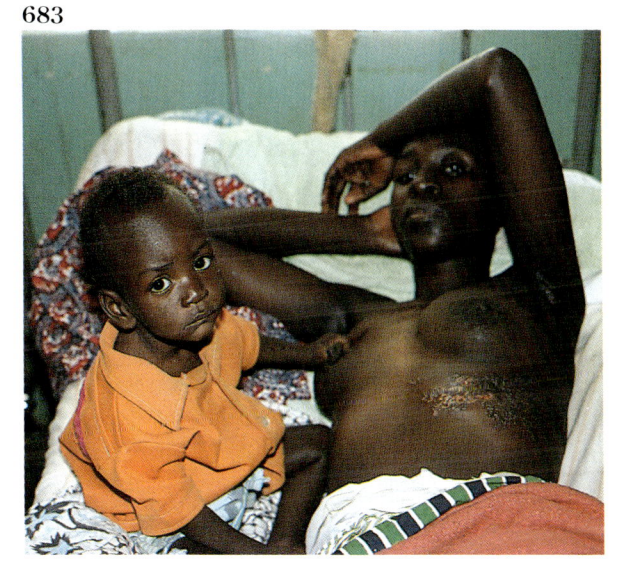

682 Kaposi's sarcoma in an African It is currently estimated by WHO that 10 million people globally are infected with HIV and 5 million in Africa alone. The global figure could rise to 100 million in a further five years. In addition to the many opportunistic viral, bacterial, fungal and parasitic infections noted throughout this Atlas (*see* **Index**) that kill victims of AIDS, many develop disseminated Kaposi's sarcoma, which is almost pathognomonic of HIV infection in the African. Severe, chronic diarrhoea due to this and a number of pathogenic agents leads to the extreme wasting condition known as 'slim disease' in East Africa. In most AIDS sufferers the terminal stages are accompanied by a plethora of different infections. (*See also* **827 & 828**.)

683 Perinatal transmission of AIDS The virus in African communities, unlike the usual situation in other areas, is transmitted mainly by heterosexual contact, perinatally from infected mothers and by parenteral infection from contaminated blood in transfusions or dirty syringes. This woman with advanced AIDS had severe herpes zoster lesions. Her infant was also HIV positive.

Rabies

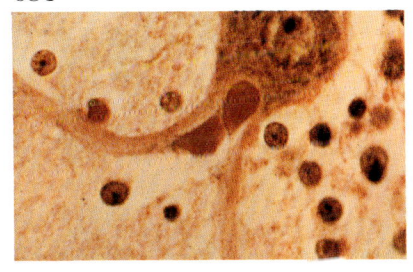

684 Negri bodies in nerve cells of rabid dog Although the dog, and to a lesser extent the cat, is the main urban transmitter of infection, foxes and other feline species as well as vampire bats are natural hosts and may also transmit the disease to man. Intracytoplasmic Negri bodies in brain cells are pathognomonic of rabies. The established clinical condition is invariably fatal. ($H\&E \times 600$)

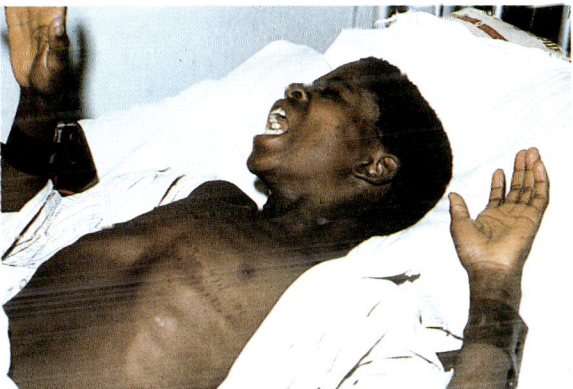

685 'Furious rabies' A 14-year-old Nigerian boy with hydrophobia following dog bites on the wrist and knee. Inspiratory spasms occurred spontaneously or were induced by the sight of water. The condition developed in spite of his receiving a 14-day course of anti-rabies vaccine.

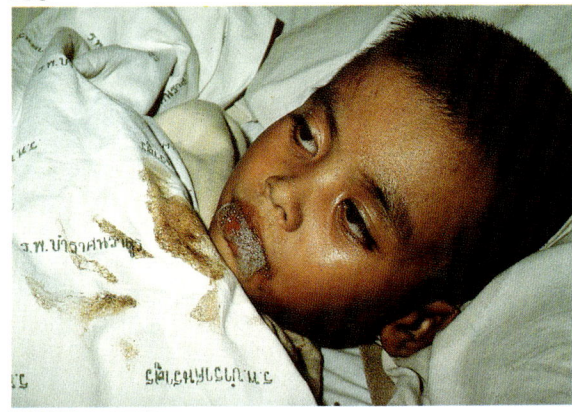

686 Autonomic nervous disorders in rabies
Hypersalivation, profuse sweating due to autonomic nervous system lesions and haematemesis characterised the infection in this Thai boy.

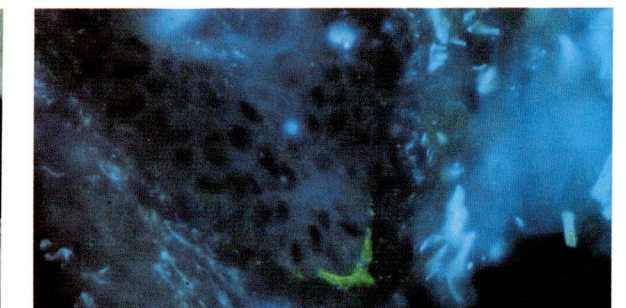

687 Fluorescent antibody staining of rabies virus
The presence of virus may sometimes be detected in a biopsy of the corneal epithelium during the incubation period, with the aid of a fluorescent antibody. Here a nerve is seen fluorescing bright green in such a specimen. ($\times 500$)

Herpes simplex

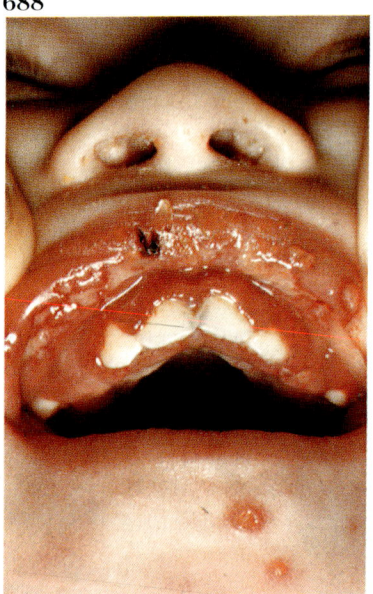

688 Acute herpetic ulcerative gingivostomatitis This condition, due to herpes simplex virus in children with severe protein-calorie malnutrition, causes a serious illness seen only uncommonly in the developed world.

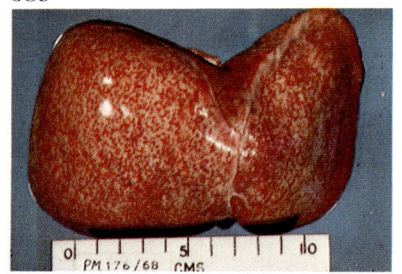

689 Liver in disseminated herpes simplex infection
Disseminated infection may affect the internal organs, e.g. liver, brain, heart, etc. This complication, which is usually fatal, occurs in patients with AIDS.

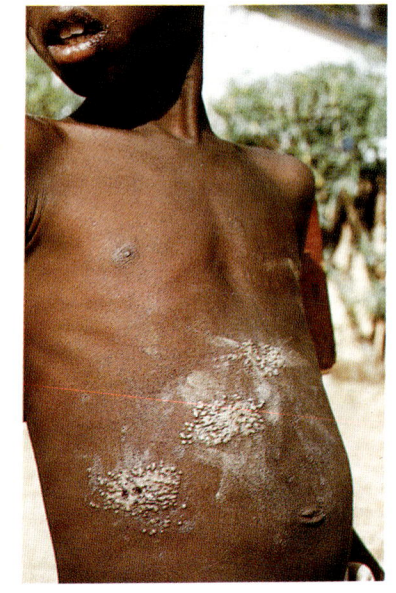

690 Herpes simplex of skin following meningitis Any debilitating illness that causes a depression of immunity may be followed by an extensive herpetic rash, as in this boy who had recovered from meningococcal meningitis.

BACTERIAL INFECTIONS
Leprosy

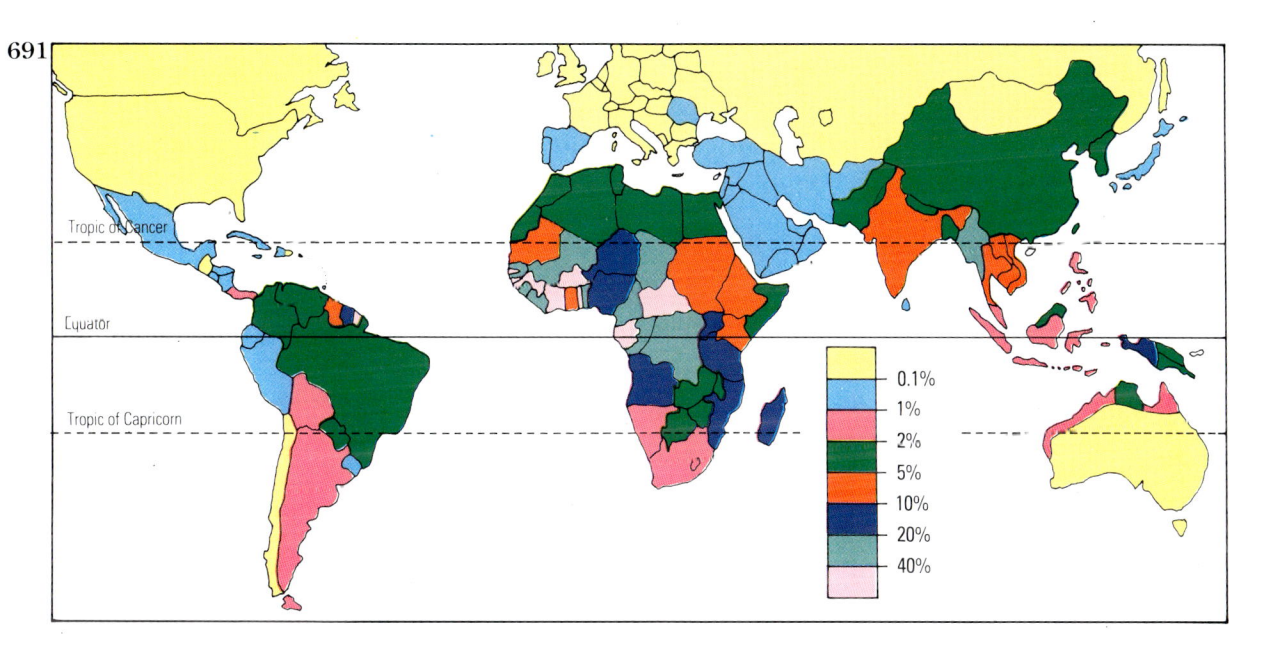

691 Distribution of leprosy Leprosy is particularly common today in Africa, the Indian subcontinent, SE Asia and South America. A vaccine against leprosy is undergoing extensive clinical trials in all these areas. Current rates per 1 000 population are shown on the figure.

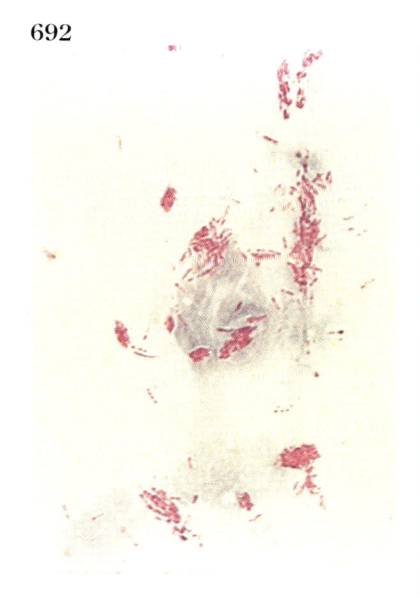

692 *Mycobacterium leprae* The acid- and alcohol-fast bacterial agent of leprosy in a smear preparation. (*Ziehl-Neelsen × 900*)

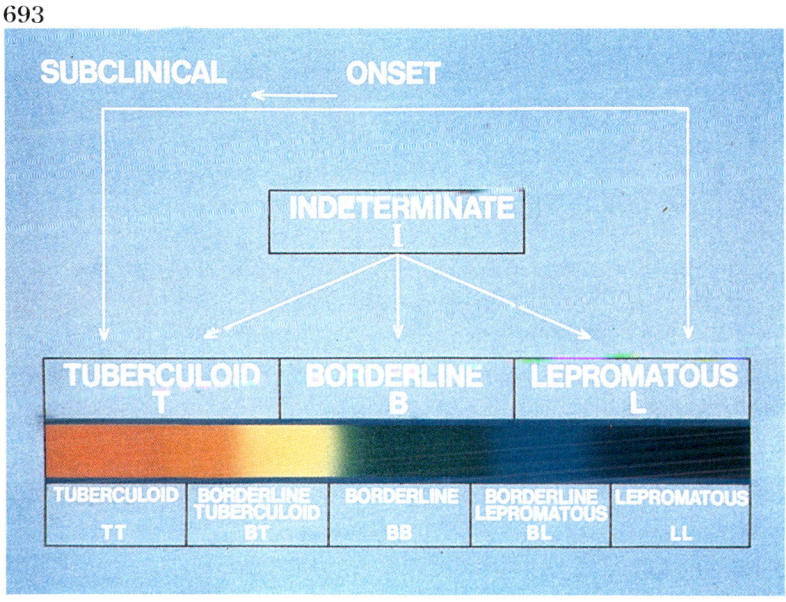

693 The clinical spectrum of leprosy The disease shows a broad spectrum depending on the patient's immune response, from healing tuberculoid at one pole to non-resolving lepromatous at the other. These responses are reflected in the histopathological picture (*see* **704-706**).

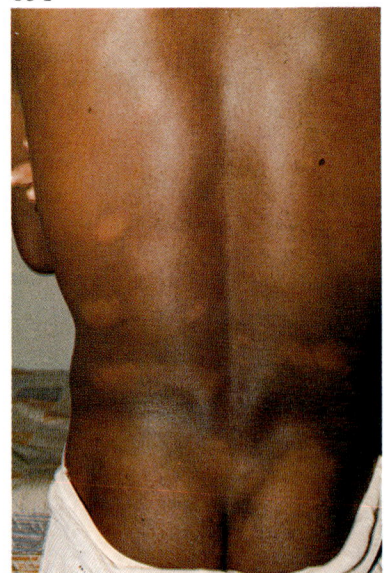

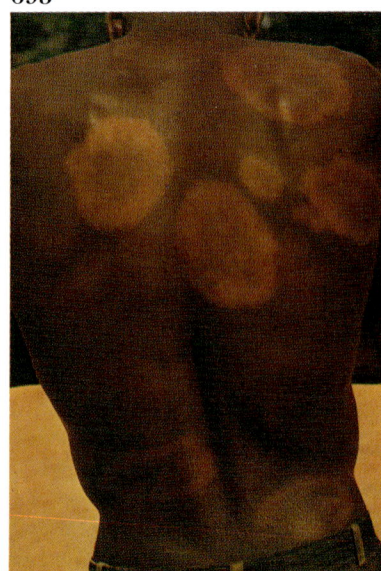

Tuberculoid leprosy

694 Early macules An early sign of leprosy, the *indeterminate* macule, is slightly hypopigmented and ill-defined. It retains tactile sensitivity, sweating function and hair growth.

695 Tuberculoid leprosy The early tuberculoid lesion is characterised by macules showing loss of sensation and hypopigmentation.

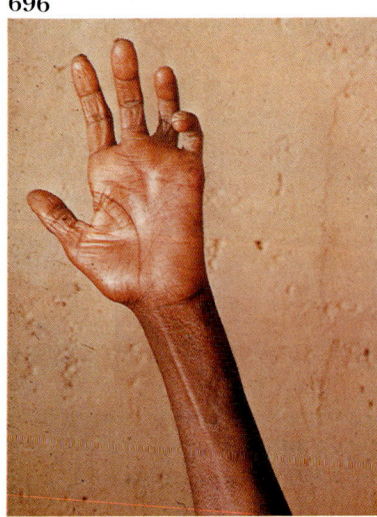

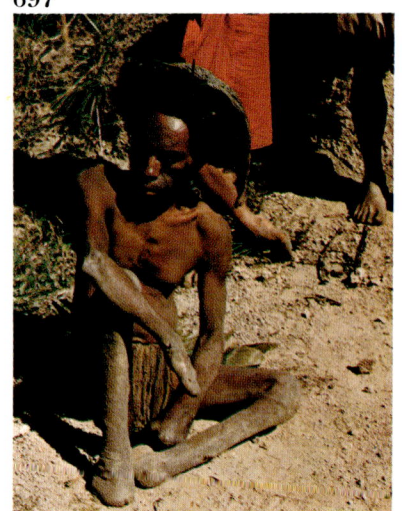

696 Ulnar nerve lesion Damage to the ulnar nerve in tuberculoid leprosy leads to weakness and wasting followed by complete paralysis and atrophy of the ulnar-innervated hand muscles, resulting in the characteristic picture of the 'main de prédicateur'.

697 Loss of extremities in late tuberculoid leprosy Neurotrophic atrophy eventually leads to the loss of phalanges, especially following trauma resulting from the anaesthesia. This man shows almost complete loss of hands and feet.

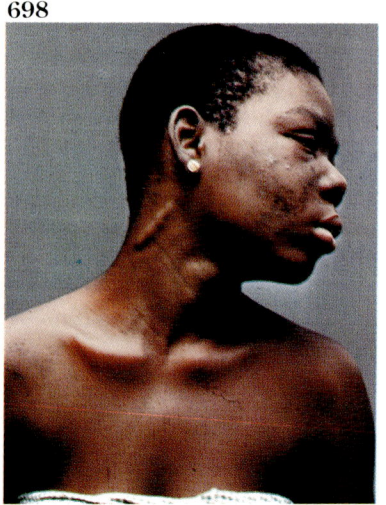

698 Nerve thickening Thickening of the great auricular nerve is also common in tuberculoid leprosy.

Lepromatous leprosy

699 Lepromatous leprosy
Lepromatous leprosy, showing extensive infiltration, oedema and corrugation causing 'leonine facies'. Note depilation of eyebrows and face, and thickening of ear.

700 Lepromatous nodule in eye
Leprosy is a common cause of blindness in the tropics.

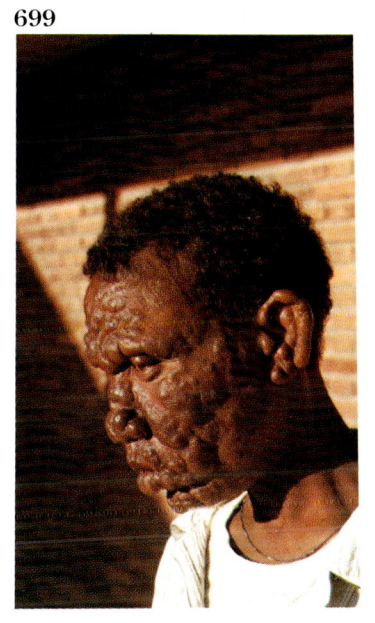

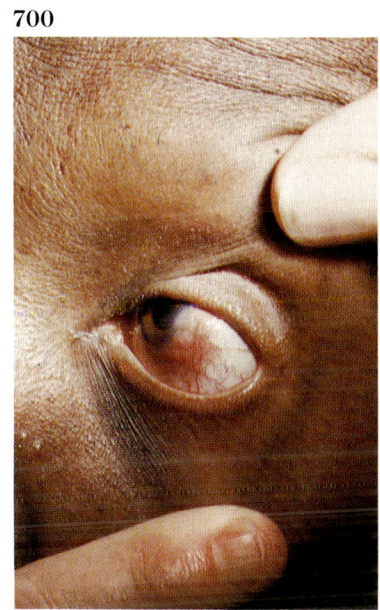

701 Gynaecomastia in leprosy This condition, which is relatively common in adult males with long-standing lepromatous leprosy, follows testicular atrophy.

702 Preparation of skin smear A biopsy is taken from a nodule and smeared for staining with Ziehl-Neelsen stain (*see* **692**).

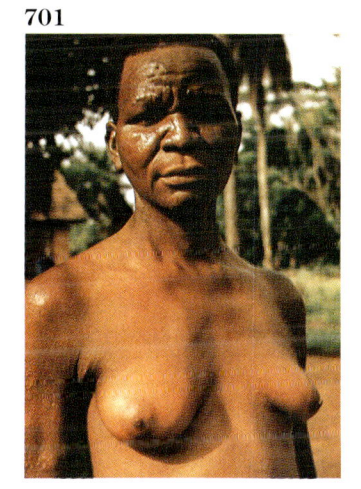

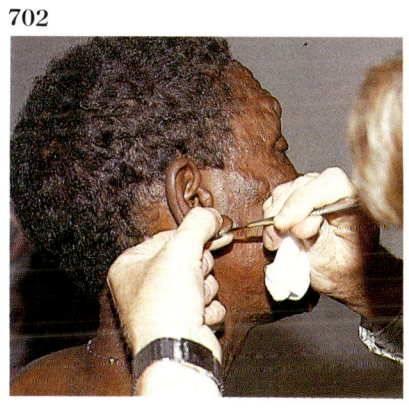

703 Organisms in skin biopsy stained by TRIFF method
Mycobacterium leprae is readily seen staining deep red in skin sections stained by this method. (*TRIFF × 200*)

173

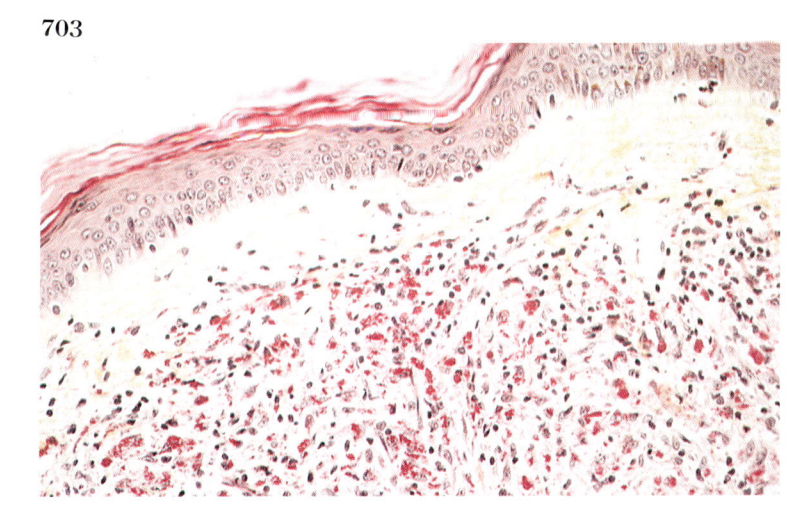

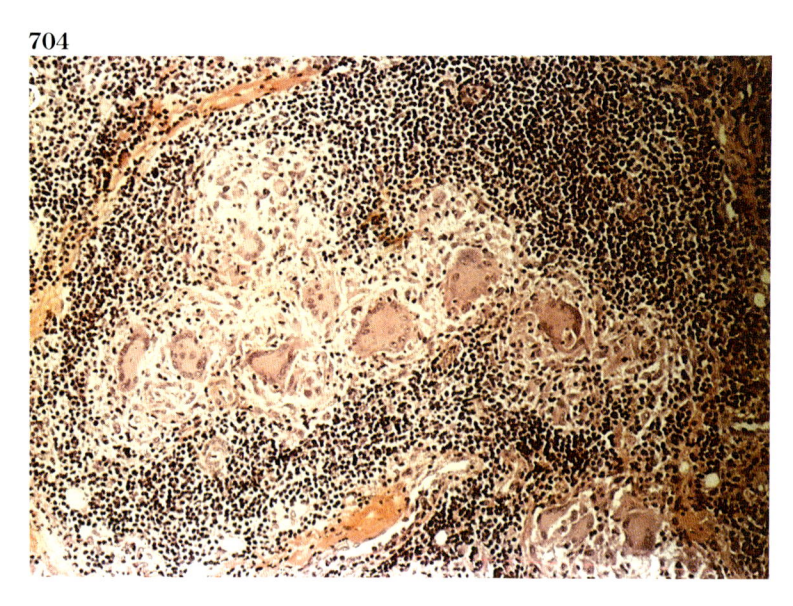

704 Histopathology of active tuberculoid leprosy The presence in this biopsy of granulomata containing numerous epithelioid cells and Langhan's giant cells is characteristic of the healing response in TT cases. No bacilli are visible. (H&E × 40)

705 Histopathology of lepromatous leprosy Very large numbers of acid-fast bacilli in vacuolated macrophages are present in this skin biopsy from a patient with lepromatous leprosy. (Ziehl-Neelsen × 500)

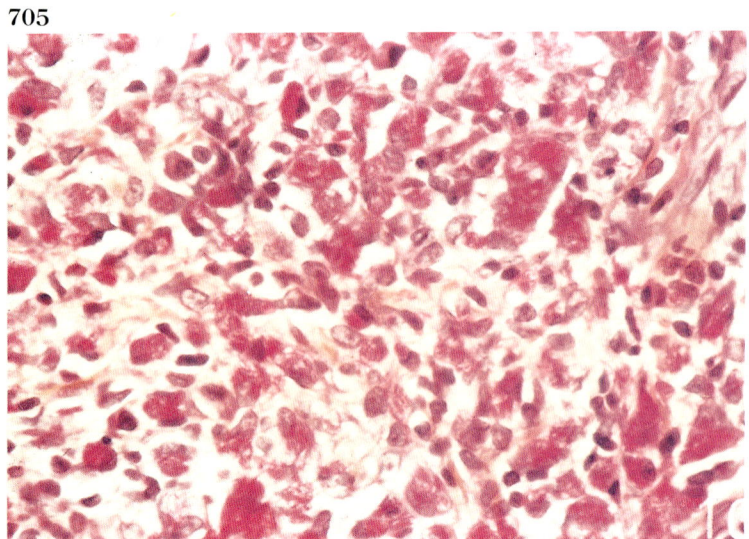

706 Biopsy of nerve in tuberculoid leprosy Cellular infiltration of the neural sheath leads to destruction of the nerve fibres which results in sensory and motor loss in the areas affected. This slide shows an epithelioid granuloma of a nerve. (H&E × 250)

707 Lepromin test The 'Mitsuda' reaction, which usually attains its maximum in four to five weeks, indicates the sensitivity of the patient to the mixture of antigens (prepared from leprosy bacilli) injected. The reaction is expressed in mm with or without ulceration and is read about the 21st day after injection. In patients with lepromatous leprosy the reaction is completely negative. In patients with tuberculoid leprosy it is variably positive.

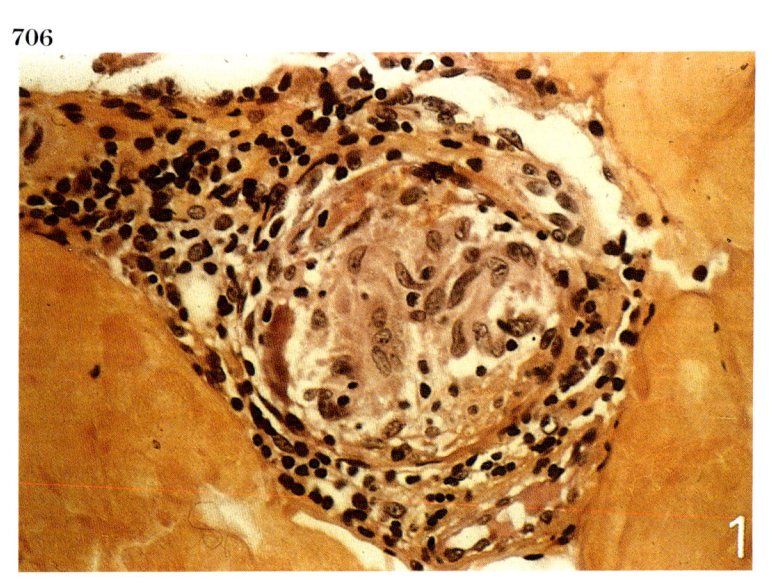

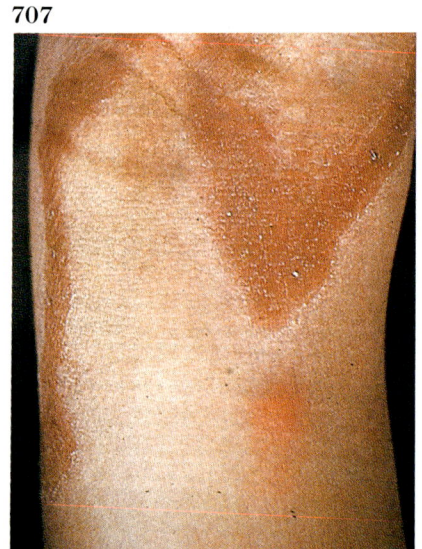

Mycobacterium ulcerans and Other Tropical Ulcers

708 Typical 'Buruli' ulcer in a Nigerian child The condition is characterised by gross, necrotising skin ulcers in which numerous acid-fast bacilli are present (*M. ulcerans*). The disease occurs in localised tropical areas in all continents.

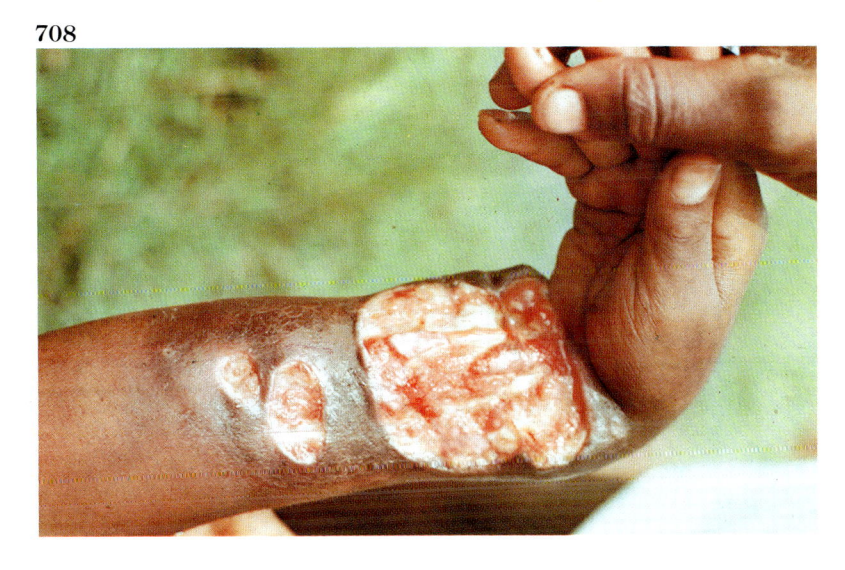

709 *M. ulcerans* in section of ulcer Acellular necrosis occurs involving the dermal layers and subcutaneous fat. Acid-fast bacilli are found in the necrotic material. (*Ziehl-Neelsen* × 900)

710 Tropical (phagedaenic) ulcer Chronic necrotising ulcers involving the skin and subcutaneous tissues are common in country areas in the humid tropics. They contain a mixed bacterial flora including *Borrelia vincenti* and a specific fusiform bacterium that has not yet been named.

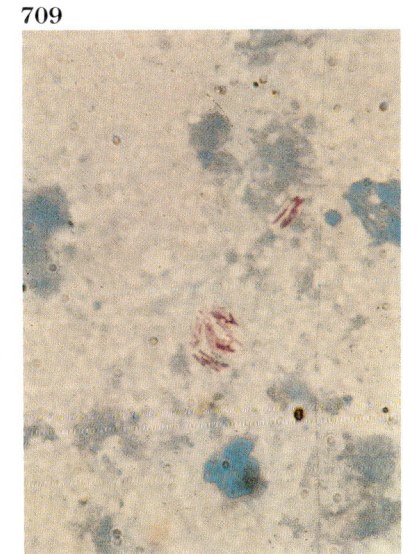

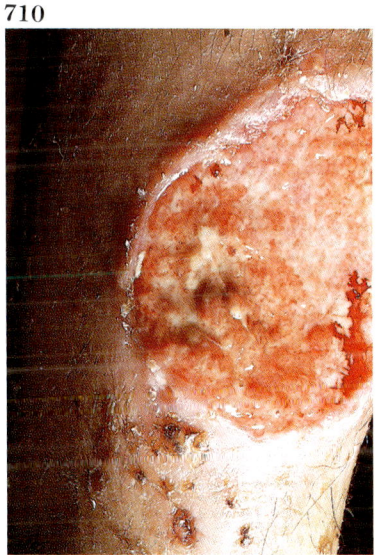

711 Bone involvement in tropical ulcer Sequestra result when bone involvement occurs.

712 Cancrum oris A gangrenous condition of the facial region associated with Vincent's organisms may follow any acute systemic disease in malnourished infants in the tropics. Gross disfigurement usually results.

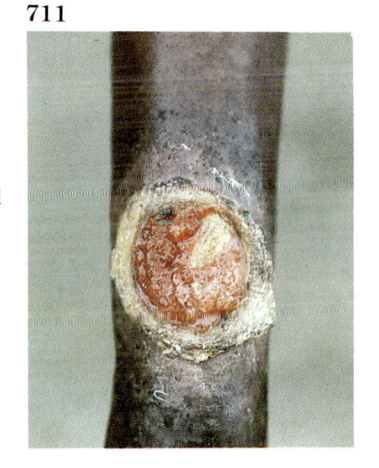

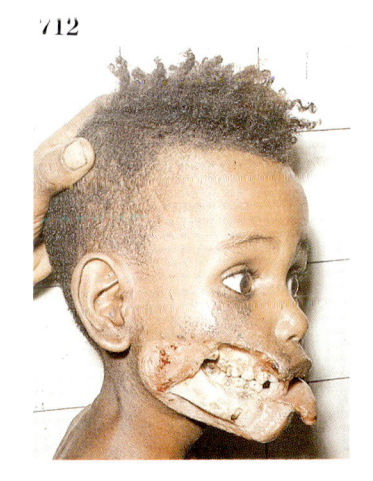

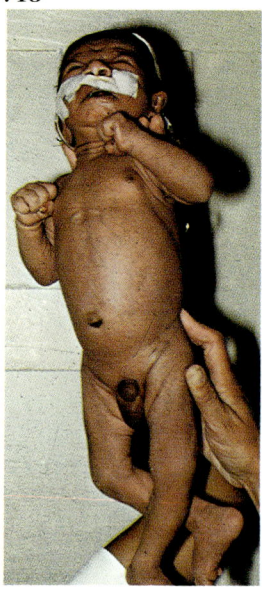

Tetanus

713 Tetanus neonatorum Tetanus is an important infection in the tropics. Infection through the umbilical cord is common in tropical conditions unless the mothers are previously immunised. One of the characteristic features is the 'risus sardonicus' resulting from spasms of the facial muscles.

Granuloma Inguinale (Donovanosis)

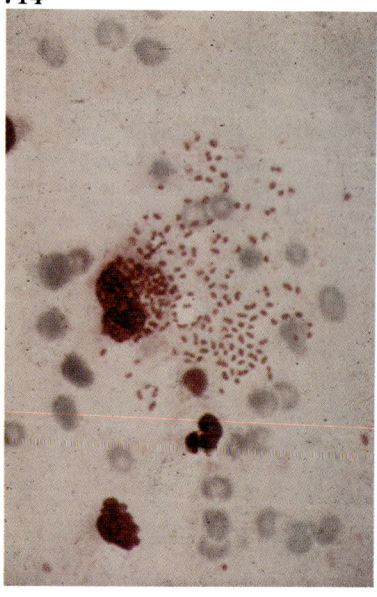

714 Donovan bodies in exudate *Donovania granulomatosis* is an encapsulated, Gram-negative coccobacillus which in lesions in man is seen within phagocytes, the 'Donovan bodies'. It is venereally transmitted (*Gram stain × 900*).

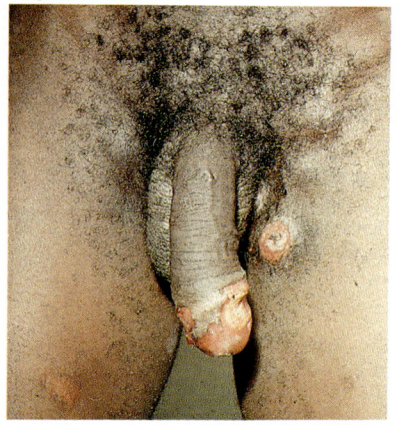

715 Donovanosis of penis and adjacent skin of leg The ulcerated lesion is deep and the floor is covered by a thick, offensive, purulent exudate. Secondary contact lesions are common.

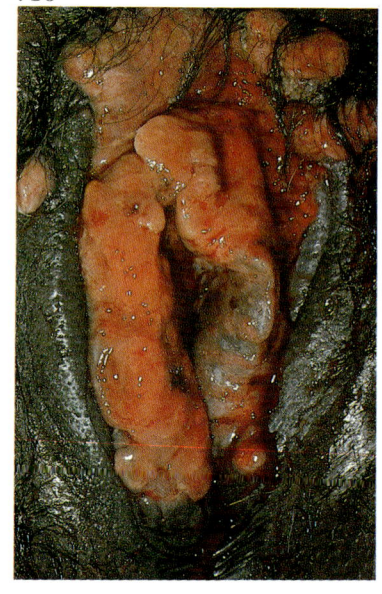

716 Donovanosis of female genitalia The disease runs a very chronic course. As in lymphogranuloma venereum, mutilating ulceration of the genitalia may occur and anorectal involvement is common. In comparison with lymphogranuloma venereum, the lymphatics are not primarily involved.

Gonorrhoea

717 Urethral discharge in gonorrhoea Gonorrhoea is widespread in the tropics where chronic gonococcal salpingitis is a common cause of infertility in women. Gonorrhoeal urethral strictures are often seen in men.

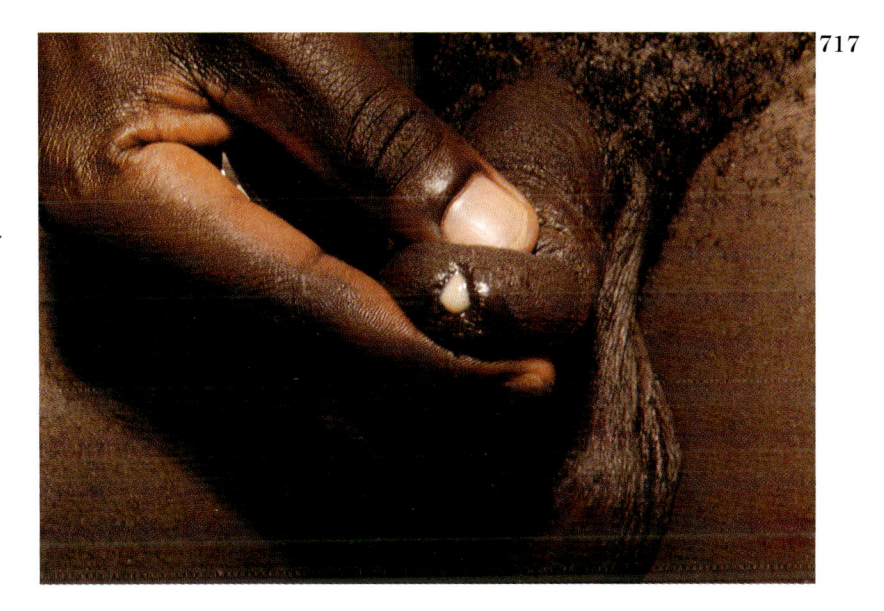

Yaws (*See also* **Table IV**)

718 Secondary framboesiform yaws Thanks to the mass penicillin-based eradication campaign of the 1950s, yaws is now a relatively rare disease in the humid tropics, although a new outbreak was recently recorded in Ghana. This Papuan child shows classical framboesiform lesions, caused by *Treponema pertenue*. Secondary lesions are frequent also at mucocutaneous junctions.

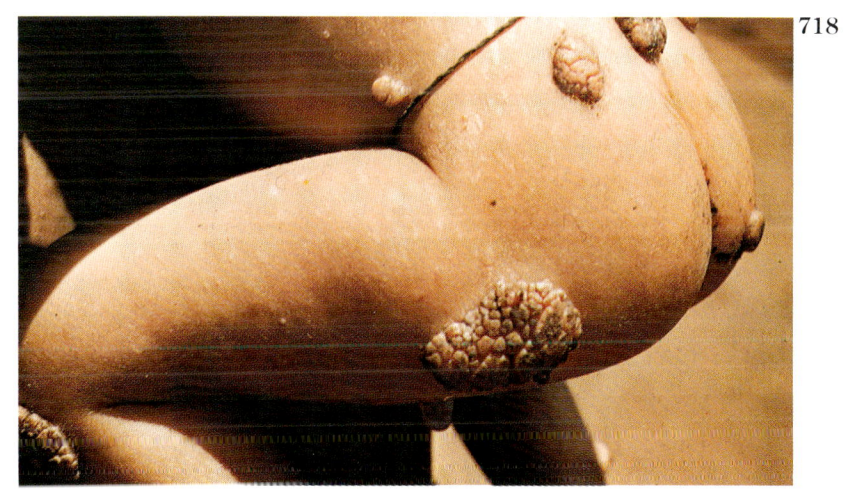

719 Plantar hyperkeratosis Hyperkeratosis of feet and hands is a common secondary phenomenon in yaws. This man's feet were seriously eroded.

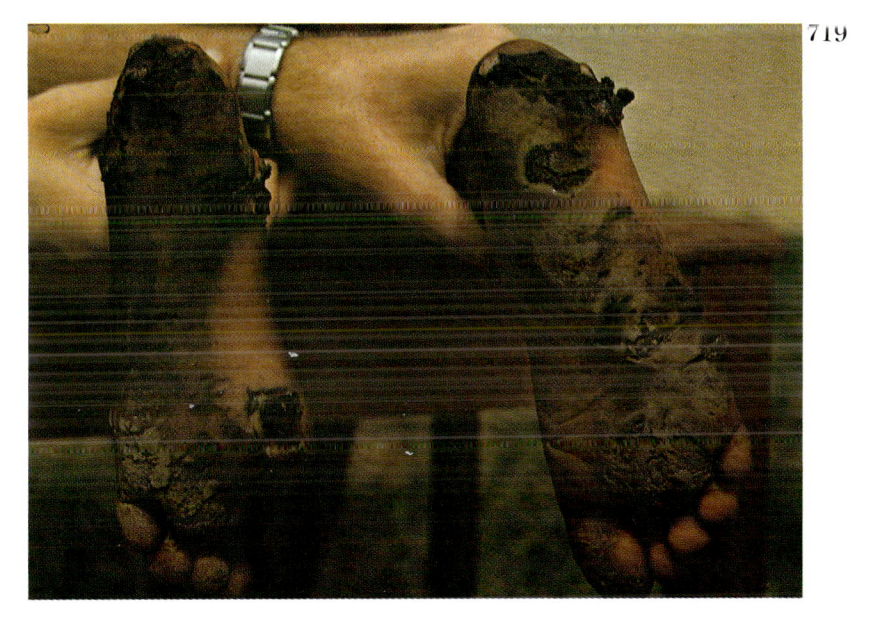

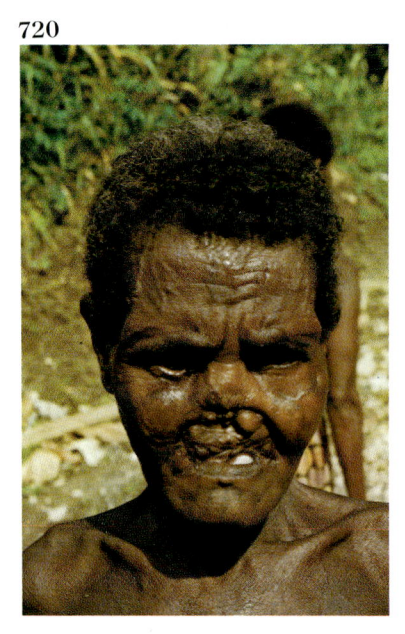

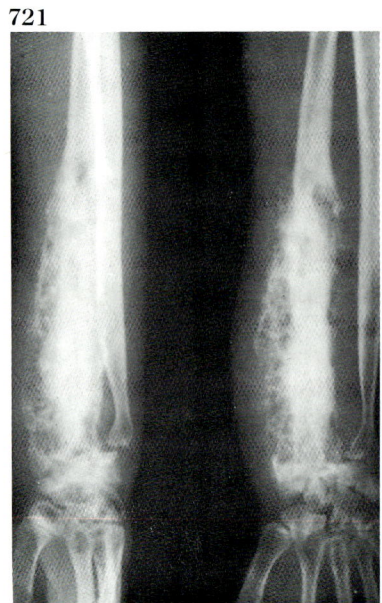

720 Gangosa The most advanced and destructive lesions affect the maxillary bones and hard palate, resulting in a condition known as 'gangosa'.

721 X-ray of forearm with yaws osteitis Focal cortical rarefaction and periosteal changes are seen, especially in the tibia ('sabre tibia'), but also in other long bones.

Syphilis

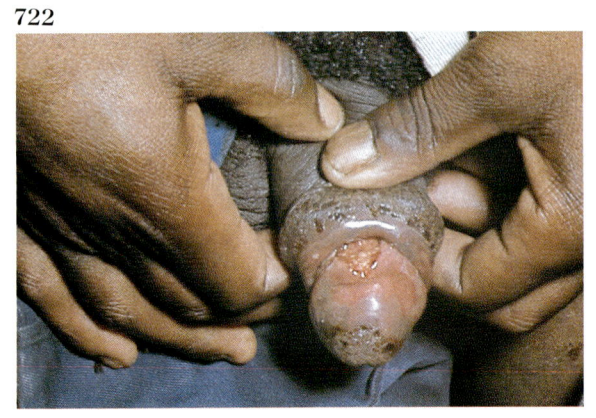

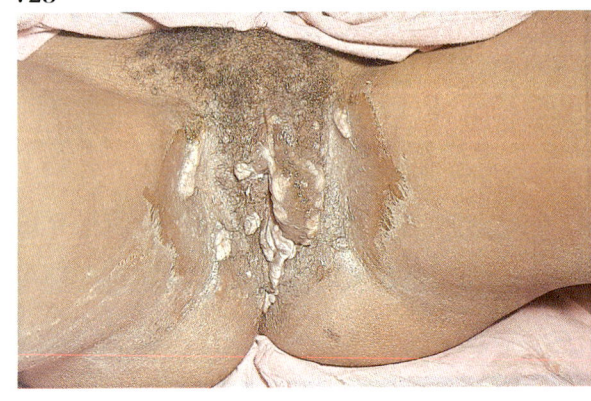

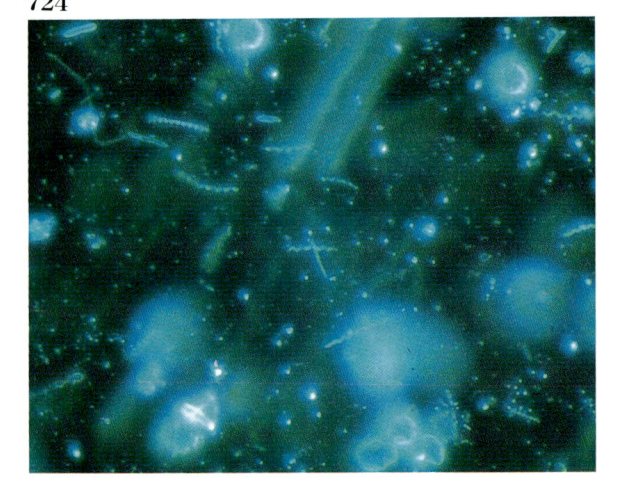

722 Primary syphilitic chancre Syphilis, the venereally transmitted treponematosis caused by *T. pallidum*, is widespread in many parts of the tropics, but did not occur where yaws was endemic. The figure shows a typical primary chancre.

723 Secondary syphilitic condylomata in the female The condition is readily diagnosed by the demonstration of spirochaetes in a dark-field preparation.

724 *Treponema pallidum* **in dark-field microscopy** ($\times 600$)

Non-venereal Treponematoses

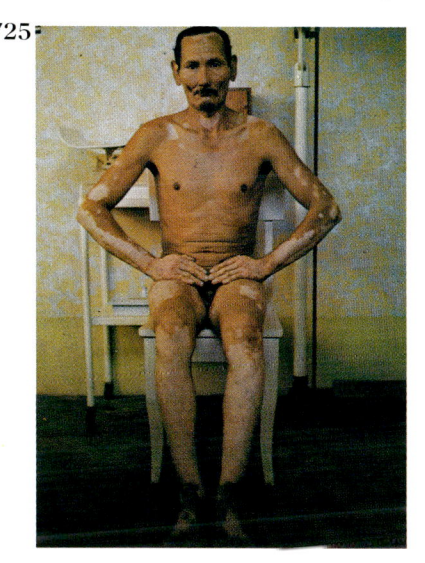

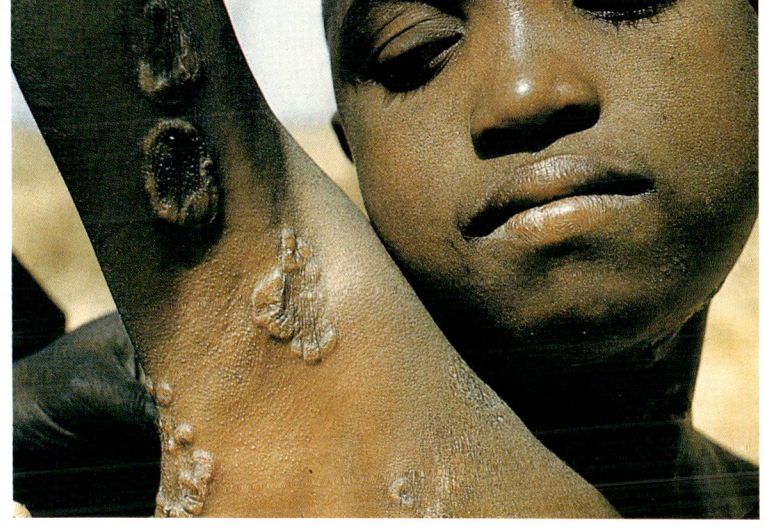

725 Depigmented lesions of pinta Pinta is endemic in the New World from Mexico to the Amazon. 'Pintids' start as small papules and develop into plaques with actively growing edges which become confluent. In the late stages the 'pintids' become depigmented. The causative organism of pinta, *T. carateum*, is morphologically indistinguishable from that of syphilis and bejel.

726 Secondary rash in endemic syphilis These non-venereal spirochaetoses ('endemic syphilis') occur mainly in dry parts of Africa, the Balkans and Australia. A florid, secondary, maculopapular eruption and associated adenitis is usually the first sign. Tertiary complications including gangosa may develop. In the Middle East the condition is known as bejel. Other forms of non-venereal 'endemic syphilides' are njovera (Rhodesia), skerlievo (Borneo), dichuchwa (Botswana) and siti (Gambia).

PROTOZOAL INFECTIONS (*See also* Table XIII)
Trichomoniasis

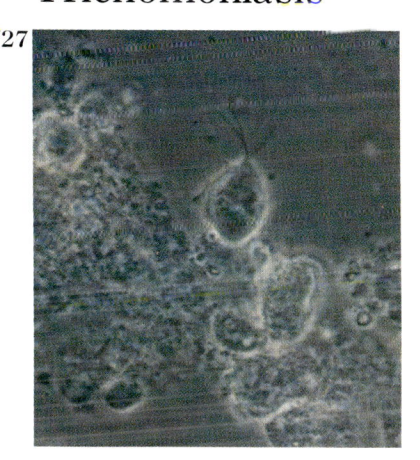

727 Living trophozoite of *Trichomonas vaginalis* The motile flagellate is found readily in the foamy vaginal discharge of trichomonal vaginitis. (*Phase-contrast × 900*) (*See also* **557**.)

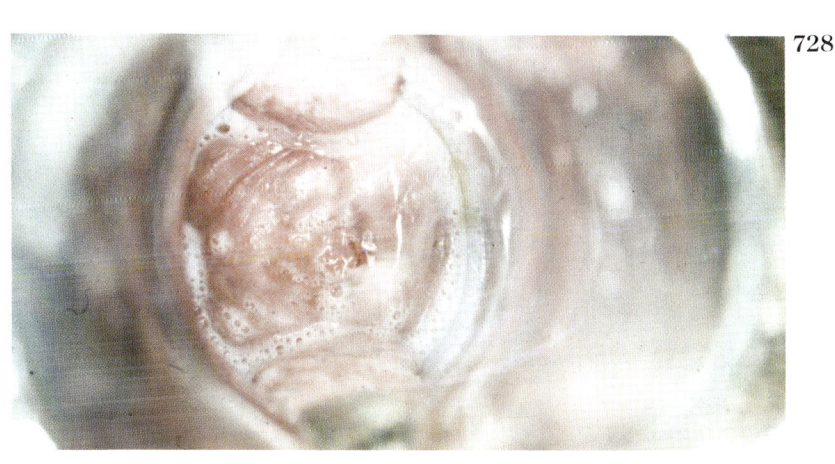

728 Trichomonal vaginitis The typical appearance of vaginitis as seen through a vaginal speculum. Note the creamy discharge which is often secondarily infected with *Candida albicans*.

Infection with 'Free-living' Amoebae

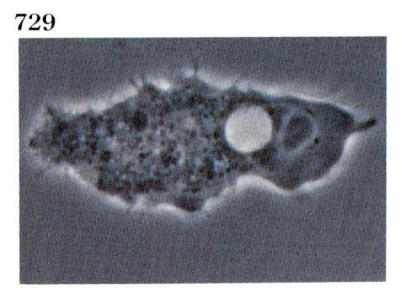

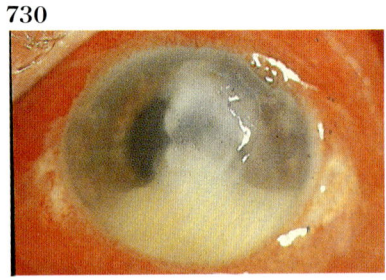

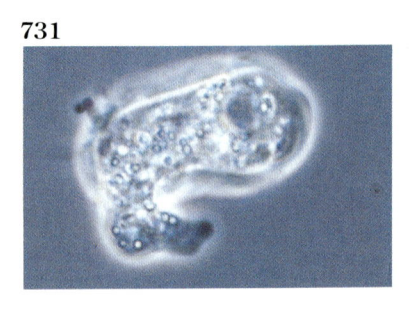

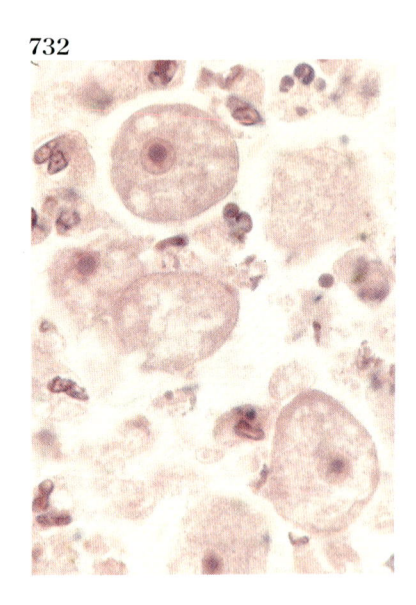

729

730

731

732

729 Living trophozoite of *Acanthamoeba culbertsoni* The 'prickly' appearance of the surface membrane from which these organisms acquire their name is seen clearly. A large vacuole is also present. Various species have been incriminated as the causative agents of chronic granulomatous encephalitis and infections of the eye (**730**), *A. culbertsoni* being the most notorious. The cysts which are resistant to desiccation are probably airborne. (*Phase-contrast × 900*)

730 Corneal infection with *Acanthamoeba species* This condition, previously rare, is increasing with the more frequent use of 'soft' contact lenses.

731 Living trophozoite of *Naegleria fowleri* Several species of *Naegleria* (Vahlkampfiidae) have been incriminated as the causative pathogens of amoebic meningoencephalitis, a condition with a high fatality rate that is usually acquired from bathing in warm water. *N. fowleri* has been isolated from such water in various swimming places, including thermal baths. As its cysts are susceptible to desiccation, its dispersal may be more restricted than that of *Acanthamoeba* species. *N. fowleri* develops a biflagellate form in water. (*Phase-contrast × 900*)

732 Section of brain containing *N. fowleri* Infection appears to be acquired through the cribriform plate of the nasal cavity following immersion in contaminated water. In this section from the brain of a Zambian who died of AIDS, the nuclear structure of the invasive trophozoites is clearly seen. (*H&E × 320*)

THE SUPERFICIAL MYCOSES (*See* Table XV)

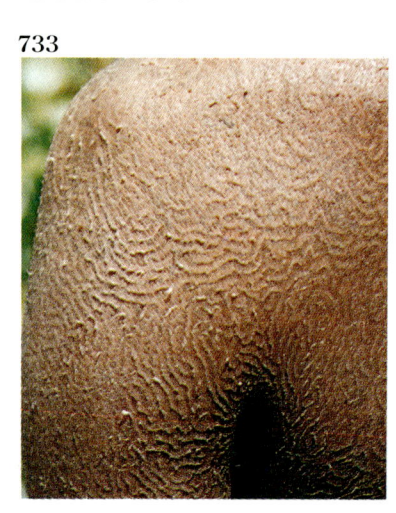

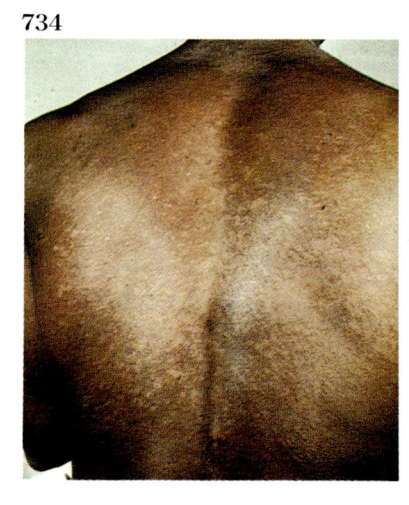

733

734

733. Tinea imbricata *Trichophyton concentricum* produces characteristic, superficial, scaly lesions in parallel lines and concentric circles. While it is common in the South Pacific and parts of the Far East, it is occasionally seen in other hot, humid areas.

734 Pityriasis versicolor This infection with *Malassezia furfur* is a common cause of hypopigmentation in dark-skinned young adults. Fluorescence of the patches in Wood's light helps to differentiate the condition from vitiligo and other depigmenting lesions.

THE SYSTEMIC MYCOSES (See Table XV)

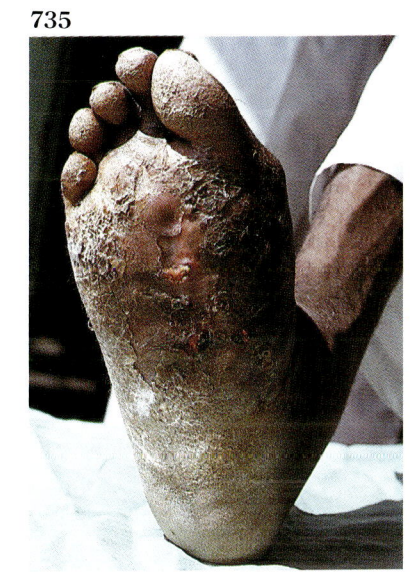

735 Mycetoma ('Madura foot') This chronic and disabling condition may be caused by a wide variety of organisms ranging from *Actinomycetes* to various *Fungi imperfecti*. This patient was seen in the Sudan where mycetoma is common.

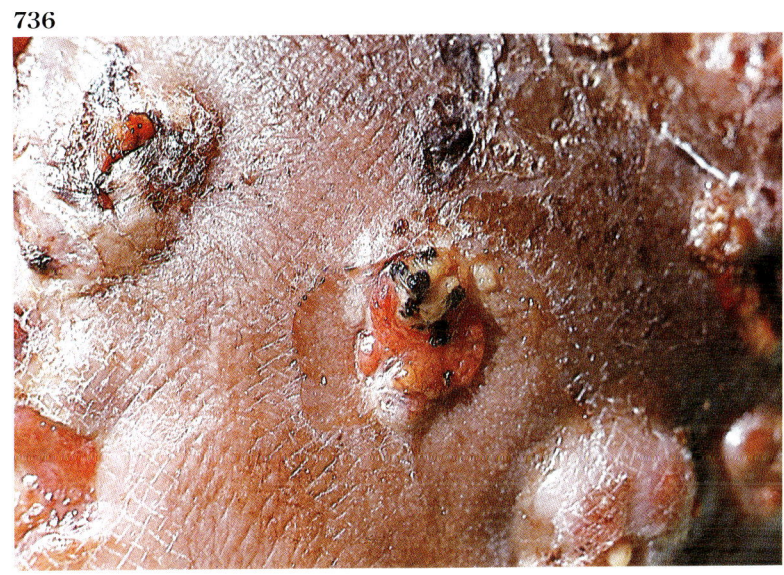

736 Fungal grains discharging Close-up of **735**, showing the coloured fungal grains being discharged from multiple sinuses.

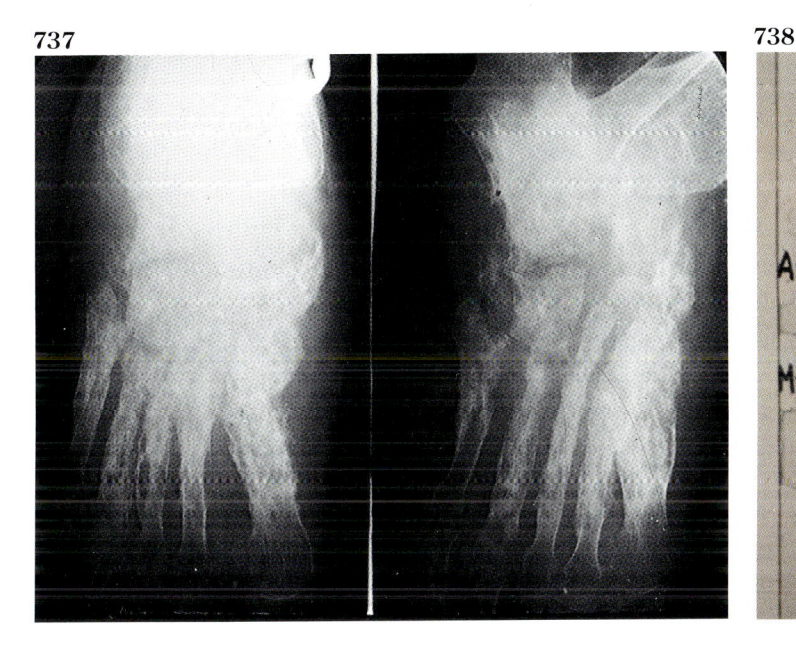

737 X-ray of Madura foot Infiltration of the tarsals and metatarsals occurs in late cases.

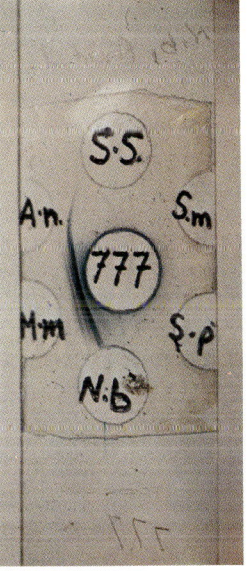

738 Serological diagnosis Fungal species identification can be made serologically. This serum contains antibodies to *Madurella mycetomae*.

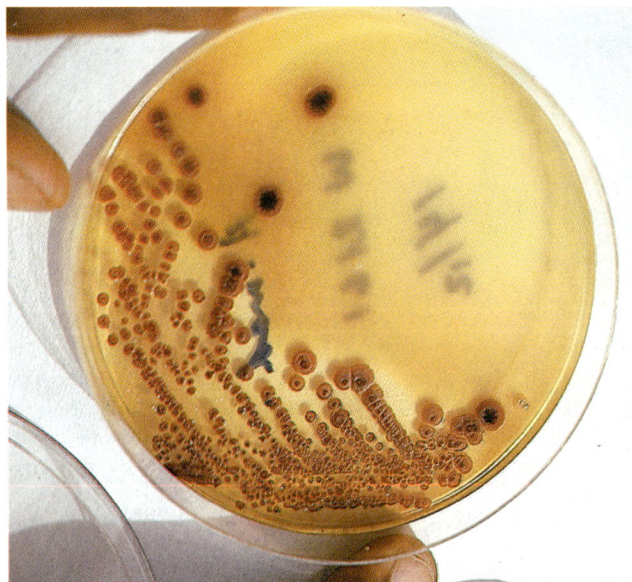

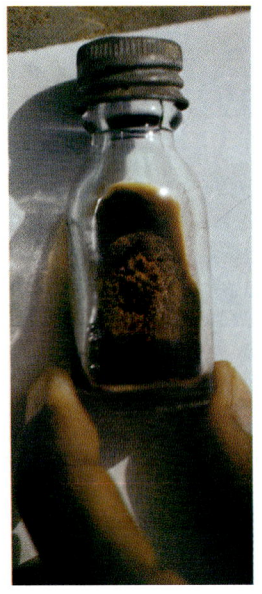

739 & 740 Culture diagnosis *M. mycetomae* (**739**) and *Streptomyces pellietieri* (**740**) on Sabouraud medium show typically shaped and pigmented colonies.

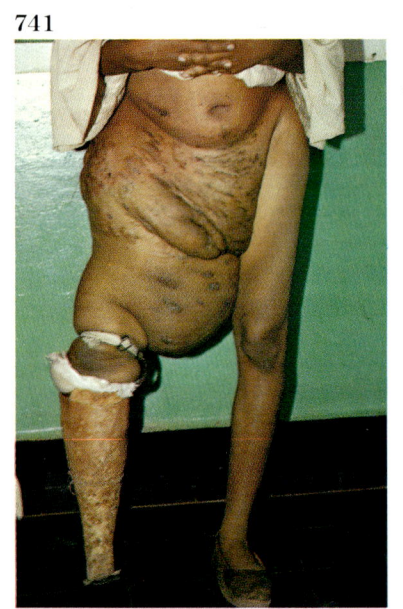

741 Chronic maduromycosis due to *S. somaliensis* infection Extensive sinus formation and osteitis have led to gross disfigurement in this Sudanese man.

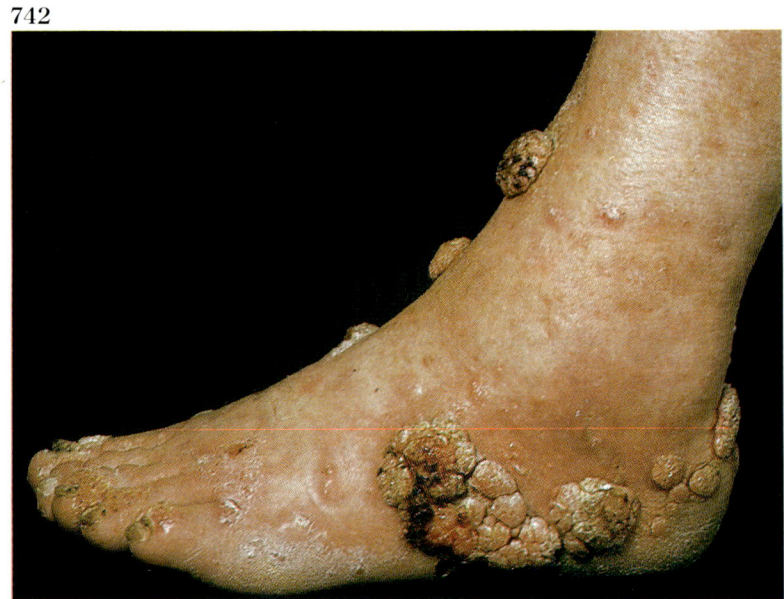

742 Early chromoblastomycosis The early lesions show a violet discoloration. The primary ulcer spreads slowly and is followed by verrucous lesions. This condition is seen in many tropical areas, including Queensland where this man was infected.

743 Verrucous dermatitis This is the late stage of chromoblastomycosis. The lesions are very chronic, usually painless but irritating. Lymphoedema follows lymphatic stasis.

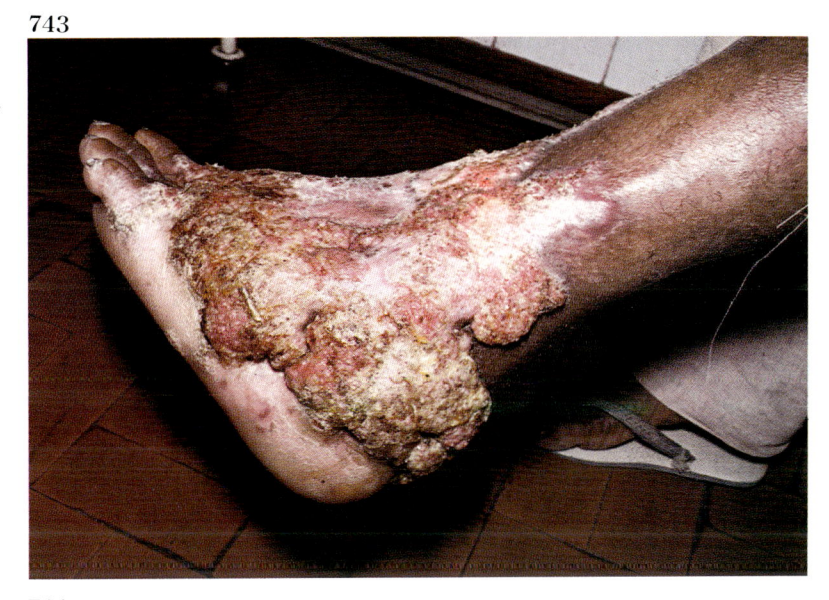

744 Lôbo's disease This condition, usually presenting with shiny, keloid-like lesions, produces a general picture similar to late chromoblastomycosis and occurs in the northeast of Brazil. It is caused by *Lôboa lôboi*.

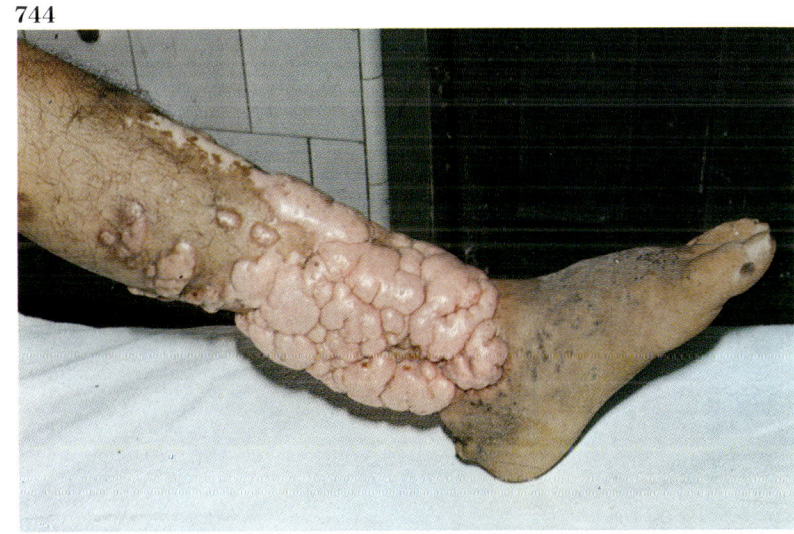

745 *Lôboa lôboi* The typical spores of this fungus are seen in this biopsy specimen from the keloidal lesions. (*H&E × 350*)

746 Mucocutaneous lesions in paracoccidioidomycosis Gross infiltration of mucocutaneous and mucous surfaces by *Paracoccidioides brasiliensis* may spread to the pharynx and larynx.

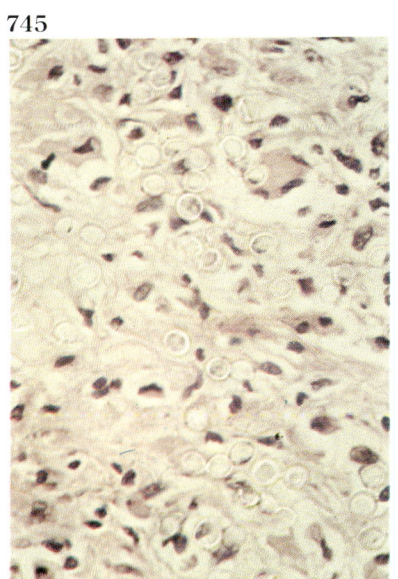

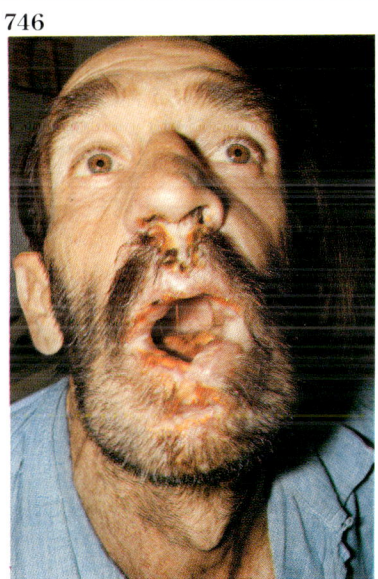

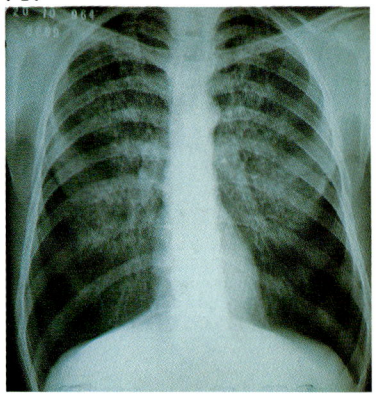

747 X-ray of chest in paracoccidioidomycosis Chronic pulmonary infiltration may result in fibrosis and eventual death from respiratory insufficiency in infections with *P. brasiliensis*.

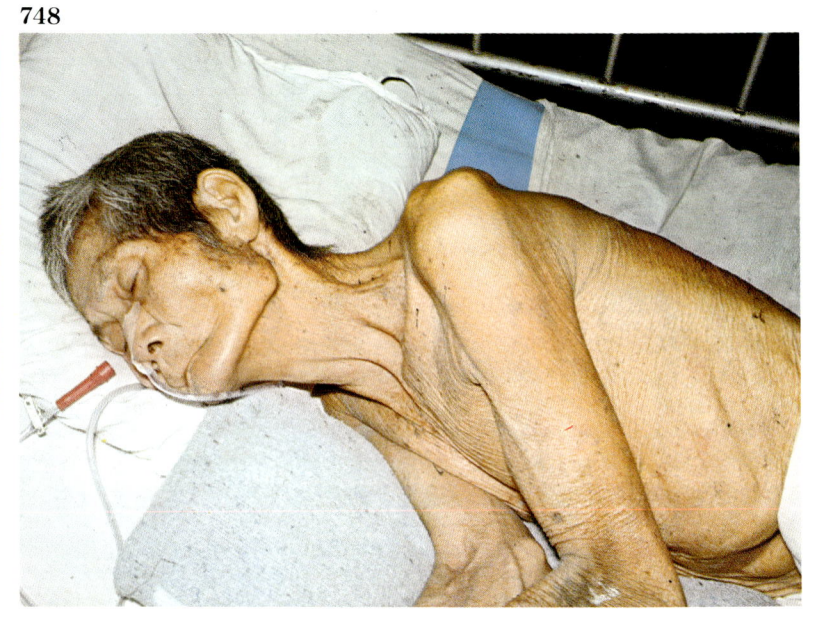

748 Cryptococcal meningitis

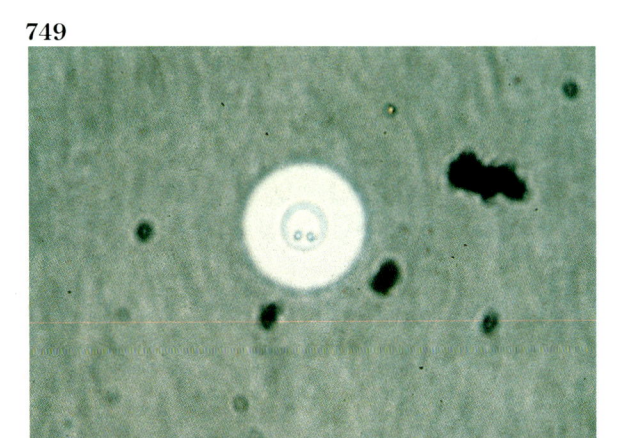

749 *Cryptococcus neoformans* in CSF The organisms are readily visualised in Indian ink preparations of infected cerebrospinal fluid from patients with meningitic infection. (× 500)

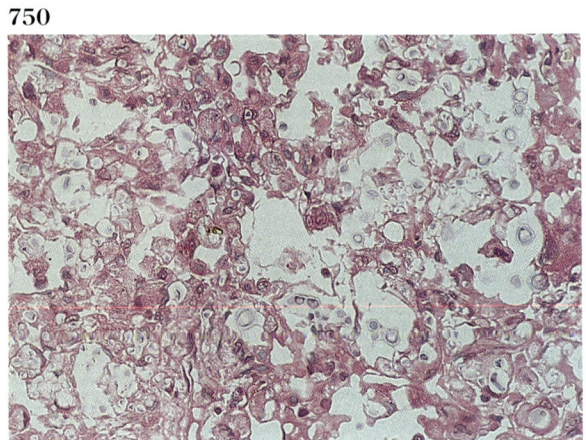

750 Lung in disseminated cryptococcosis This deep mycosis is one of the common opportunistic infections in Africans with AIDS. Numerous spores of *C. neoformans* are seen in this post-mortem section. (*PAS* × 40)

751 Lesions of sporotrichosis
The typical lymphatic spread with ulceration of secondary nodules is well shown in this figure of a patient seen in Belo Horizonte, Brazil.

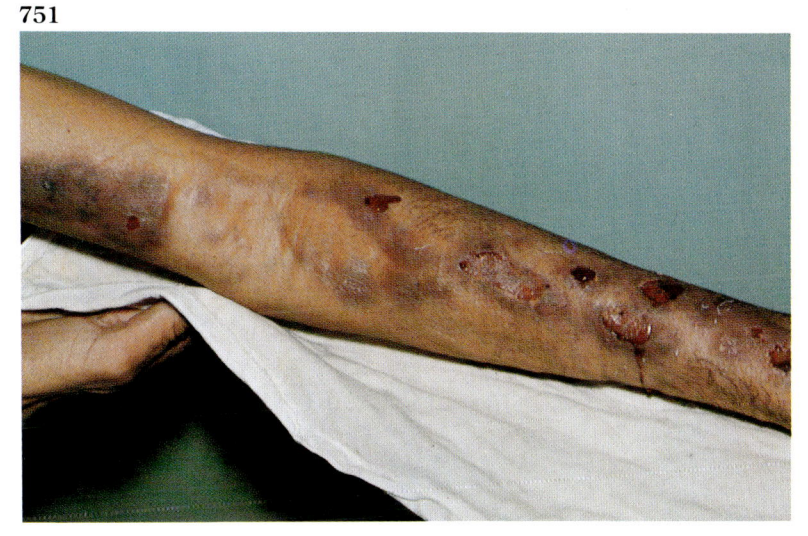

752 Sporotrichosis of the wrist
This patient was infected in Queensland. Like other deep mycoses, this infection occurs in a number of tropical regions.

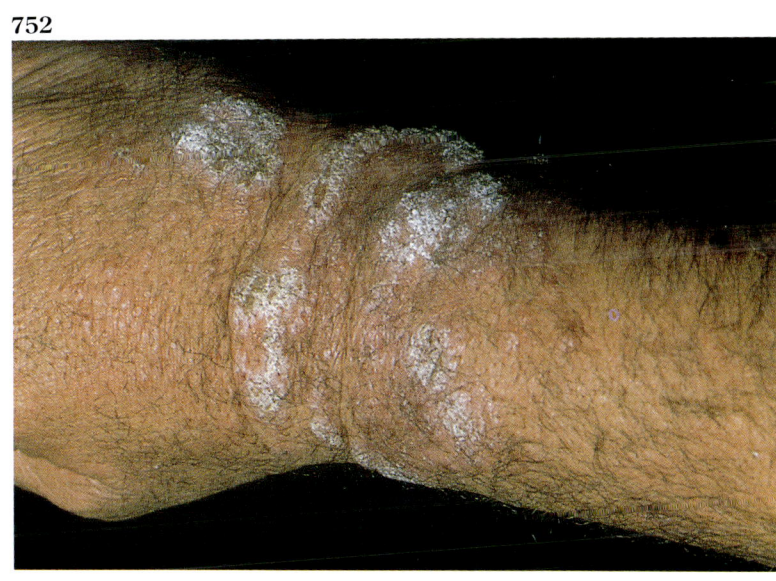

753 African histoplasmosis
Histoplasmosis caused by *Histoplasma duboisii* commonly produces large destructive lesions of the skin and subcutaneous tissues. Bones are often involved in the invasive process. Histoplasmosis has been reported as an opportunistic infection in AIDS sufferers in the Caribbean.

754 *H. duboisii* in biopsy The typical giant cell reaction to the presence of *H. duboisii* spores is seen here. (*H&E × 350*)

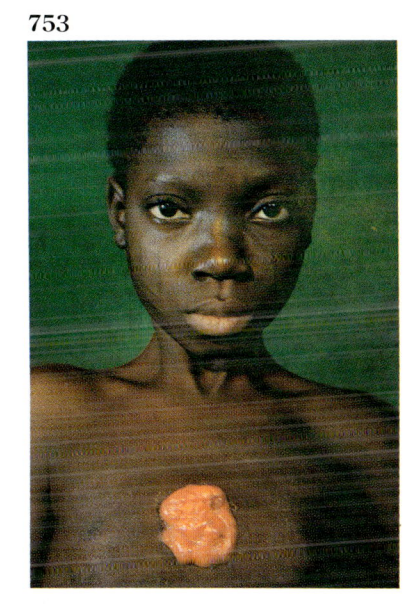

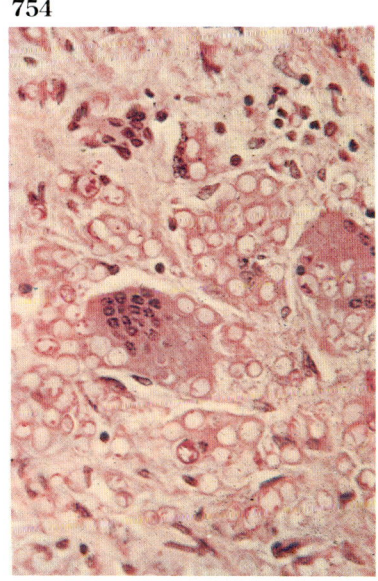

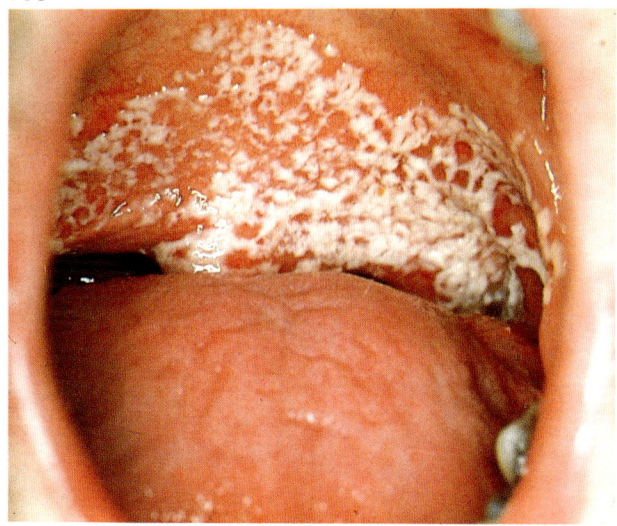

755 *Candida albicans* of the palate Severe candidiasis of the mouth and gastrointestinal tract is commonly seen in AIDS patients.

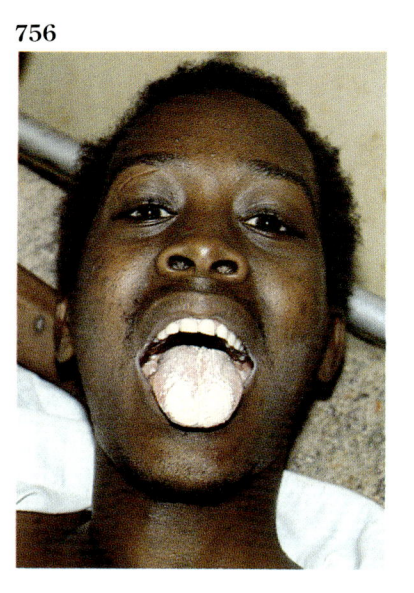

756 Oral candidiasis in an African with AIDS This patient with 'slim disease' had a very heavy *C. albicans* infection of his buccal cavity.

ECTOPARASITIC ARTHROPODS

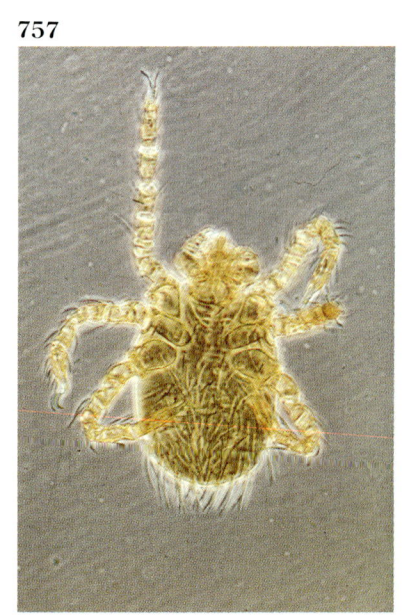

757 Larval *Trombicula autumnalis* These 'harvest mites' are common in grassland in temperate climates. The larvae, which normally feed on small mammals and birds, also attack man causing intense irritation. ($\times 90$) (See also **30**.)

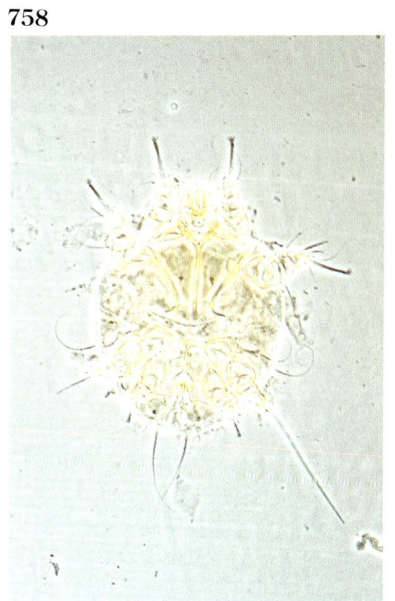

Scabies

758 & 759 Male and female scabies mites The gravid female *Sarcoptes scabiei* (**759**) burrows into the epidermis, lays its eggs and dies at the end of the tunnel. It is cosmopolitan in distribution. (*Ventral views* $\times 90$)

760 Infected scabies in a Papuan boy Intense local pruritus and dermatitis appear within a few days of infection. The tortuous tunnels may extend for several centimetres.

761 Secondary erythema in scabies Secondary infection is common and erythema may be associated with bacterial invasion of the sarcoptic tracks.

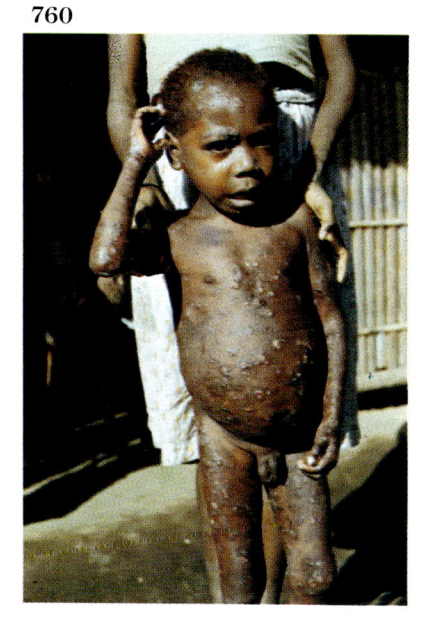

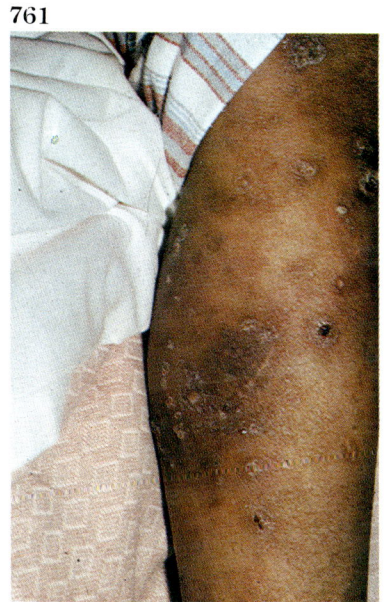

Tungiasis

762 & 763 Male and female *Tunga penetrans* The 'jigger' or 'chigger' flea occurs in tropical areas of South America and Africa. The gravid female buries itself in the skin, often under the toenails, and swells up to the size of a small pea. Eggs are laid through the entry hole. ($\times 20$)

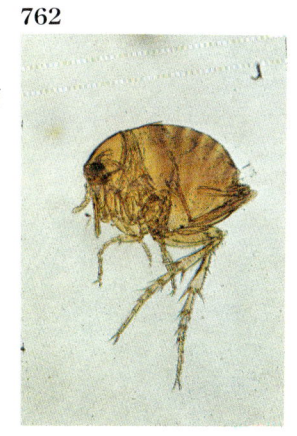

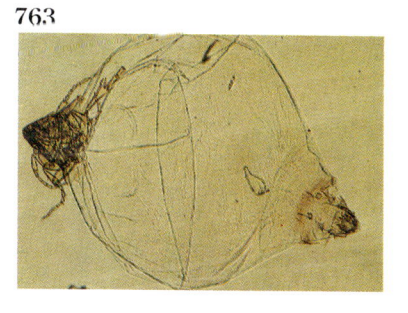

764 Jigger flea being removed from toe Habitual sufferers shell the gravid females out of the skin with a pin or sliver of bamboo, usually scattering eggs in the process. Tetanus is a common sequel to this type of self-treatment. The larvae mature to adulthood on the ground.

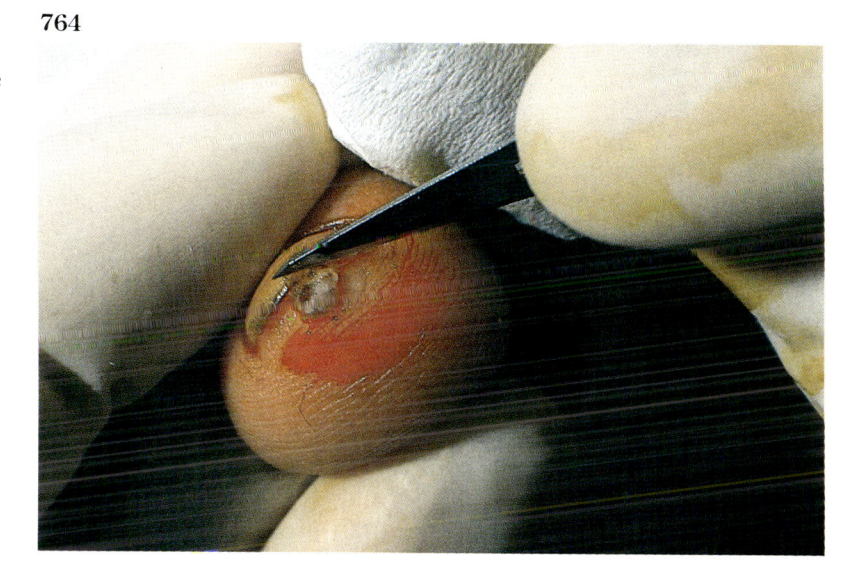

Myiasis (*See* **Table XVI**)

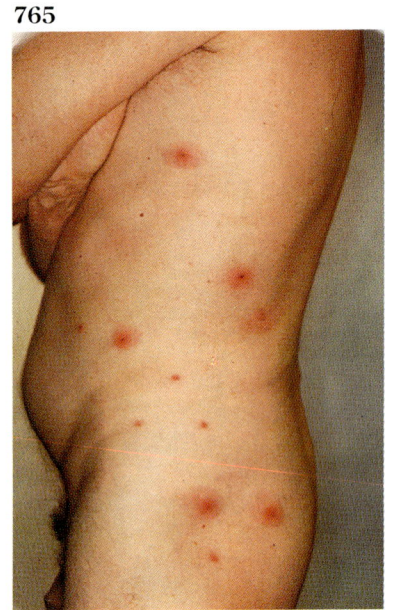

765 Tumbu fly lesions Multiple infections with larvae of *Cordylobia anthropophaga* caused painful boils on this man's trunk.

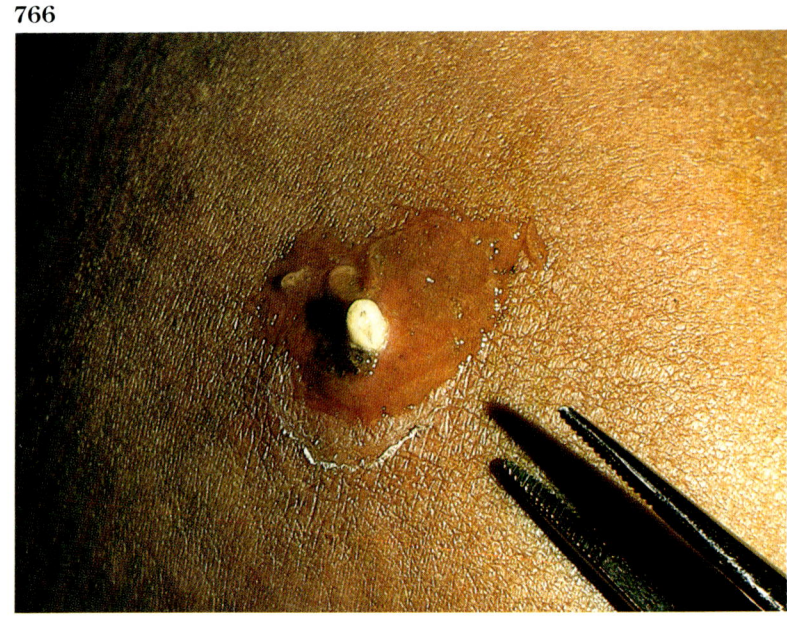

766 Extracting a larva The larva leaves the skin if it is covered in oil which blocks the spiracles. It can then be removed easily with forceps.

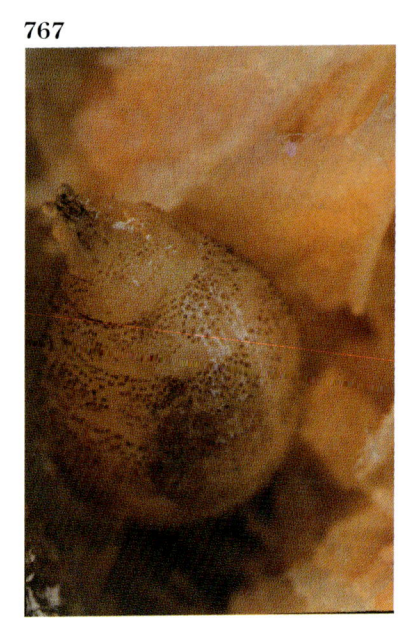

767 Larva of Tumbu fly The figure shows the powerful hooks with which the larvae feed inside the skin. (× 20)

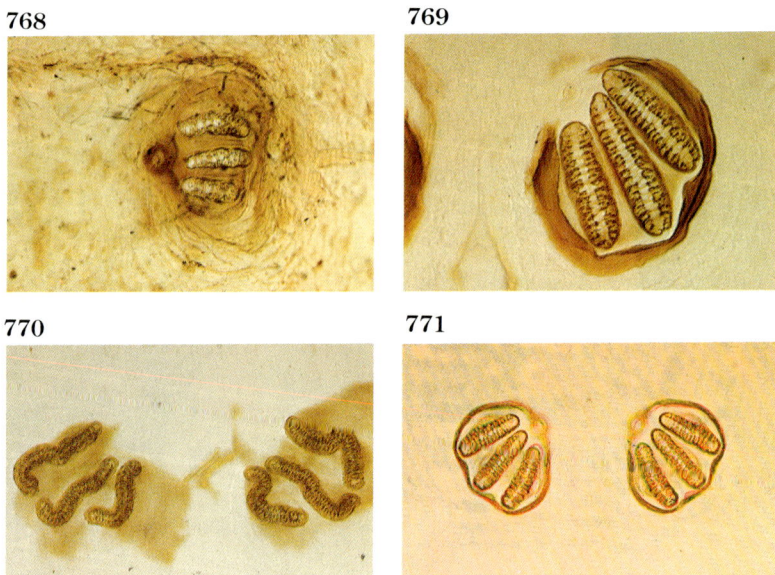

768-771 Larval spiracles of calliphorid flies *Auchmeromyia luteola* (**768**), *Chrysomyia* (**769**), *Cordylobia* (**770**), *Lucilia* or *Calliphora* (**771**). *A. luteola*, the 'Congo floor maggot', feeds on man by sucking blood nocturnally, but does not remain attached. The adult is similar to that of the Tumbu fly. The larva is separated from that of other Calliphorid flies by the distinctive posterior spiracles. (× 75)

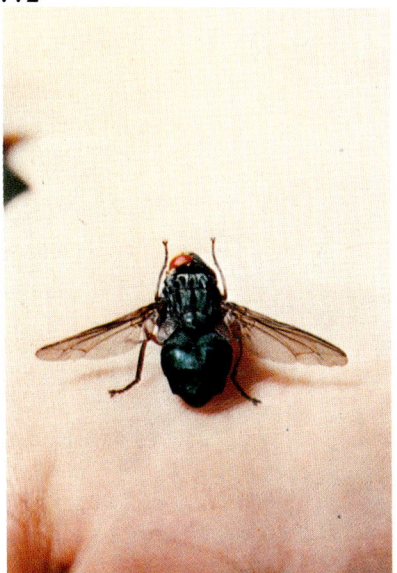

772 *Dermatobia hominis* The larvae of this fly are a cause of serious cutaneous myiasis in Brazil and other tropical areas of the New World. (*natural size*)

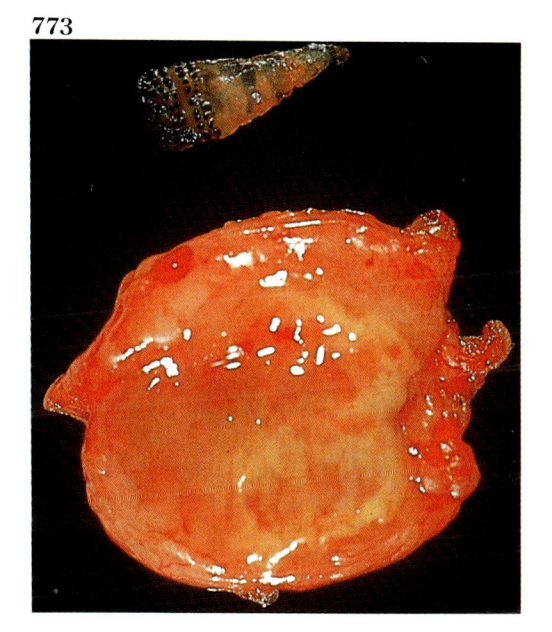

773 Larva of *D. hominis* The immature stages have characteristic rows of dark spines. This larva was extracted in Australia from the dorsum of the hand of a nine-month-old child who became infected in Venezuela.

Part VI
Airborne Infections

Infections of the upper respiratory tract are acquired mainly by the inhalation of pathogenic organisms for most of which man is the reservoir. Carriers play an important role and may represent the major part of the reservoir, e.g. meningococcal meningitis. The three main media for the transmission of airborne infections are droplets, droplet nuclei and dust.

Measles tends to be a severe disease in malnourished children, and in some epidemics in the rural tropics the mortality has been as high as 50 per cent. The infection not infrequently precipitates 'kwashiorkor'. Whooping cough is an important cause of infantile mortality in some areas of the tropics, while tuberculosis remains one of the major health problems in many tropical countries where it is being aggravated by dense overcrowding in urban slums. Tuberculosis presents a wide variety of clinical forms, but pulmonary involvement is common and is most important epidemiologically, since it is mostly responsible for the transmission of the infection. It is one of the major causes of death in Africans with AIDS.

Massive epidemics of meningococcal meningitis occur periodically in the so-called 'meningitis belt' of tropical Africa (see **778**). In this zone, the epidemics come in waves followed by periods of respite.

MEASLES

774

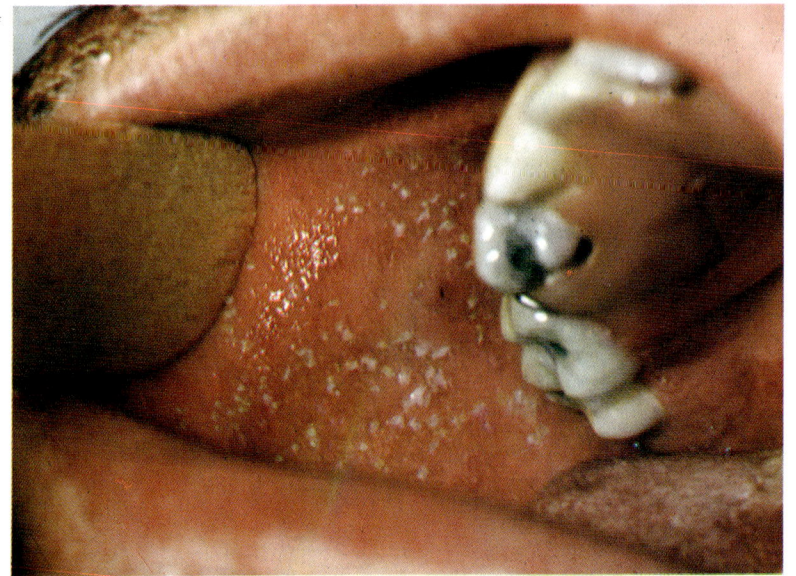

774 Koplik's spots Koplik's spots are pathognomonic of measles. They are found on mucous membranes during the prodromal stage and are easily detected on the mucosa of the cheeks opposite the molar teeth, where they resemble coarse grains of salt on the surface of the inflamed membrane. Histologically the spots consist of small necrotic patches in the basal layers of the mucosa with exudation of serum and infiltration by mononuclear cells.

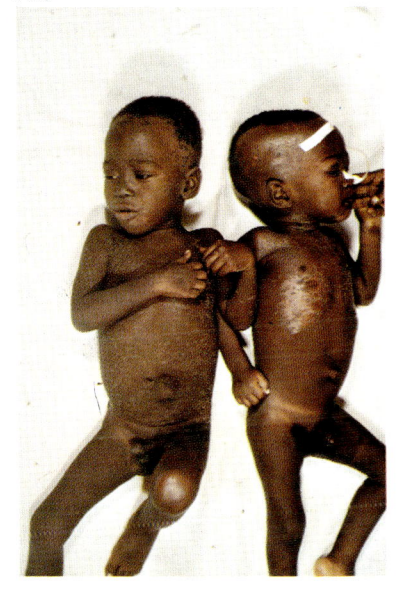

775 Measles in twins Measles is one of the most important causes of childhood mortality in the tropics. The twin on the left shows typical post-measles desquamation but is otherwise recovering. The other twin has post-measles encephalitis.

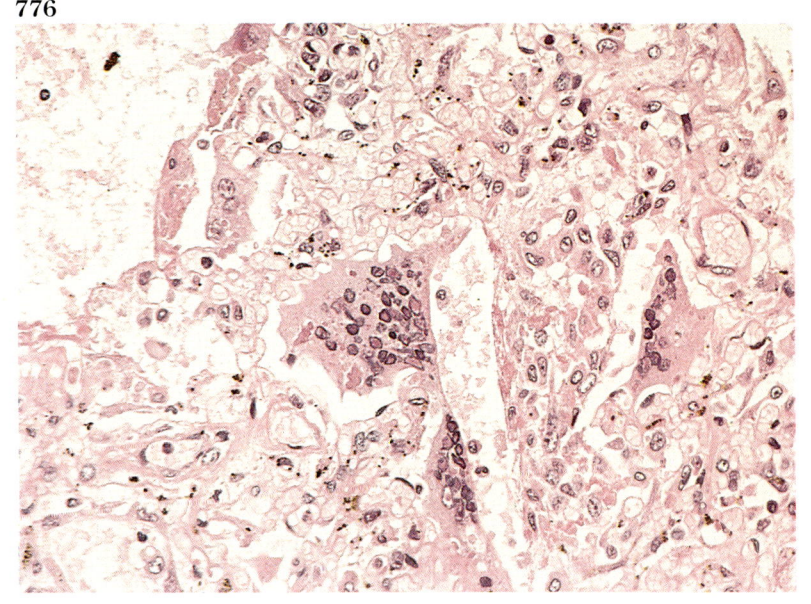

776 Lung in giant cell pneumonia Mortality is commonly associated with giant cell pneumonia during the prodromal stage. This section was from a 10-year-old girl who contracted measles while receiving steroid therapy for treatment of her nephrotic syndrome. (H&E × 500)

CYTOMEGALOVIRUS

777 Cytomegalovirus in a human hepatocyte This virus is the cause of death in up to 30 per cent of patients with AIDS in the US. One of the *Herpesvirus* group, it is present in the tissues of most normal adults, only becoming pathogenic in immuno-compromised subjects in whom it causes viral pneumonia. (× 2 100)

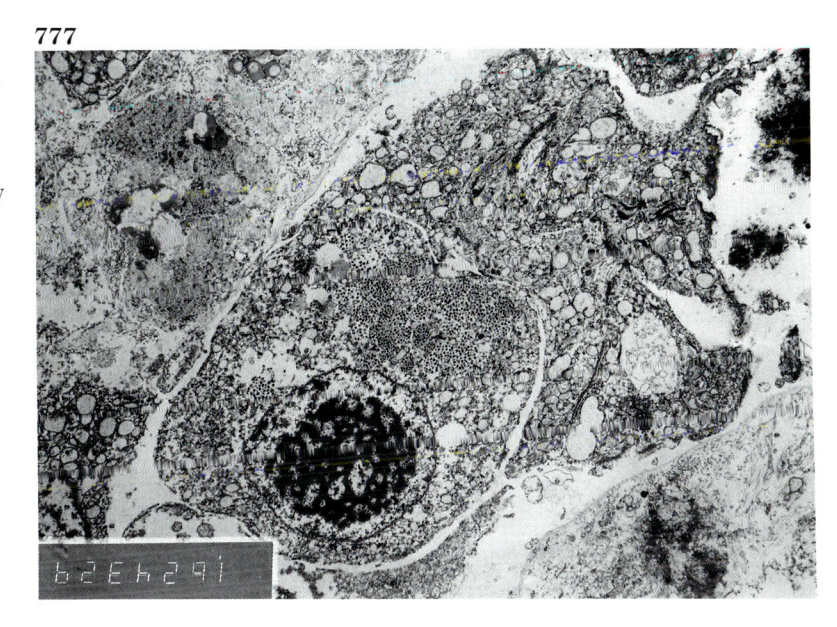

MENINGOCOCCAL MENINGITIS

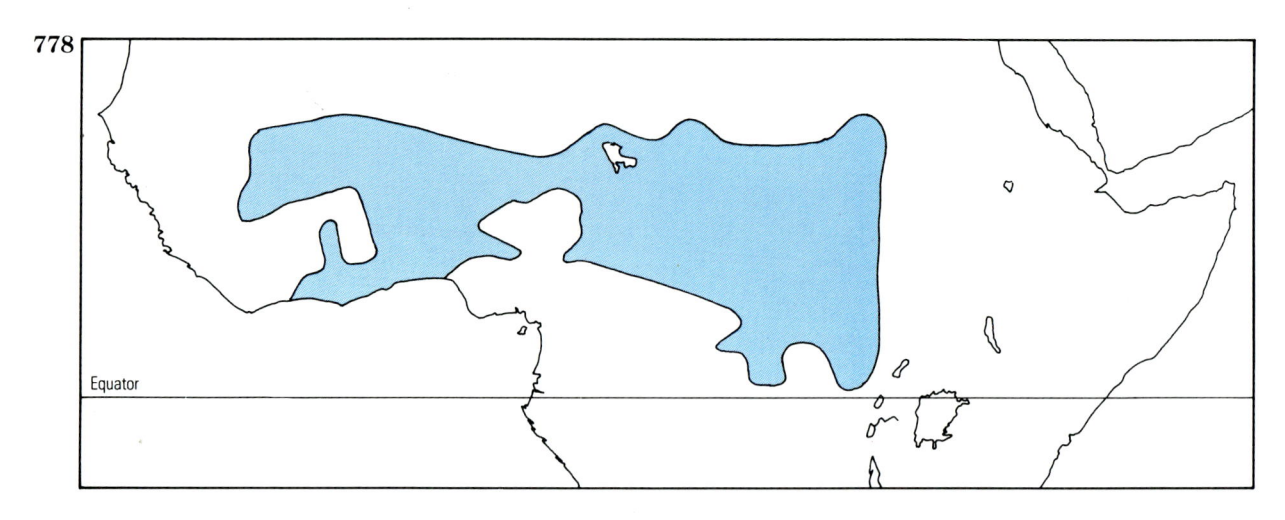

778 Distribution The 'meningitis belt' of tropical Africa, the zone lying between 5° and 15° N of the Equator, is characterised by an annual rainfall between 30 and 110 cm. The disease, however, is not limited to Africa. Overcrowding enhances the risk of acquiring the infection. Nearly 3 000 people died from meningitis in two Brazilian cities in 1974. Effective vaccines against types A and C are now available.

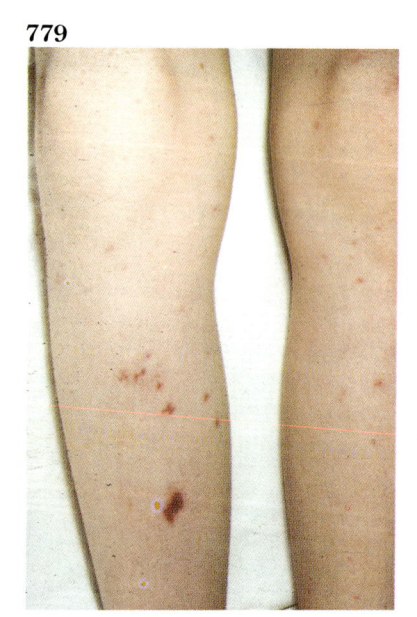

779 Rash of meningococcal meningitis The rash consists typically of irregular, scattered petechiae.

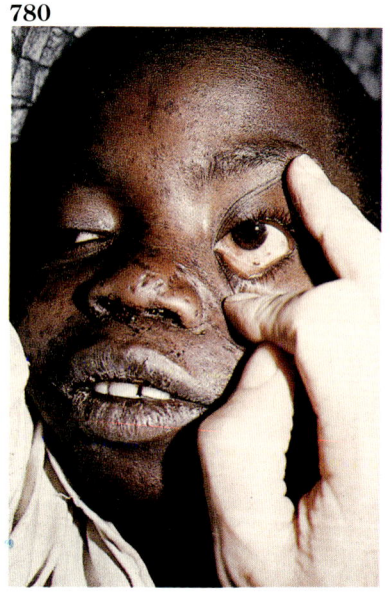

780 Petechial haemorrhages and epistaxis This Nigerian boy with meningococcal meningitis had repeated nose bleeds and conjunctival petechiae.

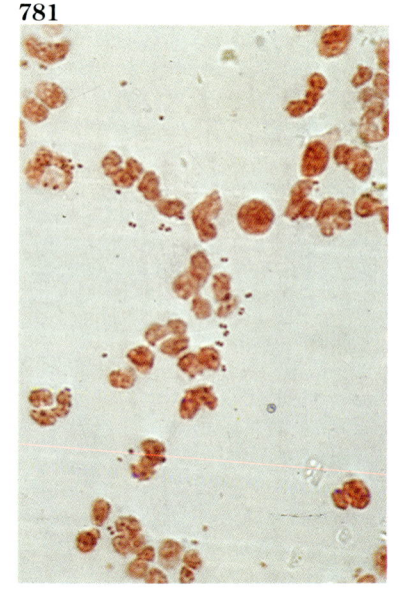

781 Smear of cerebrospinal fluid *Neisseria meningitidis* is a Gram-negative, bean-shaped diplococcal organism. In the 'meningitis belt' of Africa, type A is the causative agent of epidemics. (*Gram stain × 900*)

782 Latex agglutination test This sensitive serological test is valuable for the differentiation of meningococcal from pneumococcal and other types of meningitis.
(A - meningococcus antigen; B - pneumococcus antigen; C - *Haemophilus influenzae* antigen; D - negative control)

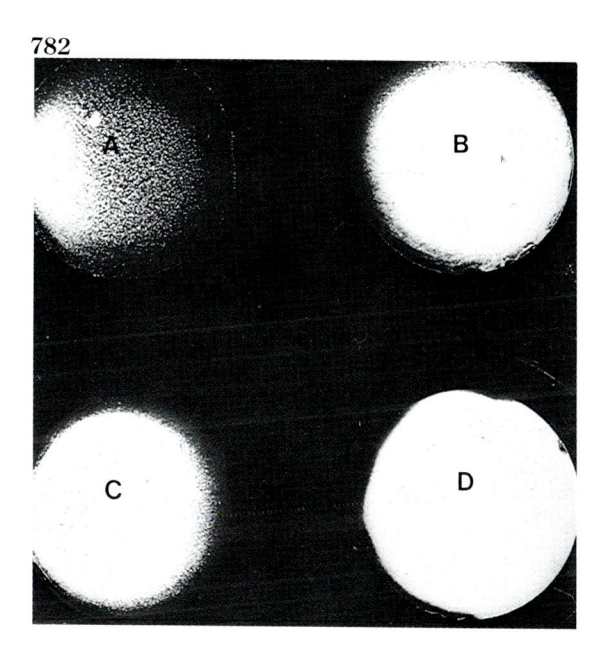

TUBERCULOSIS

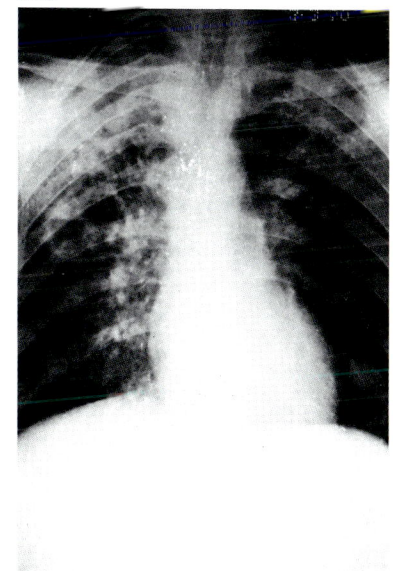

783 Acute pulmonary tuberculosis with cavitation
Tuberculosis remains one of the major health problems in the tropics. Pulmonary involvement is common and is most important epidemiologically, since it is responsible for the transmission of the infection. The incidence of fulminating tuberculosis in Africa parallels that of AIDS which is the underlying cause of the immunological breakdown in many individuals.

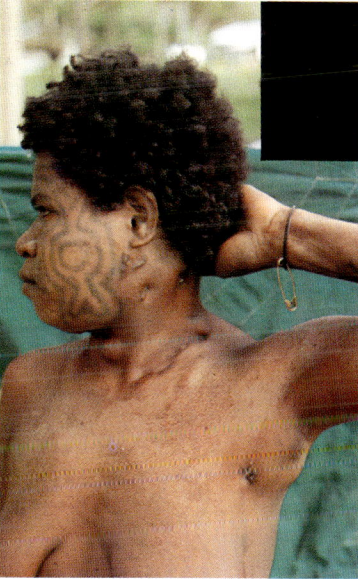

784 Tubercular glands Glandular enlargement due to human tuberculosis is not uncommon in many tropical areas. This woman is Fijian.

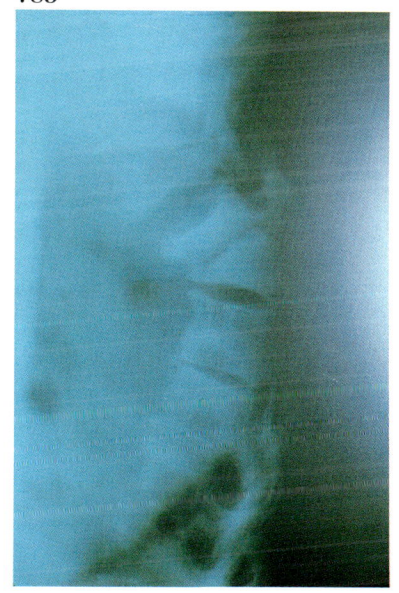

785 X-ray of spinal tuberculosis Bony lesions in the spine of this Papuan have the usual features as seen in developed countries.

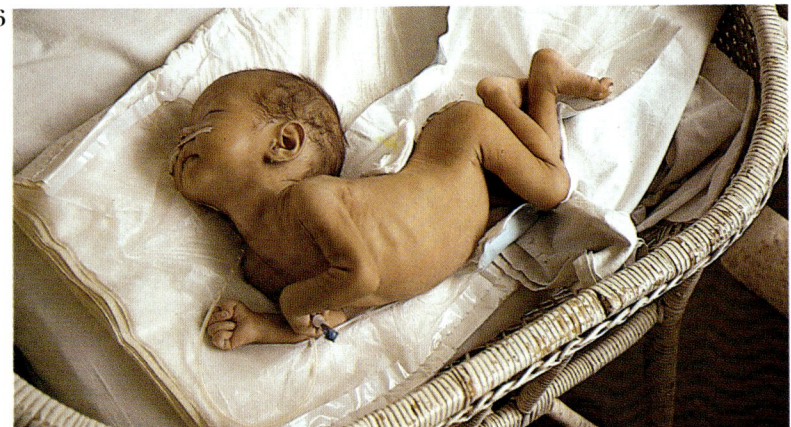

786 Tuberculous meningitis In babies, miliary tuberculosis and meningitis are killing infections. This three-month-old Nepalese infant died in spite of intensive chemotherapy.

WHOOPING COUGH

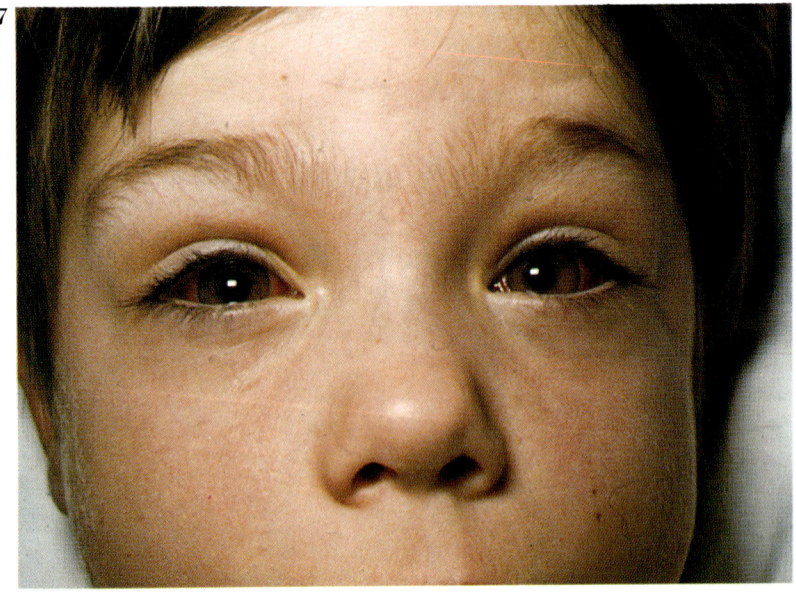

787 Child with whooping cough Whooping cough is an important cause of infantile mortality in the tropics. Subconjunctival haemorrhages are a common accompaniment of the severe coughing spasms.

Part VII
Nutritional Disorders

In large areas of the tropics, malnutrition, especially that affecting young children, is one of the principal causes of morbidity and mortality. The problem of feeding the populations of the world, and therefore maintaining an adequate status of nutritional health, is a serious one which has come to prominence, especially in parts of Africa, in recent years. Its magnitude and severity have still not received adequate attention and there is no completely reliable assessment of it in quantitative terms. Hunger, as manifest through famines or chronic undernutrition, has been recognised from prehistoric times. However, the problems related to the absence of specific nutrients have begun to be understood only relatively recently.

Human malnutrition is an ecological problem and the following intimately related factors may be involved in its pathogenesis: (1) food production and distribution; (2) food storage and processing, including contamination with aflatoxins; (3) demographic problems related to food, for example, the rate of increase of the population in most developing countries is over 2 per cent and yet the rate of increase of food production, in most areas, has not kept up with the population increase; (4) education and sociocultural factors; (5) food preparation and consumption; (6) the role of infection.

The United Nations agencies have estimated that about one third of the world's population goes to bed hungry every day, mostly in the countries of Asia, Africa and Latin America. The most 'vulnerable' groups are infants, pre-school children and pregnant and nursing mothers. Protein-calorie malnutrition is the name accepted now for a disease syndrome which includes kwashiorkor, believed to be largely due to an interaction between protein deficiency with other factors, and nutritional marasmus, which is due to a general deficiency of all nutrients, especially calories. In tropical communities one sees cases ranging from one extreme to the other.

Among adults, acute periods of undernutrition may occur in large populations because of failure of food crops, or catastrophes of one kind or another, e.g. floods, earthquakes, wars and failure of the rains.

The background of nutritional deficiency conditions is very wide and can be seen to be more dependent on the socio-economic level of the society than practically any other disease. Protein-calorie malnutrition is the most important nutritional problem of the whole world, though deficiencies of Vitamins A, B and D are also quite common. The nutritional deficiencies in many cases are complicated further by additional stress imposed by multiple parasitic infections such as intestinal helminthiases and malaria.

Many tropical diets are based on some staple carbohydrate foodstuff to which other substances are added fortuitously. These diets consist mainly of yams, cassava, rice, plantains, breadfruit and maize. Maize is a poor staple food at any time but when, in addition, the crop fails because of insect pests, famine may result. Such diets are badly balanced and lack total protein and other essential substances. They result in quantitative and/or qualitative deficiencies which are injurious to health.

KWASHIORKOR AND MARASMUS

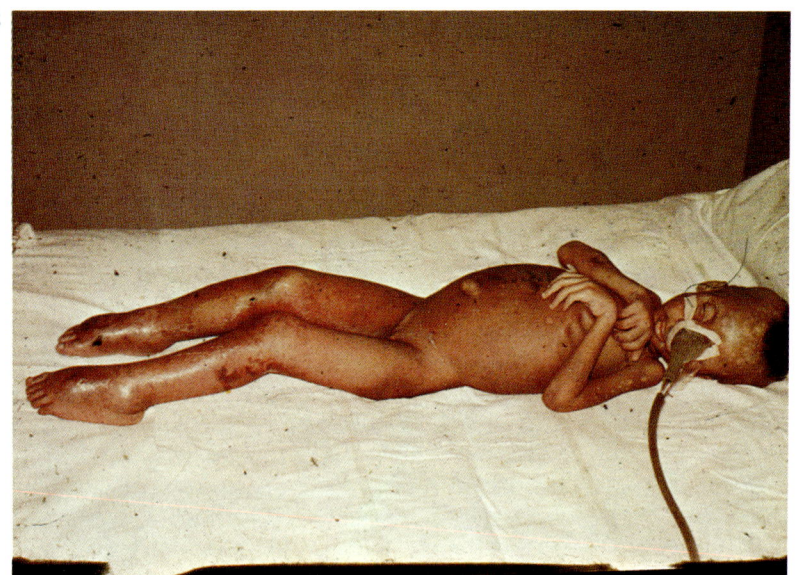

788 Oedema and hypopigmentation The presence of oedema may give a false impression that a kwashiorkor infant is well nourished. General hypopigmentation, together with some haemorrhagic skin lesions, are seen in this infant who died shortly after the photograph was taken. The exact cause of kwashiorkor is still debated. Rather than being due to simple protein-energy malnutrition, it is suggested that it is related to a deficiency in the diet of the trace element selenium which is essential to glutathione peroxidase mediated oxidation-reduction processes in the tissues. Aflatoxins and other so-far unidentified factors may also play a role.

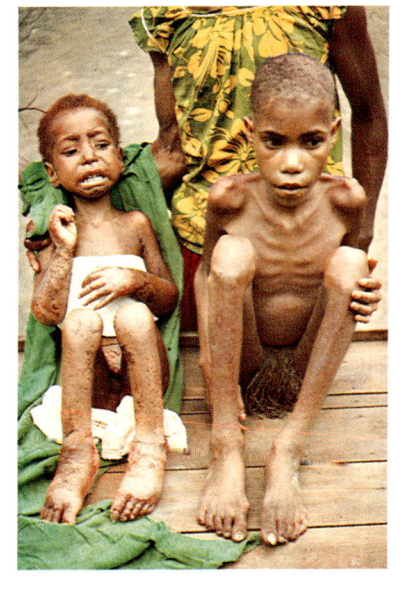

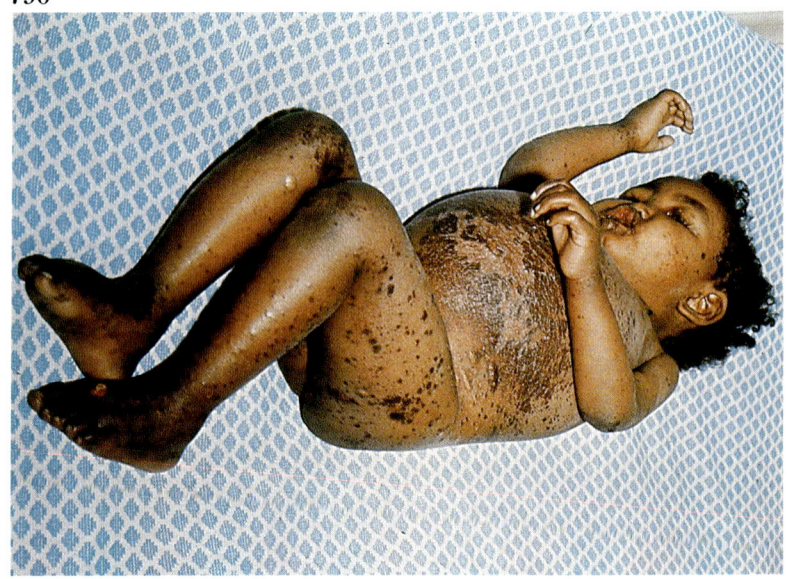

789 Kwashiorkor and marasmus in brothers Compare the miserable expression, pale hair, generalised oedema and skin changes in the child on the left with the marasmic wasting of his older brother. Kwashiorkor frequently follows acute infection and/or diarrhoea in a child during the weaning period.

790 Skin changes in kwashiorkor Serious skin changes, including erythema, followed by hyperpigmentation, 'black enamel skin' and peeling, may terminate in serious ulceration and gangrene. Note the ulceration where desquamation has occurred in this child.

NUTRITIONAL MARASMUS

791 Papuan child with nutritional marasmus Note the obvious wasting and dehydration in this marasmic infant, an all too common picture in times of famine when the total calorie intake is grossly insufficient. (The mother has tinea imbricata of the skin; *see* **733**.)

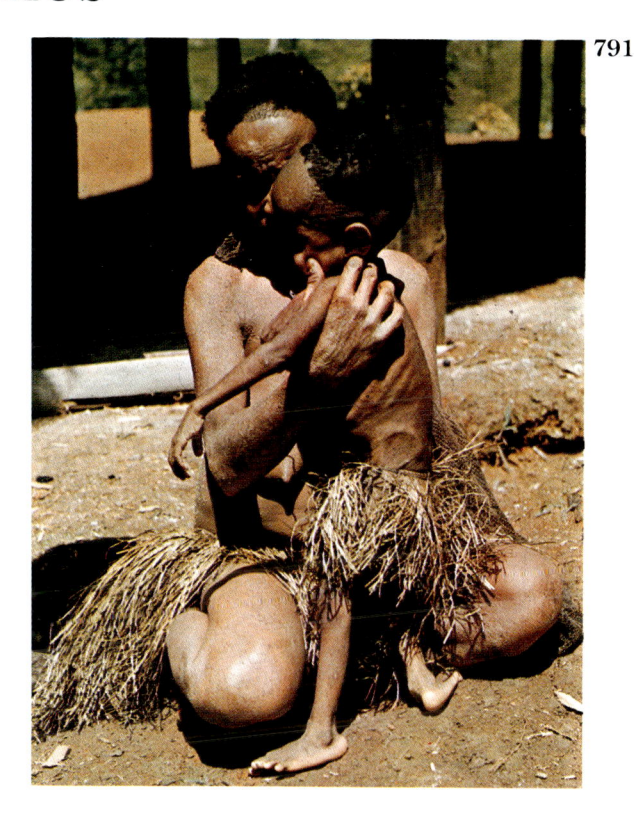

AVITAMINOSES
Vitamin A

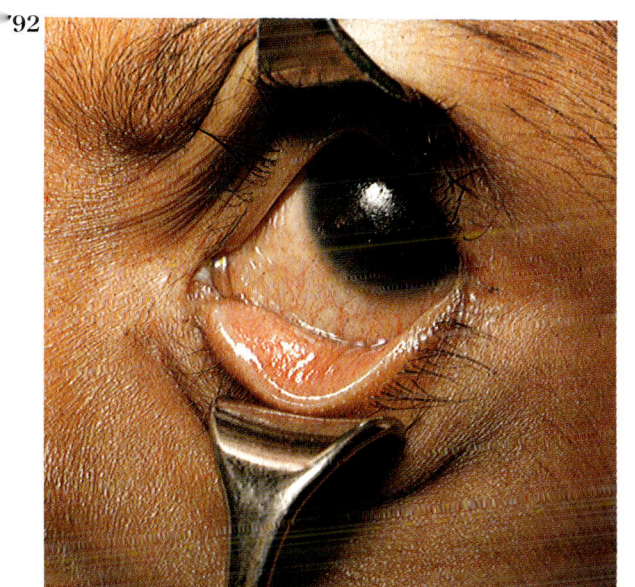

792 Xerophthalmia Vitamin A deficiency is a common cause of blindness among pre-school children in the tropics, especially in Asia. The dryness of the cornea and conjunctiva give the eye a dull, hazy appearance.

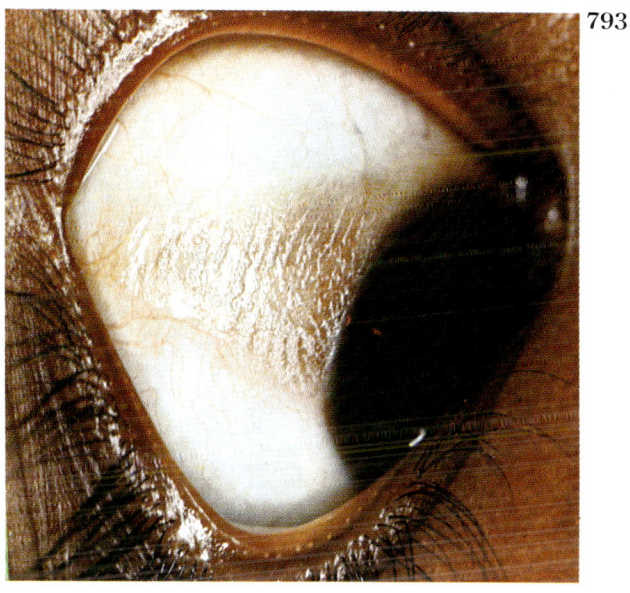

793 Bitot's spots These are silver-grey, foamy spots, usually external to the cornea and often bilateral. They are thought to be due to avitaminosis A.

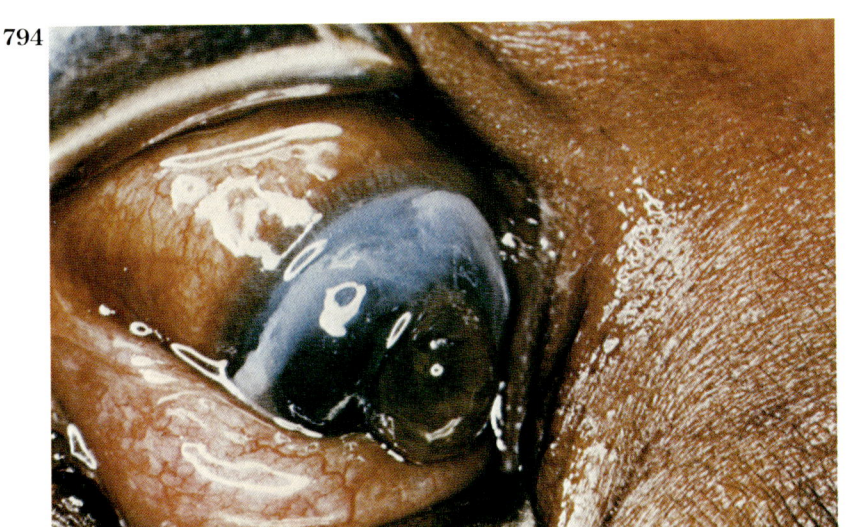

794 Keratomalacia A softening or coagulative necrosis of the cornea occurs in chronic, severe vitamin A deficiency. As for kwashiorkor, vitamin A deficiency may be precipitated by acute infections in undernourished children.

Vitamin D

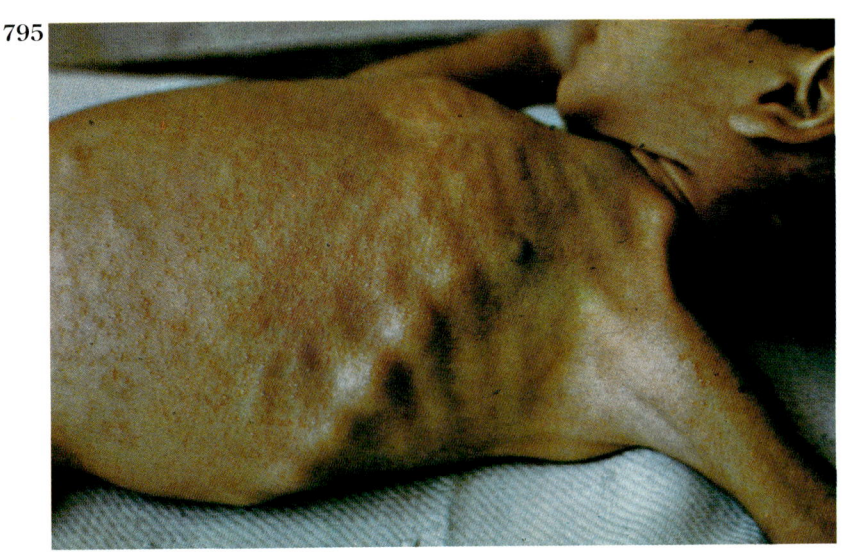

795 Infantile rickets—'Rickety rosary' This is a disease of infants and children due to insufficient vitamin D. Infants are sometimes overprotected from the sun by their mothers to avoid too rapid pigmentation of the skin and rickets occurs in this situation when it could easily be avoided. Rounded swellings that appear over the costochondral junctions near the sternum give rise to the term 'rickety rosary'.

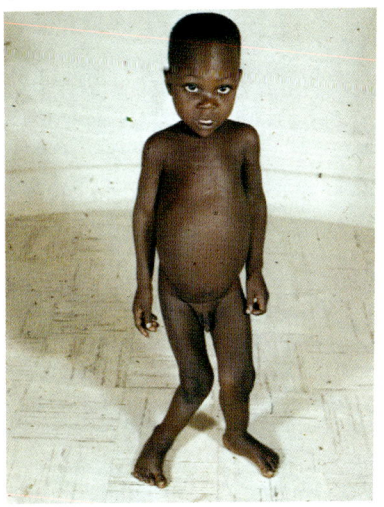

796 Infantile rickets Note the gross deformity of the legs and pigeon chest of this boy.

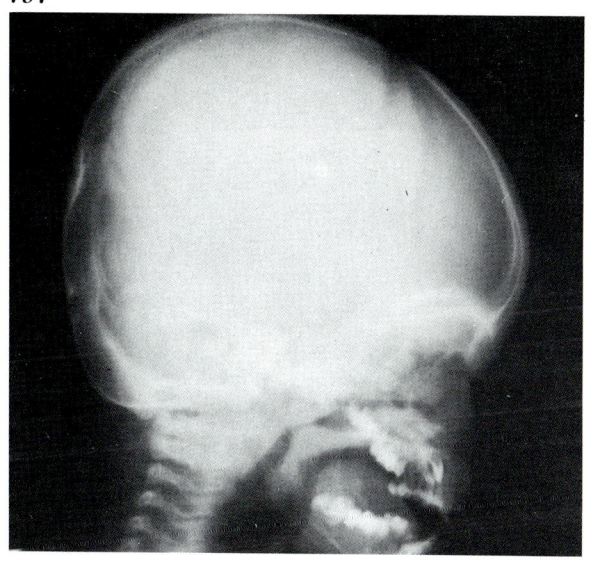

797 Skull of two-year-old infant with rickets The anterior fontanelle remains open and its edges soft.

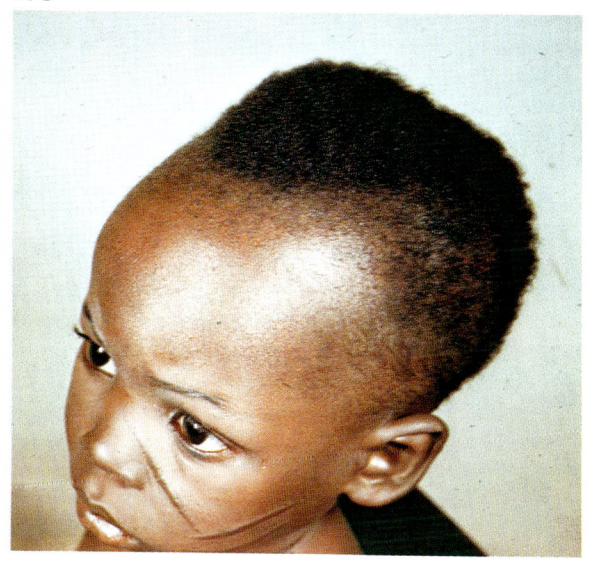

798 Bossing of the skull Bossing of the frontal and parietal eminences occurs.

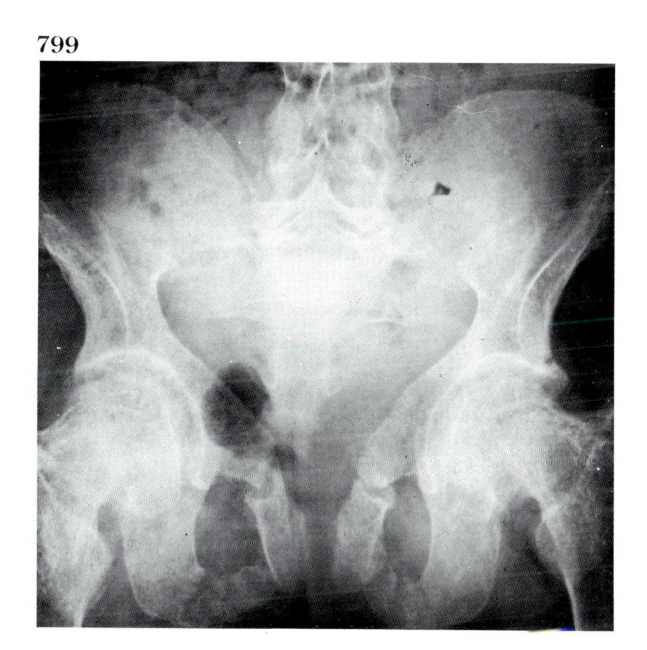

799 Osteomalacia The increased demands of pregnancy may result in gross deformity of the pelvis. This occurs, for example, in mothers kept in purdah.

The B Vitamins
Thiamine (B1)

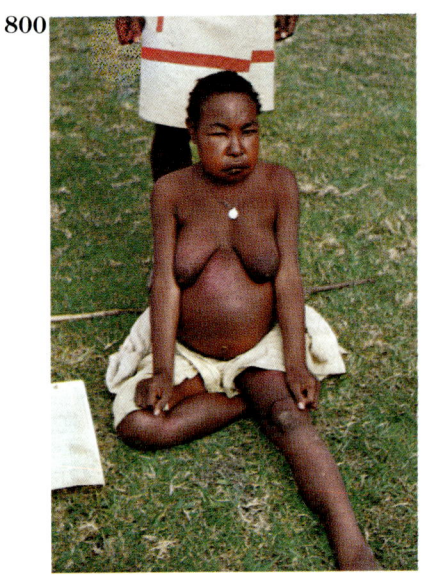

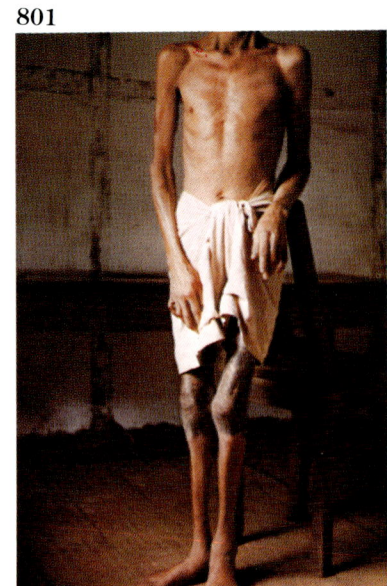

800 Beri beri oedema Beri beri is a disease characterised by generalised oedema, peripheral neuropathy and sometimes heart failure, associated with thiamine deficiency.

801 Peripheral neuropathy Wrist drop and marked wasting of the lower extremities occur in some patients.

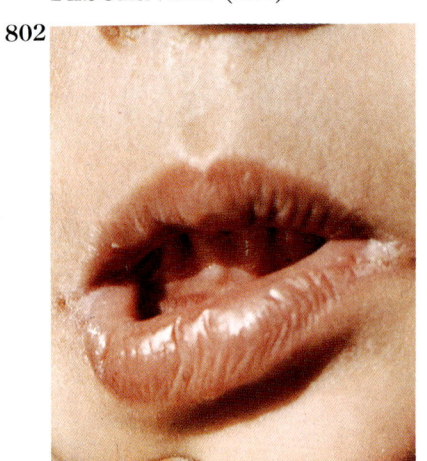

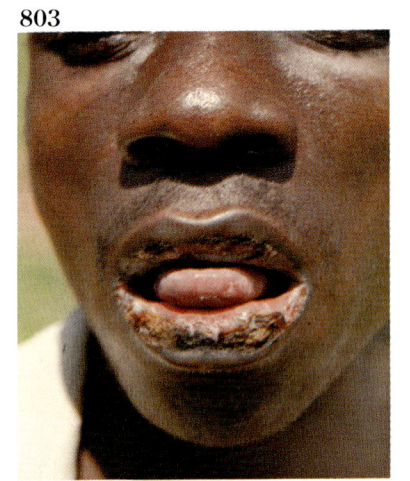

Riboflavine (B2)

802 Angular stomatitis This consists of grey-white fissures at both angles of the mouth due to riboflavine deficiency.

803 Cheilosis A sore, cracked condition of the lips occurs in association with riboflavine deficiency.

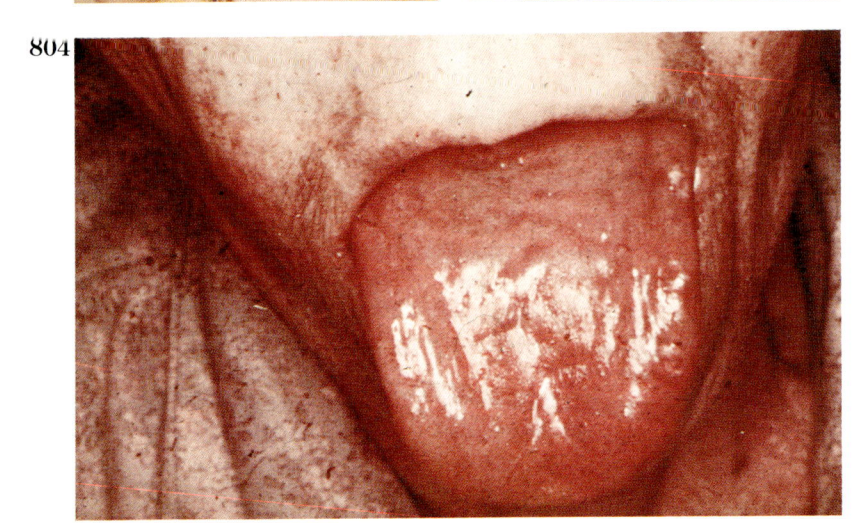

804 Glossitis The tongue is sore and an abnormally deep red colour.

Folic acid

805 Anaemia of folic acid deficiency Folic acid deficiency results in a macrocytic megaloblastic anaemia (*Giemsa × 900*).

806 Bone marrow in folic acid deficiency The appearance in this marrow is characteristic of folic acid deficiency. (*Giemsa × 900*)

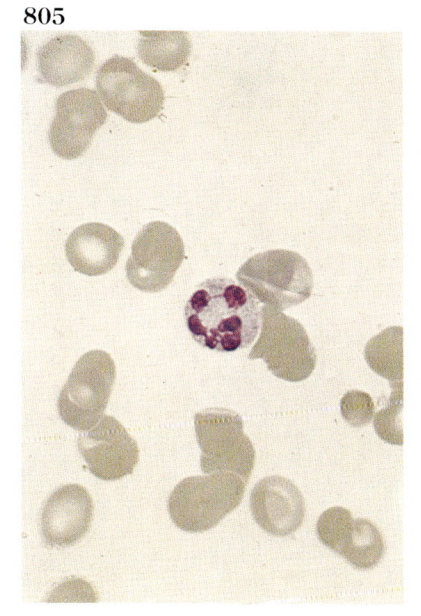

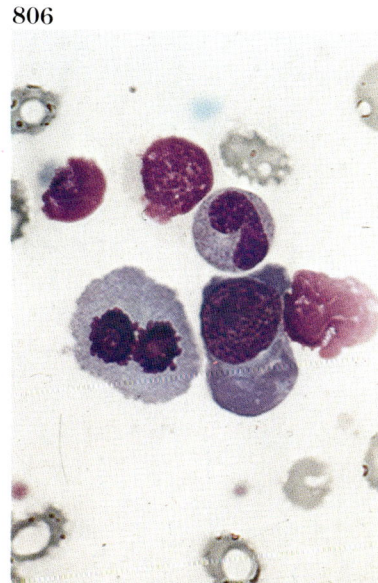

Nicotinic acid (PP)

807 Pellagra The diagnostic triad of the rash of pellagra is a combination of symmetrical skin lesions, sharp demarcation, and distribution in parts exposed to the sun. It is relatively common in people whose diet is composed predominantly of maize.

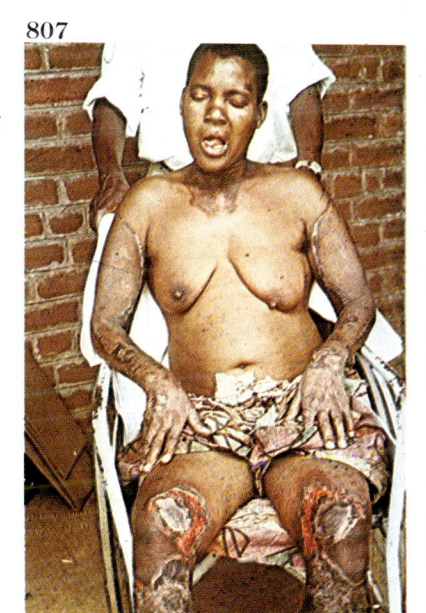

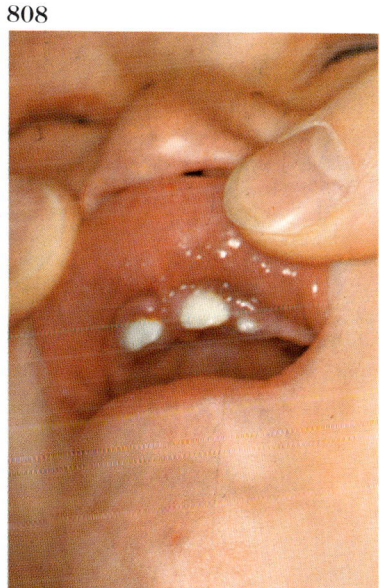

Vitamin C

808 Scurvy Vitamin C deficiency is rare in the tropics. Severe gingivitis and loosening of the teeth occur in scurvy.

Part VIII
Miscellaneous Disorders

In this section are grouped some common conditions that occur almost exclusively in the tropics, as well as a number of exotic curiosities. Diseases such as Burkitt's tumour, endomyocardial fibrosis and the abnormal haemoglobin syndromes are so well-documented elsewhere that we could not do them justice without repeating many of the illustrations already available. We felt, however, that one or two points should be included here to highlight their importance, rather than to omit them altogether from this atlas. Curiosities such as ainhum are interesting entities of limited geographical distribution, while conditions such as pneumocystosis, endemic goitre, hepatoma and venomous bites are important in many areas of the tropics.

ZOONOTIC VIRAL INFECTIONS (See Table XVII)
Lassa Fever

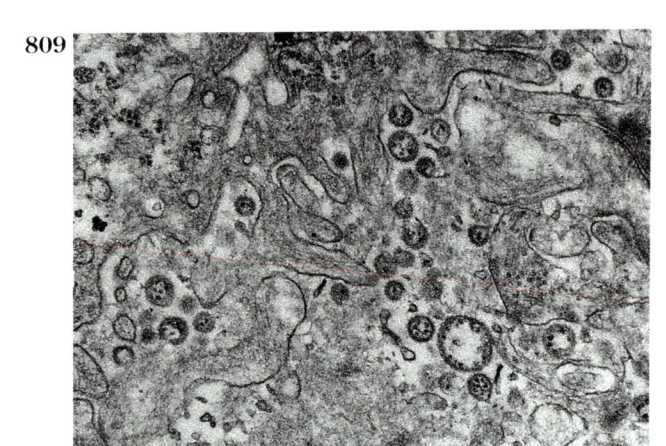

809 Virus of Lassa fever The virus of Lassa fever belongs to the arbovirus group. Its mode of transmission to man is not fully understood, but person to person infections seem common. Virus particles are seen in the perisinusoidal space in this biopsy of liver from a fatal human case. ($\times$ *18 300*) (From W. C. Winn Jr, T. P. Monath, F. A. Murphy & S. G. Whitfield 'Lassa Virus Hepatitis: Observations on a fatal case from the 1972 Sierra Leone epidemic', *Archives of Pathology* 1975, **99**, 599-604.)

810 Rodent reservoir, *Mastomys natalensis* Lassa fever occurs as an acute infectious disease in rural areas of West Africa. During the second week of infection, toxic or vascular symptoms appear: pharyngitis, serous effusions, facial oedema, haemorrhagic diathesis, disorders of the central nervous system and a state of shock. The case fatality rate is high among severe cases but benign, febrile cases of the disease also occur, as well as asymptomatic carriers. A rodent reservoir has been implicated in the epidemiology of Lassa fever.

811 Facial oedema in Lassa fever Facial oedema is a common feature of severe cases and carries a poor prognosis. The risk of man to man transmission of the virus is now considered to be less of a hazard than was originally believed and strict barrier nursing in individual isolation units is no longer used routinely.

812 Liver in Lassa fever Acellular liver necrosis is a marked feature of the hepatic lesion. (*H&E × 250*)

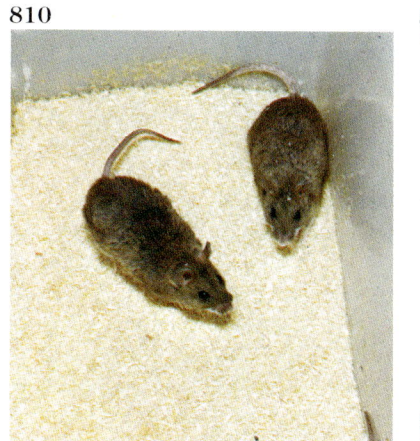

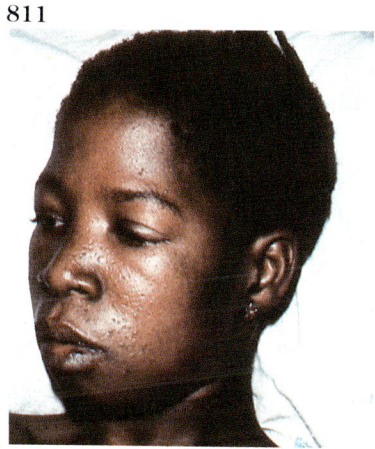

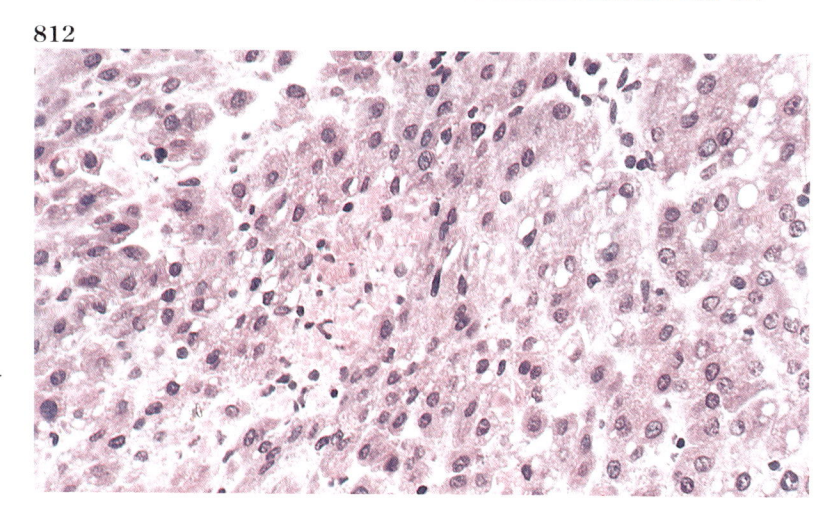

Marburg and Ebola Haemorrhagic Fevers

813 Virus of Ebola haemorrhagic fever This and the Marburg virus, which is morphologically almost identical, are the only branched viruses so far known. The virus shown here is from human liver. (× 30 000)

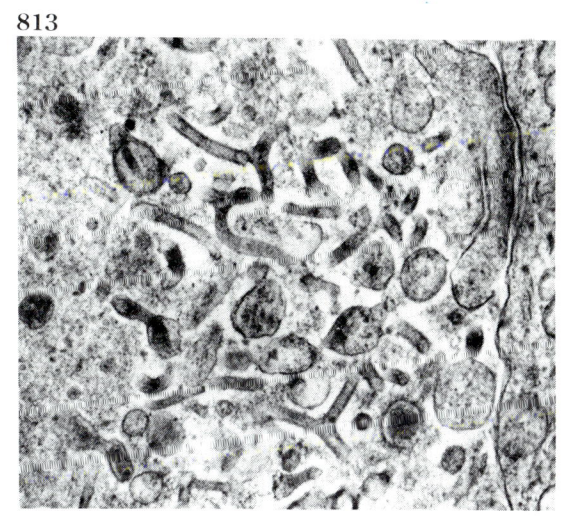

814 Ebola haemorrhagic fever Outbreaks have occurred in Zaïre and the southern Sudan with a high case fatality rate in severely ill patients. Haemorrhagic manifestations in the skin and internal organs are common. However, mild cases as well as asymptomatic carriers also occur. In these a papular rash is seen, usually around the fifth day of the illness.

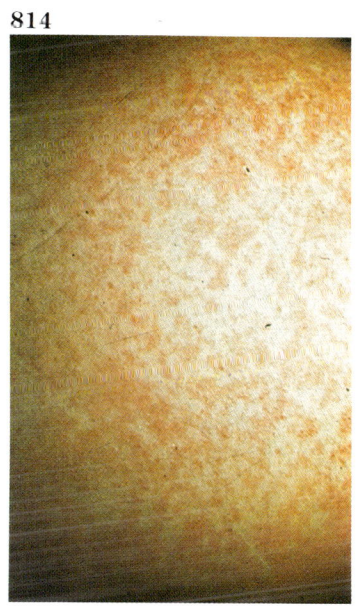

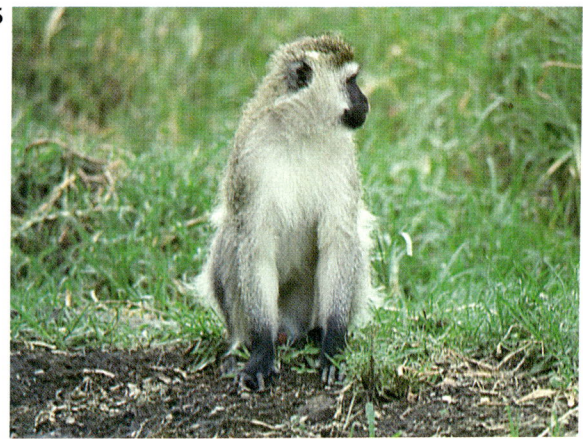

815 *Cercopithecus aethiops*, **reservoir of Marburg virus** The African Green monkey or Vervet was the source of lethal infections contracted by laboratory workers in Europe. Sporadic cases have also occurred in Africa. The causative virus closely resembles that of Ebola haemorrhagic fever (*see* **813**).

Haemorrhagic Fever with Renal Syndrome (HFRS)

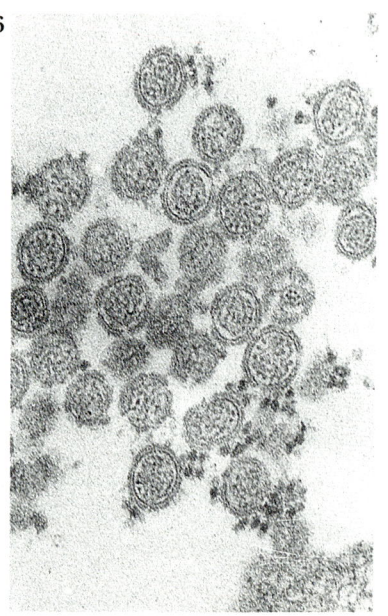

816 Ultrastructure of Hantaan virus This RNA virus of the family Bunyaviridae has been identified as the cause of a widely distributed, haemorrhagic fever which is sometimes associated with acute nephropathy and renal failure. Korean haemorrhagic fever, Scandinavian 'nephropathia epidemica' and similar syndromes all appear to be due to the same virus or related viruses. Various rodents, such as species of *Apodemus* and *Clethrionomys*, act as natural reservoirs, the virus residing in their lungs, and even laboratory rats have been found infected in several countries. Transmission may be direct or airborne or, possibly, through tickbite during epidemics. The virus particles seen here in section were grown in Vero E6 cells. (× *62 000*)

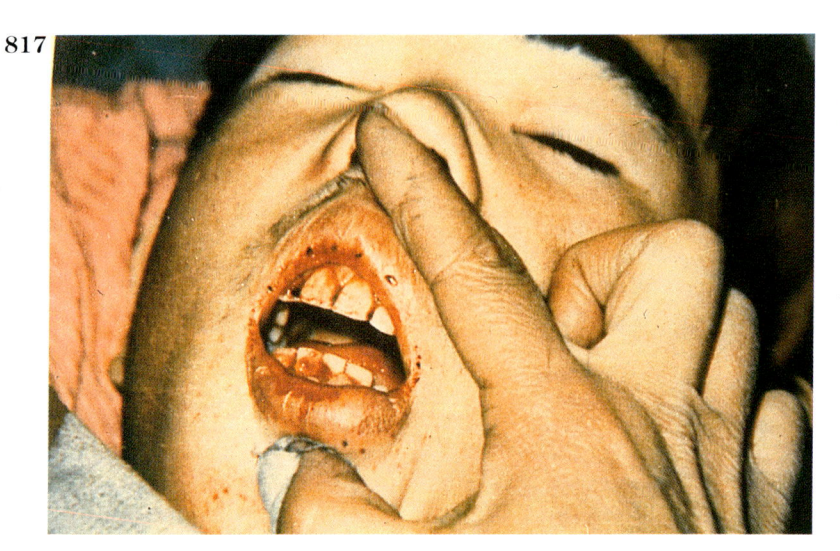

817 HFRS in a Chinese patient Severe haemorrhages occurred in the mouth of this 20-year-old man three days after the onset of his illness.

PNEUMOCYSTOSIS
Pneumocystis carinii

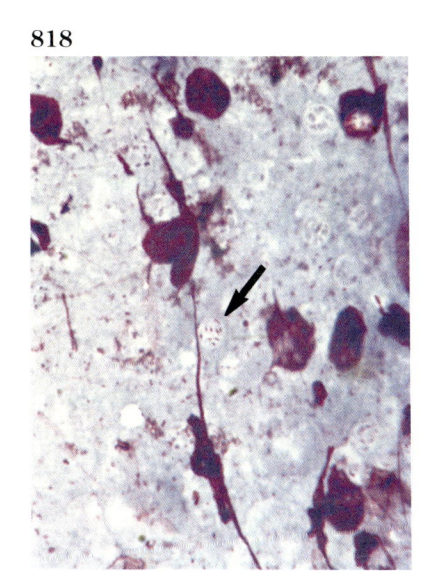

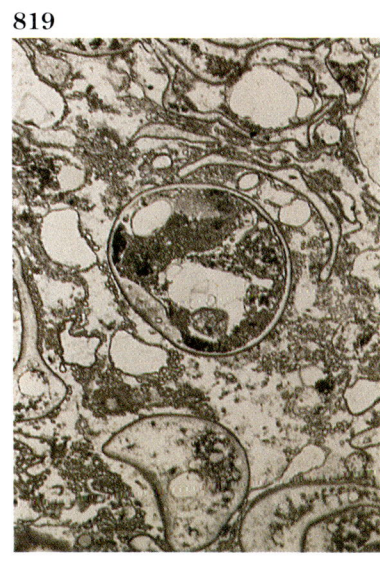

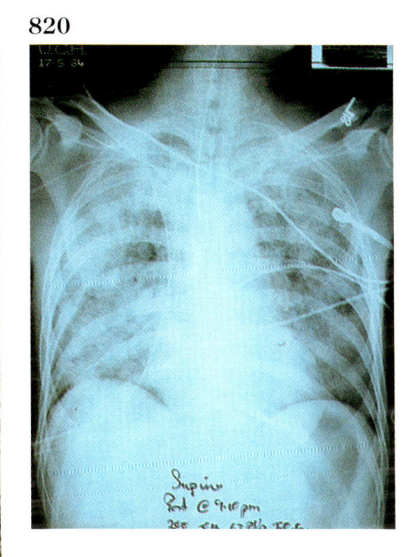

818

819

820

821

818 *P. carinii* in lung smear This organism, which is present as a commensal in many animals, is an opportunistic parasite in man. It produces eight-nucleated cysts which can be seen in smears of pulmonary aspirates. (*Giemsa × 2 500*)

819 Ultrastructure of *P. carinii* Ribosomal RNA analysis has confirmed the fungal nature of this organism. (× *30 000*)

820 *Pneumocystis* pneumonia Massive pulmonary infection is the commonest cause of death in immunocompromised patients, including more than half of those with AIDS. The response to antiprotozoal chemotherapy is generally poor or only transient. Antifungal agents await trial.

821 Silver stain of section of lung The encysted organisms are seen as black objects in the foamy exudate that fills the alveoli. (*Mallory's silver stain* x *380*)

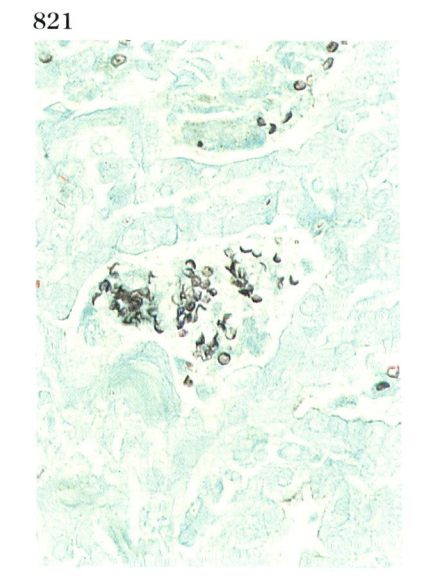

NEOPLASTIC CONDITIONS
Burkitt's Tumour

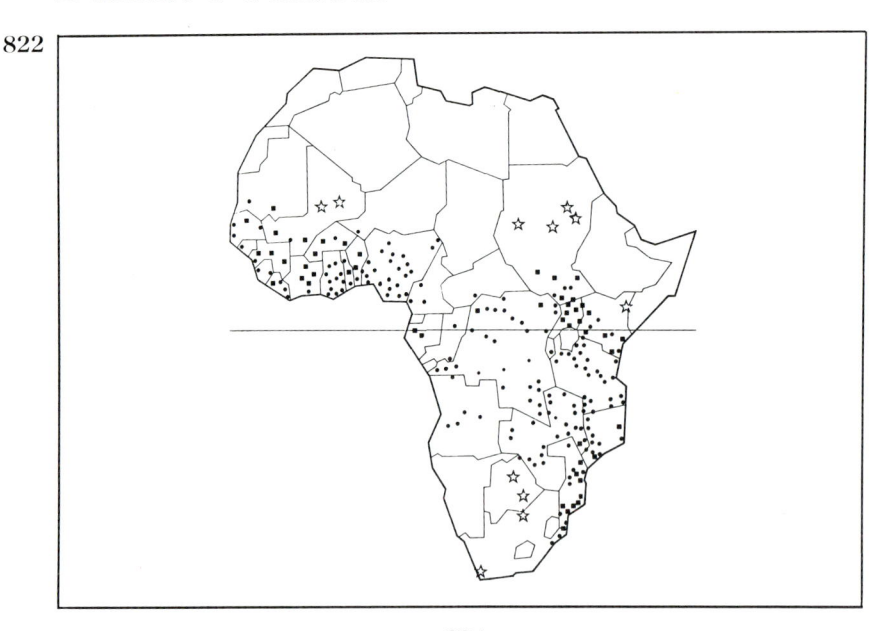

822 Distribution in Africa
The geographical distribution of Burkitt's lymphoma in high incidence is mainly controlled by two climatic parameters, temperature and humidity. In tropical Africa, as well as other continents, the distribution of Burkitt's tumour is roughly the same as that of malaria. In the map, circles indicate where numbers of cases have been reported, squares show areas of unspecified documentation and stars indicate occasional cases.

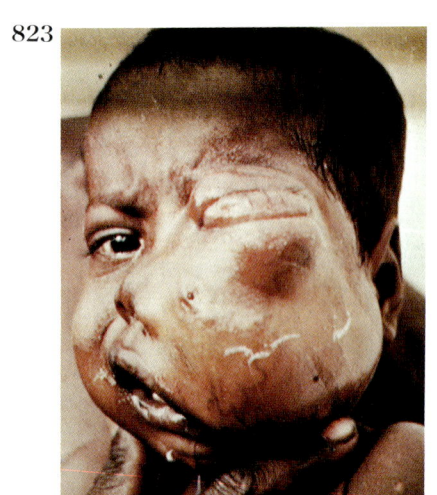

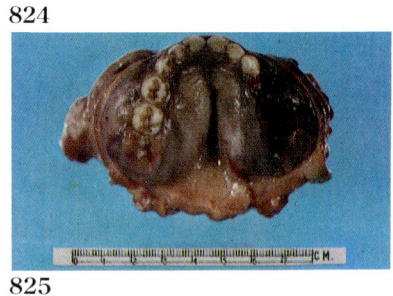

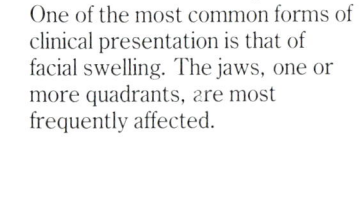

823 & 824 Maxillary tumour
One of the most common forms of clinical presentation is that of facial swelling. The jaws, one or more quadrants, are most frequently affected.

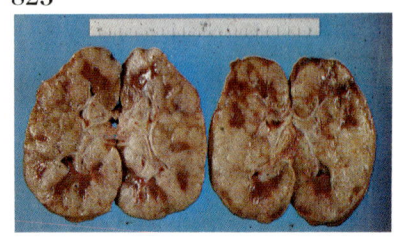

825 Kidneys with Burkitt's tumour Massive replacement of both kidneys with tumour cells is apparent in this figure. Any organ can be affected.

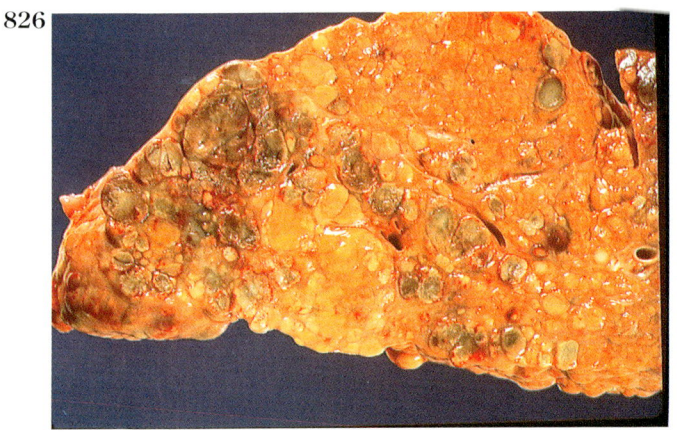

Hepatoma

826 Macroscopic appearance of liver Primary carcinoma of the liver is unusually common in the tropics. Coarse nodular changes can be seen in this figure. Aflatoxins in certain diets appear to be an important contributory factor.

Kaposi's Sarcoma

827 Kaposi's sarcoma and AIDS Reference has already been made to the high frequency of this tumour, often in disseminated form, in patients with AIDS. It was known to occur commonly in Africans, often as a relatively benign tumour but, in HIV-positive cases, it develops the fulminating form shown in **682**.

828 Biopsy of Kaposi's sarcoma with associated *Leishmania* amastigotes Large numbers of amastigotes were found in a biopsy taken from a lesion of Kaposi's sarcoma on the leg of a 35-year-old male who was HIV positive. Subsequently a heavy infection was found in a marrow biopsy and the organisms were typed biochemically as *L. infantum*. The infection was probably acquired in Greece. He was afebrile but had an enlarged spleen and liver. (*Giemsa-colophonium* × 350)

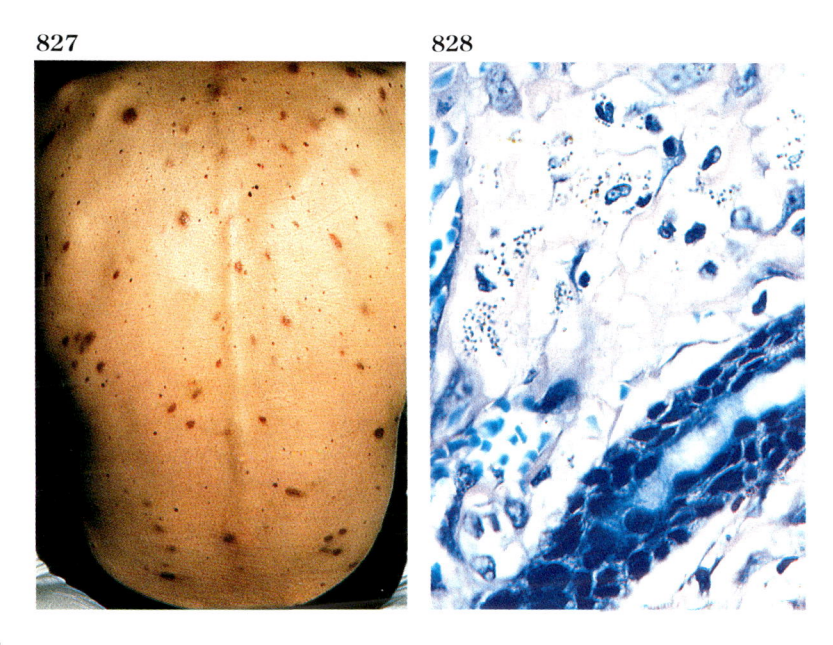

GENETIC BLOOD DYSCRASIAS

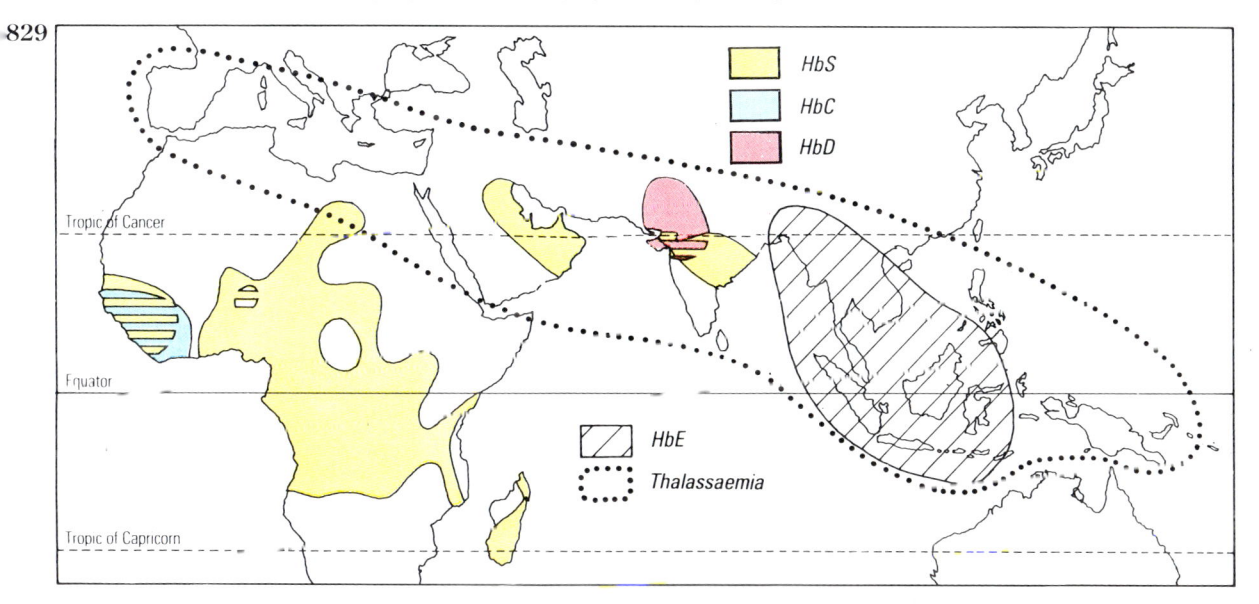

829 Distribution of haemoglobinopathies The most important abnormal haemoglobins in the tropics are Hb S, C and E. Thalassaemia, which is a failure of foetal haemoglobin synthesis, is also widespread. Hb D has a limited distribution and is clinically mild. The abnormal haemoglobins also occur in Central and South America and among blacks in the US. The haemoglobin AS phenotype favours the survival of the gene in tropical Africa where falciparum malaria is holoendemic, but the SS phenotype increases host mortality. This is known as 'balanced polymorphism'. Alpha and β thalassaemia, HbE and G6PD deficiency also afford relative protection against severe *P. falciparum* infection in heterozygotes (*see* **69**).

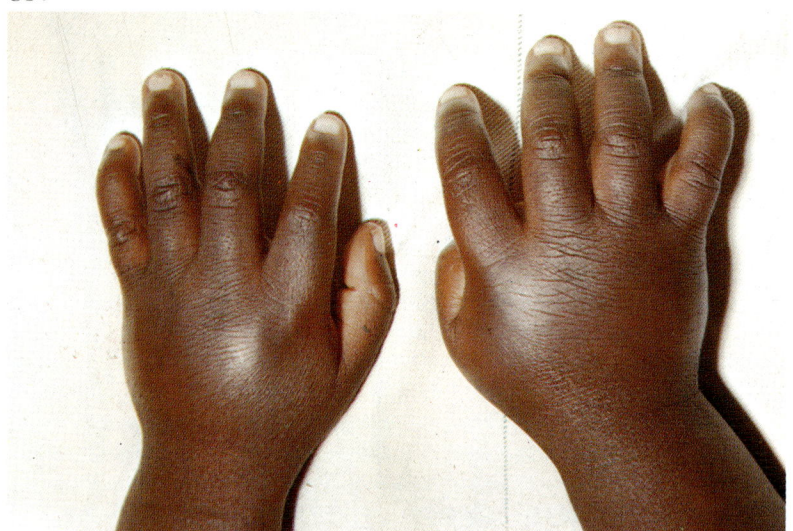

830 Dactylitis due to sickle cell disease Severe bilateral dactylitis is a common presentation of sickle cell disease in children.

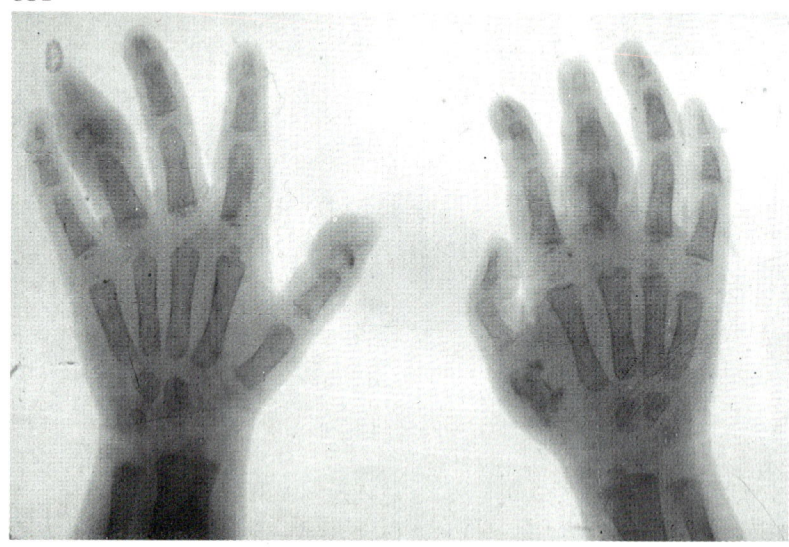

831 X-ray of hands in sickle cell disease Note destructive changes in small bones, the result of multiple infarction complicated by infection (in this case by a *Salmonella* species).

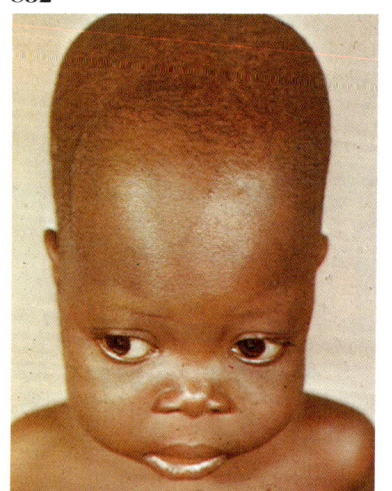

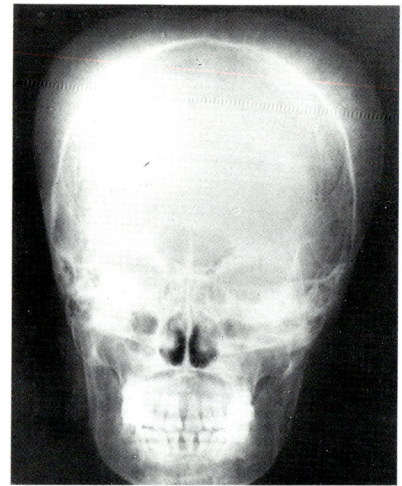

832 Bossing of skull Bossing of the skull due to hyperplasia of the marrow is another feature of sickle cell disease. Similar appearances may be seen in thalassaemia and in any other severe, congenital haemolytic anaemia.

833 X-ray of skull in thalassaemia Haemoglobin E disease produces this typical 'hair-on-end' appearance of the skull in X-rays.

VENOMOUS BITES AND STINGS
Snake Bite Poisoning

Venomous snakes include members of three families: sea snakes (*Hydrophiidae*), cobras and mambas (*Elapidae*) and vipers (*Viperidae*).

834 Elapidae—the cobra *Naja naja* Cobras such as that shown here, and other Elapids, produce both neurotoxins and tissue necrotoxins.

835 Viperidae—venom emerging from poison fang The *Viperinae* and *Crotalinae* (pit vipers) mainly produce toxins affecting the blood and blood vessels.

836 Myoglobinuria following sea snake bite The figure shows rapid clearance of myoglobinuria following administration of life-saving, sea snake antivenom.

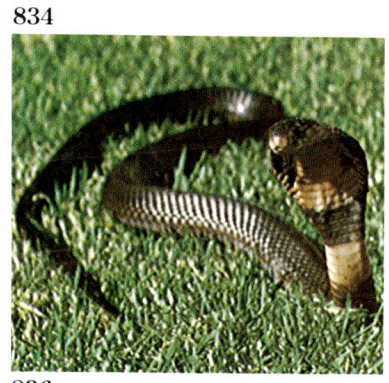

837 Ptosis due to elapid bite Elapid venom produces a neuromuscular block, especially of cranial nerves, thus affecting vision, swallowing and respiration.

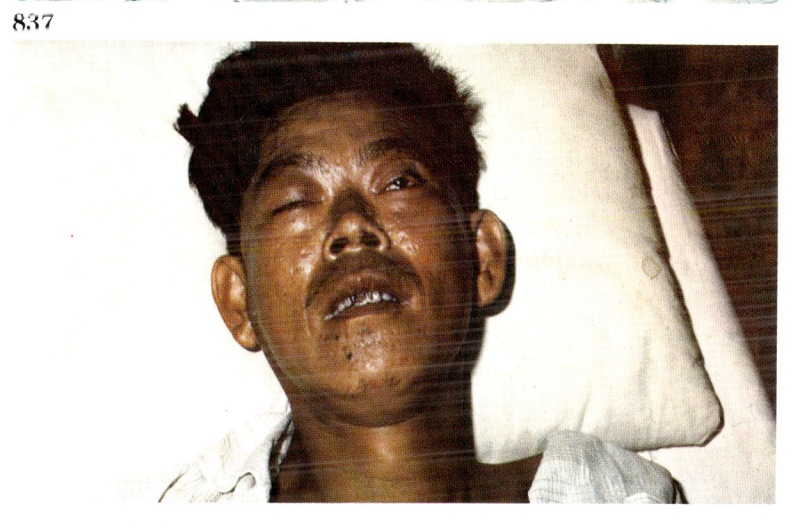

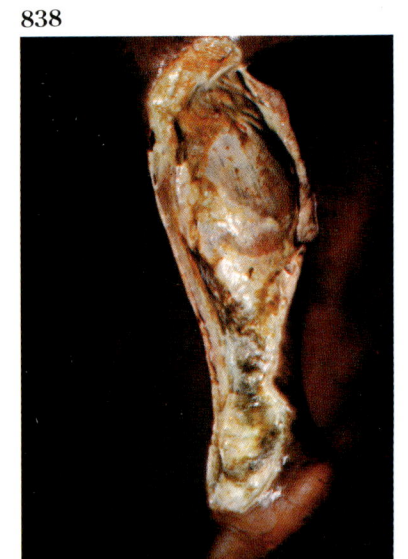

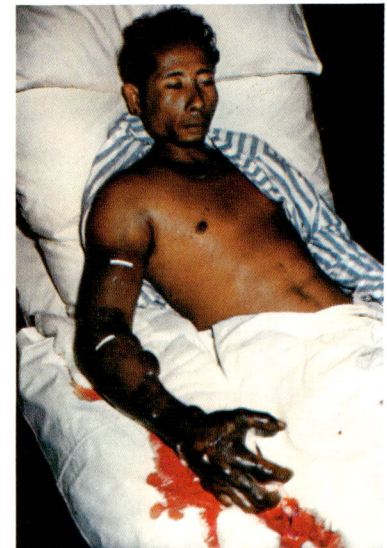

838 Extensive necrosis after cobra bite on leg This patient was bitten several days previously by a cobra.

839 Viper bite causing shock Severe shock associated with serious local tissue damage and haemorrhage.

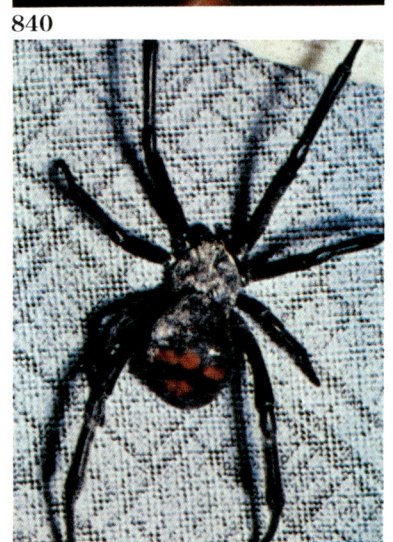

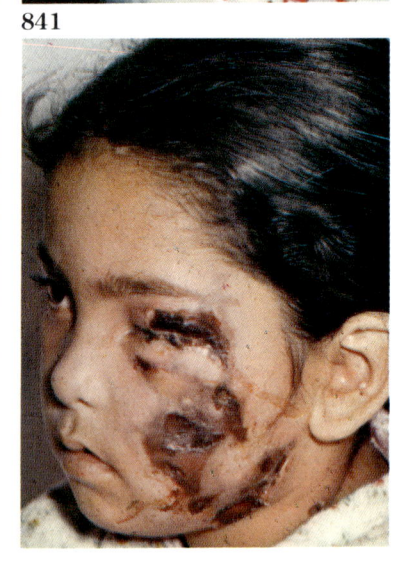

Spider Bites

840 'Black Widow' spider The best-known poisonous spider is the 'Black Widow', *Latrodectus mactans*. Humans are bitten only by the females.

841 Sloughing of skin following spider bite This Chilean child was bitten by a *Loxosceles laeta*. Necrosis and sloughing followed severe blistering at the site of the bite and generalised facial oedema.

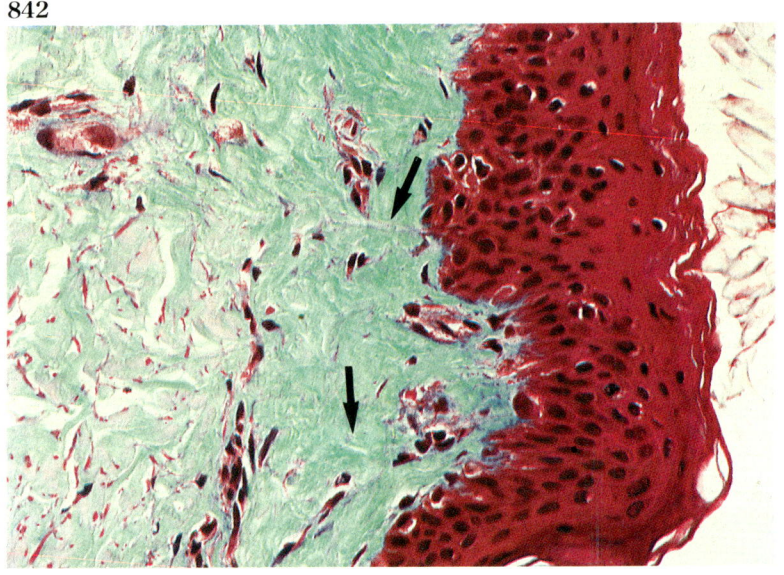

Jelly Fish Envenomation

842 Nematocysts of the 'Sea wasp' in subcutaneous tissue The section shows the beaded tracks (arrows) made by the highly venomous nematocysts of the Cubomedusid jelly fish, *Chironex fleckeri* (the 'North Queensland marine stinger'). Stings by this coelenterate can kill a human adult within minutes. These and other venomous jelly fish are common in the tropical waters of Australasia and parts of the Indian Ocean. (*H&E × 300*)

DISEASES OF UNCERTAIN AETIOLOGY OR EPIDEMIOLOGY

Endomyocardial Fibrosis

843 Fibrotic changes in heart of African Endomyocardial fibrosis is a common cause of heart disease in the tropics. It presents in three clinical forms: mainly left-sided as mitral incompetence; right-sided with features suggestive of constrictive pericarditis; and the third form involving both sides of the heart presenting as congestive cardiac failure.

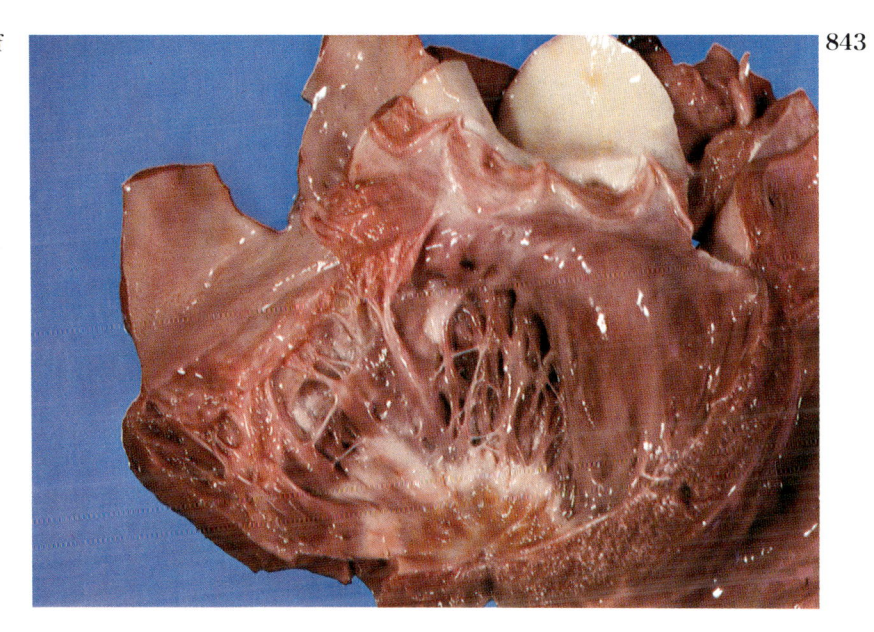

Endemic Goitre

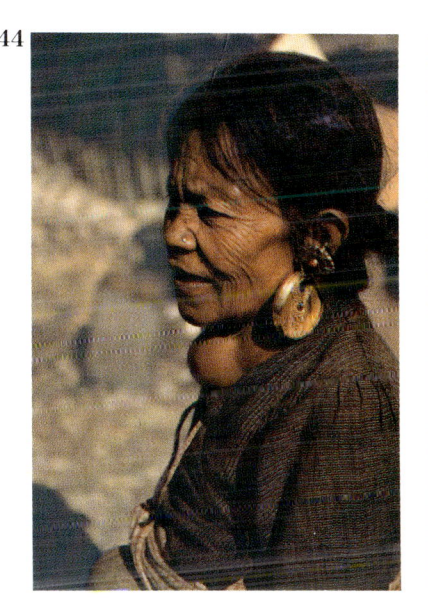

844 Nepalese woman with goitre Endemic goitre, which is common in many parts of the tropics, especially in mountainous areas, is probably due directly or indirectly to iodine deficiency.

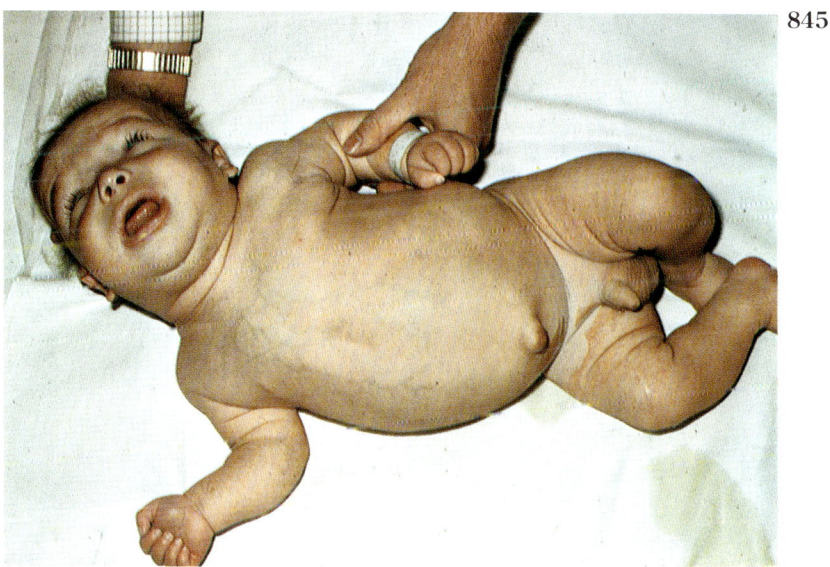

845 Cretin Endemic cretinism is often seen in areas where endemic goitre occurs.

Ainhum

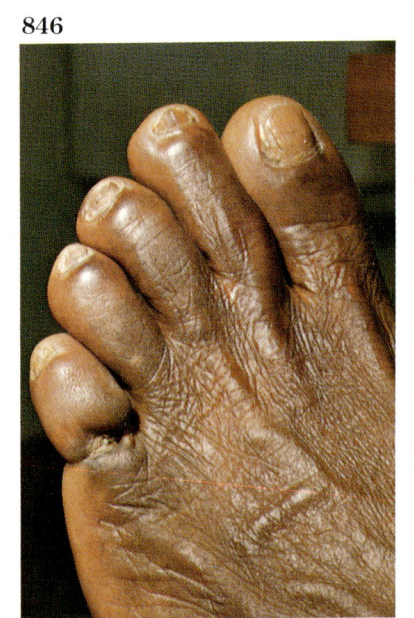

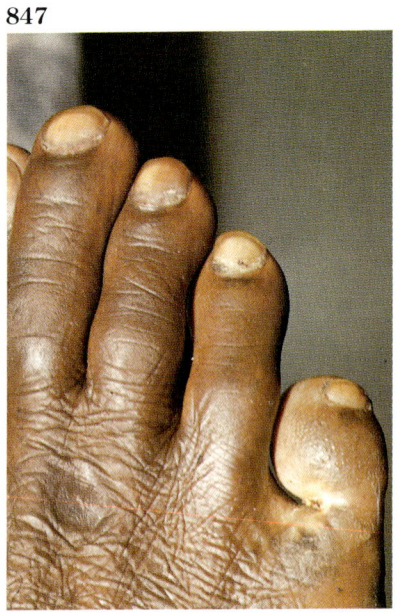

846 & 847 Bilateral ainhum of small toe This condition of unknown aetiology is a progressive encircling fibrosis of a toe, usually the fifth.

Brazilian Foliaceus Pemphigus

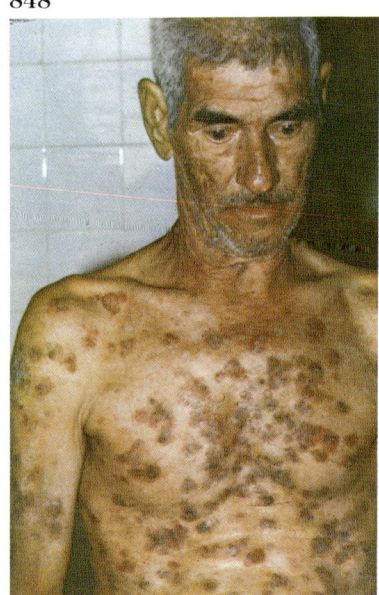

848 Adult Brazilian with 'fogo selvagem' A chronic form of pemphigus is endemic in a number of localities in Central Brazil. The causative agent and mode of transmission are unknown.

Sprue

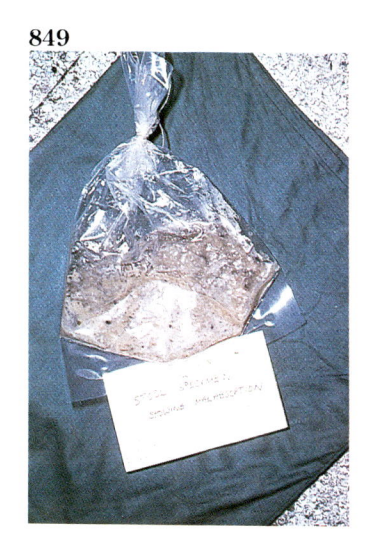

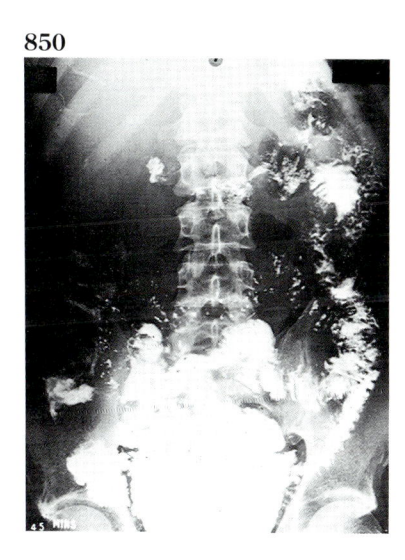

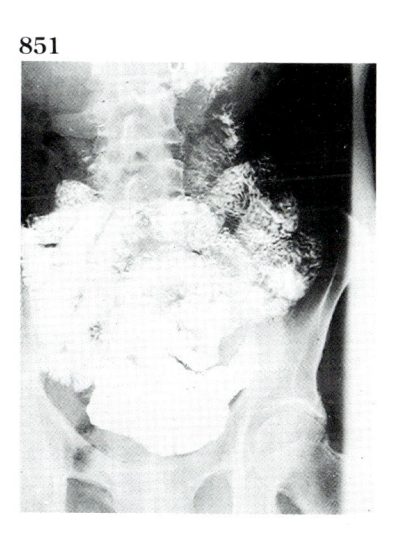

849

850

851

849 Faeces from a patient with sprue Sprue is characterised by chronic steatorrhoea with associated abdominal symptoms, glossitis and anaemia.

850 & 851 X-rays of patient with sprue The figures show loss of normal intestinal pattern before (**850**) and recovery after three months of treatment (**851**).

Vesical Calculi

852 Collection of bladder stones Bladder stones are very common in children in northeast Thailand and parts of the Middle East. The aetiology is unknown but nutritional factors are implicated. Inadequate phosphate consumption may be one important factor.

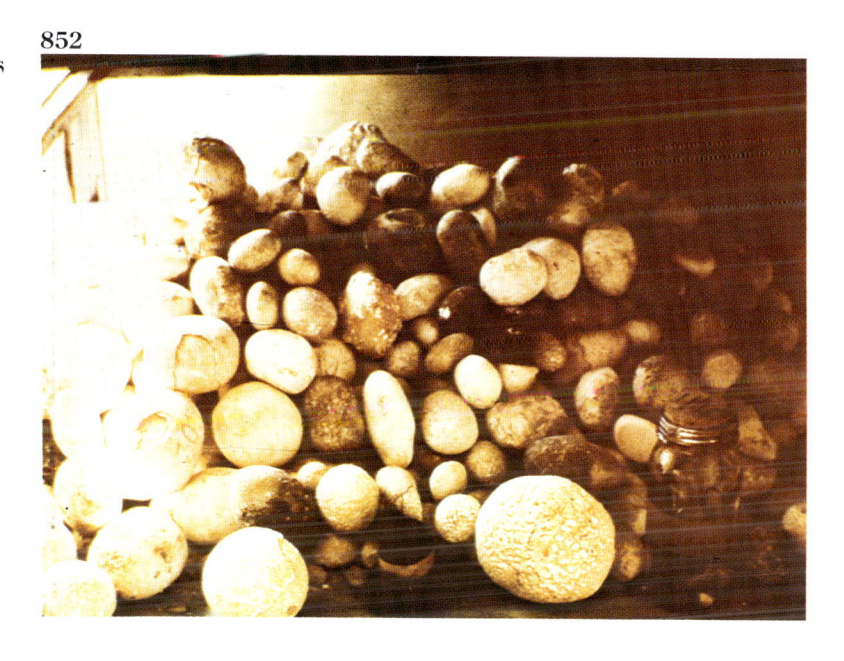

852

List of Tables

I	Arthropod Vectors of Disease	215
II	Arboviruses Infecting Man	216, 217
III	The Rickettsial Diseases	218
IV	Pathogenic Spirochaetes	219
V	The Protozoa (Phylum Apicomplexa) of Medical Importance	220
VI	The Protozoa (Class Zoomastigophorea) of Medical Importance	221
VII	Trypanosomes of Medical and Veterinary Importance	222
VIII	The Genus *Leishmania* and the Leishmaniases	223, 224
IX	The Nematodes of Medical Importance and their Prevalence	225
X	The Microfilariae Occurring in Man	226
XI	The Digenetic Trematodes of Medical Importance and their Prevalence	227
XII	Snails and Other Molluscs of Medical Importance (Class Gastropoda)	228
XIII	The Protozoa (Phyla Ciliophora and Sarcomastigophora) of Medical Importance	229
XIV	The Cestodes of Medical Importance and their Prevalence in Man	229
XV	The Superficial and the Systemic Mycoses	230
XVI	The Myiasis-producing Diptera of Medical Importance	231
XVII	Classification and Causes of Haemorrhagic Fevers	232

TABLE I   ARTHROPOD VECTORS OF DISEASE

Class	Order	Vector	Disease Transmitted
CRUSTACEA	COPEPODA	*Cyclops* spp. (water fleas)	guinea worm, fish tapeworm
	DECAPODA	crayfish, freshwater crabs	paragonimiasis
ARACHNIDA	ACARINA	hard ticks	spotted and Q fevers, virus encephalitides, Lyme disease
		Ornithodorus spp. (soft ticks)	endemic relapsing fever
		mites	scrub typhus, rickettsial pox, scabies
INSECTA	ANOPLURA	*Pediculus humanus* (body louse)	epidemic typhus, epidemic relapsing fever
	MALLOPHAGA	chewing lice	*Dipylidium caninum* (dog tapeworm)
	BLATTARIA	cockroaches	*Hymenolepis diminuta* (rat tapeworm)
	HEMIPTERA	Reduviidae (assassin bugs)	Chagas' disease
	DIPTERA	*Anopheles*	malaria, filariasis (*W. bancrofti, B. malayi*)
		culicines	filariasis (*W. bancrofti, B. malayi*), arboviruses (incl. yellow fever, dengue)
		Culicoides	filariasis (*M. ozzardi, M. perstans, M. streptocerca*)
		Simulium	filarial blindness (*O. volvulus*)
		Chrysops	filariasis (*Loa loa*)
		Phlebotomus Lutzomyia	sandfly fever, Bartonellosis, the leishmaniases
		Glossina	African trypanosomiasis
	SIPHONAPTERA	fleas	plague, murine typhus, rat and dog tapeworms
	COLEOPTERA	beetles	rat tapeworms
	LEPIDOPTERA	grain moths	rat tapeworms

(*see also* Part V, Ectoparasites)

TABLE II ARBOVIRUSES INFECTING MAN

Family	Genus	Virus or disease	Vectors	Reservoir hosts	Amplifier hosts
Togaviridae	*Alphavirus*	Chikungunya	*Aedes*	Baboons	
		Eastern equine encephalitis	*Aedes*	Birds	Horses
		Mayaro	*Aedes, Anopheles*	?	
		Mucambo	Culicines	?	
		O'Nyong-Nyong	*Anopheles*	?	
		Semliki Forest	mosquitoes	?	
		Ross River	*Aedes*	?	
		Sindbis	Culicines	Birds	
		Venezuelan equine encephalitis	*Aedes, Anopheles*	Rodents, birds	Horses
		Western equine encephalitis	*Culex*	Birds	Horses
	Flavivirus (mainly mosquito-borne)	Banzi	Culicines	?	
		Bussuquara	Culicines	Rodents	
		Dengue 1,2,3,4	*Aedes*	?	? Monkey
		Ilheus	Culicines	Birds	
		Japanese B encephalitis	*Culex, Anopheles*	Birds, bats	Pigs
		Kunjin	Culicines	Birds	
		Murray Valley encephalitis	Culicines	Birds	
		Rocio	Mosquitoes	?	
		St. Louis encephalitis	Culicines	Birds, bats	
		Spondweni	Culicines	?	
		Wesselbron	Culicines	Rodents	
		West Nile	*Culex*, Ixodids, Argasids	Rodents, birds, bats	
		Yellow fever	*Aedes aegypti*	Monkeys	
		Zika	Culicines	?	

TABLE II (continued)

Family	Genus	Virus or disease	Vectors	Reservoir hosts	Amplifier hosts
	Flavivirus (mainly tick-borne)	Absettarov	Ixodids	?	
		Hanzalova	Ixodids	?	
		Hypr	Ixodids	Rodents	
		Kumlinge	Ixodids	Rodents, birds	
		Kyasanur Forest disease	Ixodids Argasids	Rodents	Monkeys
		Louping ill	Ixodids	Rodents, birds	
		Negishi	Ixodids	?	
		Omsk haemorrhagic fever	Ixodids	Rodents	
		Powassan	Ixodids	Rodents	
		Russian spring-summer encephalitis	Ixodids	Rodents, birds	
		Dakar bat virus	?	Bats	
Reoviridae	*Orbivirus*	Colorado tick fever	Ixodids Argasids	Rodents	
Bunyaviridae	*Nairovirus*	Crimea-Congo haemorrhagic fever	Ixodids	Cattle	
	?	Hantaan virus*	? Ticks	Rodents	
	Bunyavirus	California encephalitis	*Aedes*	Rodents, rabbits	
		Oropuche	Biting midges	Monkeys	
		Brazilian group	Mosquitoes	?	
		Bunyamwere group	Culicines	?	
	Phlebovirus	Rift Valley fever	*Anopheles*	Cattle, sheep	
		Sandfly fever	*Phlebotomus*	?	

? Not yet known
* Cause of Korean haemorrhagic fever, Nephropathia epidemica, Haemorrhagic Fever with Renal Syndrome (HFRS).
See also Table XVII.

TABLE III   THE RICKETTSIAL DISEASES*

Group	Disease	Causative Agent	Vector	Animal reservoir
TYPHUS	Epidemic	*Rickettsia prowazeki*	*Pediculus humanus*	None
	Brill–Zinser disease	*R. prowazeki*	*P. humanus*	None
	Murine	*R. mooseri*	*Xenopsylla cheopis*	Rat
SPOTTED FEVERS	Rocky Mountain, Eastern, Western, South American	*R. rickettsi*	Various tick species	Many small mammals
	Fièvre boutonneuse	*R. conori*	*Rhipicephalus sanguineus*	Dog
	Siberian tick typhus	*R. siberica*	*Dermacentor* spp. *Haemaphysalis* spp.	Farm animals
	Queensland tick typhus	*R. australis*	*Ixodes holocyclus*	Marsupials
	Rickettsial pox	*R. akari*	Mites	Mice
	Scrub typhus	*R. tsutsugamushi*	Trombiculid mites	Small mammals mice. field rats
	Trench fever	*R. quintana*	*P. humanus*	None
	Q fever	*Coxiella burnetii*	Ticks**	Cattle, sheep, goats, wild animals

*Identification is usually confirmed by serological typing (Weil-Felix reaction).
**Transmission is mainly from dairy animals or their products, sometimes by inhalation of infectious organisms in aerosol form.

TABLE IV PATHOGENIC SPIROCHAETES

Genus	Species	Mode of Transmission	Reservoir	Disease
Leptospira	serotypes *icterohaemorrhagiae*	Water	Rats	Leptospirosis, Weil's disease,
	canicola	Water	Dogs, pigs, cattle	Canicola fever
	many other serotypes			
Borrelia	*recurrentis*	*Pediculus humanus*	None	Louse-borne relapsing fever
	duttoni	*Ornithodorus moubata*	None	Tick-borne relapsing fever
	burgdorferi	*Ixodes*	Rodents	Lyme disease
	other spp.	*Ornithodorus* spp.	Various mammals, birds, etc.	Asiatic, African, S. American relapsing fevers
Treponema	*pallidum*	Venereal, congenital.	None	Syphilis
		Endemic	None	Bejel
	pertenue	Contact	None	Yaws
	carateum	Contact	None	Pinta
	vincenti[*]	Contact	? None	Vincent's angina, 2^e infections
Spirillum	*minus*[**]		Rodents, other small mammals	Rat-bite fever

[*]Placed by some authors in the genus *Borrelia*
[**]Not strictly a spirochaete as it is flagellated.

TABLE V   THE PROTOZOA (PHYLUM APICOMPLEXA) OF MEDICAL IMPORTANCE

Phylum etc.	*Family*	*Genus & Species*
SARCOMASTIGOPHORA (see Tables VI and XIII)		
CILIOPHORA (see Table XIII)		
MICROSPORA (see **579**, **580**)		
APICOMPLEXA		
Subclass PIROPLASMASINA	BABESIIDAE[1]	*Babesia microti*
		B. bovis
		B. divergens
		Babesia spp.
Subclass COCCIDIASINA		
Order EUCOCCIDIORIDA		
Suborder HAEMOSPORORINA	PLASMODIIDAE	*Plasmodium vivax*
		P. ovale
		P. malariae
		P. (Laverania) falciparum
Suborder EIMERIORINA	SARCOCYSTIDAE	*Toxoplasma gondii*
		Sarcocystis hominis[2]
		S. suihominis[3]
		Sarcocystis spp.[4]
	EIMERIIDAE	*Isospora belli*
	CRYPTOSPORIDIIDAE	*Cryptosporidium* spp.
Subclass NOT DETERMINED		*Pneumocystis carinii*[5]
ORDER NOT DETERMINED		*Blastocystis hominis*[6]

[1]All rare in man.
[2]Man definitive, cattle intermediate host.
[3]Man definitive, pig intermediate host.
[4]'*Sarcocystis lindemanni*' consists of a number of unidentified species for which man is an intermediate host.
[5]Just identified as analogous to the fungi on the basis of its ribosomal RNA.
[6]Recently recognised to be an anaerobic protozoan, order Amoebida.

TABLE VI THE PROTOZOA (CLASS ZOOMASTIGOPHOREA) OF MEDICAL IMPORTANCE

Phylum	Subphylum etc.	Order	Genus & Species
APICOMPLEXA (see Table V)			
CILIOPHORA (see Table XIII)			
SARCOMASTIGO-PHORA	SARCODINA (see Table XIII)		
	MASTIGOPHORA		
	[Class] ZOOMASTIGOPHOREA (No vector)	RETORTAMONADIDA	*Chilomastix mesnili*
		DIPLOMONADIDA	*Giardia lamblia*
		TRICHOMONADIDA	*Trichomonas vaginalis* *T. hominis* *Dientamoeba fragilis**
	(Invertebrate vector)	KINETOPLASTIDA	*Leishmania* spp. (see Table VIII)
			Trypanosoma spp. (see Table VII)

*This parasite is now considered to be a flagellate and not an amoeba.

TABLE VII   TRYPANOSOMES OF MEDICAL AND VETERINARY IMPORTANCE

Genus (subgenus)	Species	Host Species	Disease
in Africa			
SALIVARIA			
Trypanosoma (Duttonella)	*vivax*	antelopes, ruminants, equines, dogs	Souma
	uniforme	antelopes, ruminants	(pathogenic)
T. (Nannomonas)	*congolense*	antelopes, ruminants, equines, pigs, dogs	(pathogenic)
	simiae	pigs, warthogs, camels	(pathogenic)
T. (Trypanozoon)	*brucei brucei*	antelopes, domestic mammals	Nagana
	b. rhodesiense	antelopes, man	Sleeping sickness (acute form)
	b. gambiense	man, pigs	Sleeping sickness (chronic form)
	*evansi**	bovines, equines, camels, dogs, etc.	Surra
	*equiperdum***	equines	Dourine
T. (Pycnomonas)	*suis*	domestic and wild pigs	(pathogenic)
in South America			
SALIVARIA			
Trypanosoma (Duttonella)	*vivax****	bovines	(pathogenic)
T. (Herpetosoma)	*rangeli*****	many wild animals, man	(non-pathogenic)
STERCORARIA			
T. (Schizotrypanum)	*cruzi*****	man, armadillos, opposums, dogs, etc.	Chagas' disease

All species transmitted by tsetse flies except:
 *by tabanid flies
 **by coitus
 ***by various biting flies
 ****by reduviid bugs

TABLE VIII THE GENUS *LEISHMANIA* AND THE LEISHMANIASES*

Type of Disease	Species	Localities	Main Vectors	Main Reservoirs
VISCERAL LEISHMANIASIS				
KALA-AZAR (60% between 10 and 20 years old)	*L(L)donovani*	India, China (N. of Yangtze R.)	*P. argentipes* *P. chinensis*	man dog, ? jackal
	? L(L)donovani	Kenya	*P. martini*	? man
	L(L)archibaldi	Sudan	*P. orientalis*	serval cat, genet
INFANTILE KALA-AZAR (80–90% under 10 years old)	*L(L)* sp.	Saudi Arabia Yemen Ethiopia	? ? ?	? ? ?
	L(L)infantum	USSR China Iraq France and Italy Mediterranean basin	*P. major* ? *P. major* *P. ariasi* *P. perfiliewi* *P. perniciosus* *P. major*	fox, wolf, dog "raccoon dog" ? jackal dog, fox *Rattus rattus* dog
	L(L)chagasi	Brazil Colombia Venezuela Mexico Paraguay Ecuador Honduras El Salvador Bolivia Guatemala	*Lu. longipalpis* *Lu. longipalpis* ?	fox, dog dog ?
ORONASAL K-A	*L(L)infantum*	France	(as classical Kala-azar)	
POST K-A DERMAL LEISHMANIASIS (PKDL)	*L(L) donovani*	India China	(as classical Kala-azar)	
	? L(L) donovani	Kenya		
CUTANEOUS LEISHMANIASIS (OLD WORLD)				
ORIENTAL SORE and RECIDIVA	*L(L)tropica*	India USSR (urban) Iran Mediterranean basin Saudi Arabia	*P. sergenti* *P. sergenti* *P. ansarii* *P. sergenti* *P. perfiliewi* *P. sergenti*	dog man dog man ?
ORIENTAL SORE and ORONASAL	*L(L)major*	USSR (rural) Saudi Arabia Central Asia Mediterranean basin Sudan Senegal India	*P. papatasi* *P. papatasi* *P. papatasi* *P. papatasi* ? *P. papatasi* *P. duboscqi* *P. salehi*	gerbils gerbils, merions gerbils, merions gerbils, merions rodents rodents rodents
	L(L)tropica complex	Namibia	*P. rossi*	hyrax
SINGLE SORE and DIFFUSA	*L(L)aethiopica*	Ethiopia Kenya	*P. longipes* *P. pedifer*	hyrax hyrax *Cricetomys*

TABLE VIII (continued)

Type of Disease	Species	Localities	Main Vectors	Main Reservoirs
NEW WORLD CUTANEOUS				
SIMPLE CUTANEOUS and DIFFUSA	L(L)mexicana	Mexico Guatemala Belize	Lu. olmeca	forest rodents
	L(L)pifanoi	Venezuela	? Lu. flaviscutellata	?
	L(L)amazonensis	Brazil (Amazon basin)	Lu. flaviscutellata	forest rodents
	L(L)venezuelensis	Venezuela	? Lu. olmeca bicolor	?
	L(L)garnhami	Venezuela	? Lu. townsendi	opposum
	L(L)mexicana complex	Belize Trinidad São Paulo State Dominican Republic Texas	? Lu. flaviscutellata ? ? ?	? forest rodents ? ? ?
	L(L) lainsoni	Brazil (Pará)	?	?
	L(V) spp.	Belize C. America	? Lu. ovallesi ? Lu. crucians	?
ESPUNDIA	L(V)braziliensis	Brazil**	Lu. wellcomei ? Lu. migonei ? Lu. anduzei ? Lu. intermedia	forest rodents ? paca
		Ecuador Peru Bolivia Venezuela Paraguay Colombia	? ? ? ? ?	? ? ? ? ?
PIAN BOIS	L(V)guyanensis	Guyanas N.Brazil	Lu. umbratilis Lu. whitmani Lu. anduzei	sloths, ant-eaters ? rodents
SIMPLE SORE or PIAN BOIS	L(V)panamensis	Panama Costa Rica Colombia	Lu. trapidoi Lu. ylephiletor ? Lu. gomezi ? Lu. panamensis	sloths monkeys kinkajou olingo
UTA	L(V)peruviana	Peru (W. of Andes) Argentine	? Lu. verrucarum ? Lu. peruensis	dog ?

*This genus has been divided into *Leishmania (Leishmania)*, type species *L(L)donovani* and *Leishmania (Viannia)*, type species *L(V) braziliensis*.
**Forested areas east of the Andean chain.

TABLE IX THE NEMATODES OF MEDICAL IMPORTANCE AND THEIR PREVALENCE*

Subclass	Order (Suborder)	Superfamily	Genus & Species	Probable Prevalence in Man
ADENOPHOREA	ENOPLIDA	TRICHUROIDEA	Trichinella spiralis	49 million
			Trichuris trichiura	670 million
			Capillaria hepatica	rare
			C. philippensis	thousands
SECERNENTEA	RHABDITIDA	RHABDITOIDEA	Strongyloides stercoralis	70 million
	STRONGYLIDA	ANCYLOSTO-MATOIDEA	Ancylostoma duodenale	} 900 million
			Necator americanus	
			Ancylostoma caninum	thousands
			A. braziliense	thousands
			A. ceylanicum	rare
			Ternidens deminutus	thousands
			Oesophagostomum apiostomum	rare
			Syngamus laryngeus	rare
		TRICHOSTRON-GYLOIDEA	Trichostrongylus spp.	10 million
		METASTRON-GYLOIDEA	Metastrongylus elongatus	rare
			Angiostrongylus cantonensis	thousands
	OXYURIDA	OXYUROIDEA	Enterobius vermicularis	360 million
	ASCARIDIDA	ASCARIDOIDEA	Ascaris lumbricoides	1233 million
			Toxocara canis	thousands
			Toxocara cati	thousands
			Lagochilascaris minor	rare
			Anisakis spp.	rare
			Pseudoterranova decipiens	thousands
	SPIRURIDA (SPIRURINA)	SPIRUROIDEA	Gongylonema pulchrum	rare
		GNATHOSTOMA-TOIDEA	Gnathostoma spinigerum	rare
		THELAZOIDEA	Thelazia callipaeda	rare
		FILARIOIDEA	Wuchereria bancrofti	} 90 million
			Brugia malayi	
			B. timori	thousands
			Loa loa	33 million
			Onchocerca volvulus	40 million
			Mansonella perstans	65 million
			M. streptocerca	? millions
			M. ozzardi	15 million
			Dirofilaria spp.	rare
	SPIRURIDA (CAMALLANINA)	DRACUNCU-LOIDEA	Dracunculus medinensis	98 million

*Updated in part from Le Riche (1967) in *Health of Mankind*, CIBA Symposium (Churchill, London) p. 38 to allow for increase in world population and reductions due to control measures.

TABLE X   THE MICROFILARIAE OCCURRING IN MAN

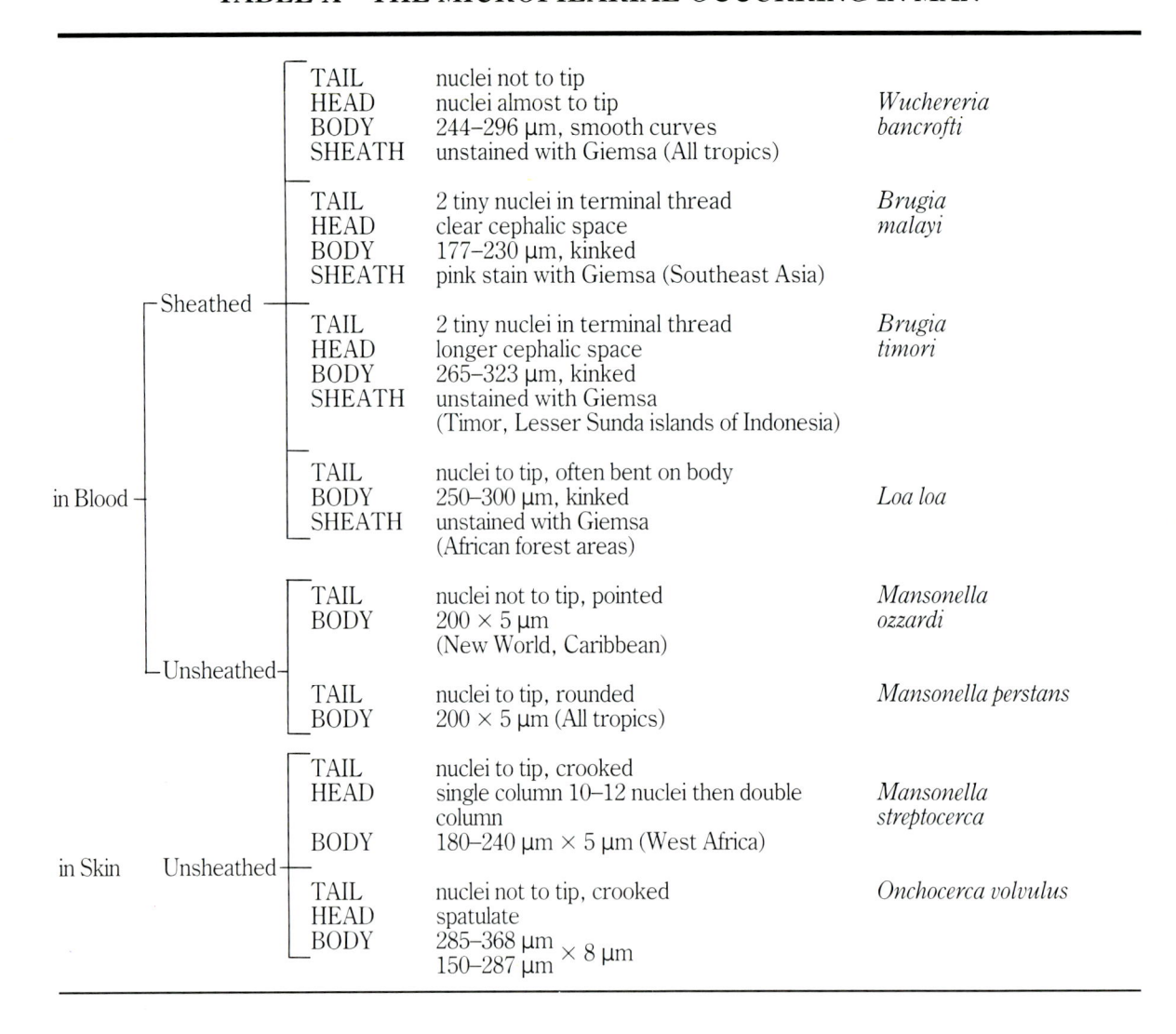

in Blood
- Sheathed
  - TAIL: nuclei not to tip
  - HEAD: nuclei almost to tip
  - BODY: 244–296 µm, smooth curves
  - SHEATH: unstained with Giemsa (All tropics)

  Wuchereria bancrofti

  - TAIL: 2 tiny nuclei in terminal thread
  - HEAD: clear cephalic space
  - BODY: 177–230 µm, kinked
  - SHEATH: pink stain with Giemsa (Southeast Asia)

  Brugia malayi

  - TAIL: 2 tiny nuclei in terminal thread
  - HEAD: longer cephalic space
  - BODY: 265–323 µm, kinked
  - SHEATH: unstained with Giemsa (Timor, Lesser Sunda islands of Indonesia)

  Brugia timori

  - TAIL: nuclei to tip, often bent on body
  - BODY: 250–300 µm, kinked
  - SHEATH: unstained with Giemsa (African forest areas)

  Loa loa

- Unsheathed
  - TAIL: nuclei not to tip, pointed
  - BODY: 200 × 5 µm (New World, Caribbean)

  Mansonella ozzardi

  - TAIL: nuclei to tip, rounded
  - BODY: 200 × 5 µm (All tropics)

  Mansonella perstans

in Skin — Unsheathed
  - TAIL: nuclei to tip, crooked
  - HEAD: single column 10–12 nuclei then double column
  - BODY: 180–240 µm × 5 µm (West Africa)

  Mansonella streptocerca

  - TAIL: nuclei not to tip, crooked
  - HEAD: spatulate
  - BODY: 285–368 µm / 150–287 µm × 8 µm

  Onchocerca volvulus

TABLE XI THE DIGENETIC TREMATODES OF MEDICAL IMPORTANCE AND THEIR PREVALENCE

Superorder	Order	Super-family	Genus & Species	Estimated Cases (min.)	No.
ANEPITHELIO-CYSTIDA	STRIGEATOIDEA	SCHISTOSO-MATOIDEA	*Schistosoma mansoni*	57 million	1
			S. haematobium	78 million	2
			S. japonicum	69 million	3
			S. intercalatum	thousands	4
			S. mattheei	thousands	5
			S. mekongi	thousands	6
	ECHINOSTOMIDA	PARAMPHISTO-MATOIDEA	*Gastrodiscoides hominis*	rare*	7
			Watsonius watsoni	rare	8
		ECHINOSTO-MATOIDEA	*Fasciola hepatica*	thousands	9
			F. gigantica	rare	10
			Fasciolopsis buskii	15 million	11
			Echinostomum ilocanum	rare**	12
EPITHELIO-CYSTIDA	PLAGIOCHIIDA	PLAGIOR-CHIOIDEA	*Dicrocoelium dendriticum*	rare	13
			Troglotrema salmincola	rare	14
			Paragonimus westermanni	5 million	15
			P. africanus	rare	16
			P. uterobilateralis	thousands	17
	OPISTHORCHIIDA	OPISTHOR-CHIOIDEA	*Opisthorchis felineus*	1 million	18
			O. viverrini	10 million	19
			*Clonorchis sinensis****	28 million	20
			Heterophyes heterophyes	thousands	21
			Metagonimus yokogawai	thousands	22

(Note: The numbers in the right-hand column refer to Table XII in which are indicated the molluscs that serve as intermediate hosts for these trematodes.)

*Said to be common in Assam
**Said to be common in the Philippines
***Now referred to as *Opisthorchis sinensis*

TABLE XII   SNAILS AND OTHER MOLLUSCS OF MEDICAL IMPORTANCE (CLASS GASTROPODA)

(The relation of the genera to the helminths that infect them is indicated by reference to the numbers in Table XI. The most important helminths are in bold type.)

Subclass	Order	(Suborder)	Family	Genus & Species	Helminths
STREPTO-NEURA	PROSOBRAN-CHIATA	fresh water	BITHYNIIDAE	*Bithynia* spp. *Parafossularis* spp.	**18, 19, 20** **20**
			POMATIOPSIDAE	*Oncomelania* spp. *Tricula aperta*	**3** **6**
			THIARIDAE	*Thiara granifera*	**15**, 22
			PLEUROCERIDAE	*Semisulcospira libertina*	**15**, 22
			PILIDAE	*Pila conica*	12
		brackish and sea water	POTAMIDIDAE	*Cerithidia cingulata* *Pirenella conica*	21 21
EUTHY-NEURA	PULMONATA	BASOMATOPHORA fresh water	PLANORBIDAE	*Biomphalaria* spp. *Bulinus (Bulinus)* spp. *Bulinus (Physopsis)* spp. *Segmentina hemisphaerula* *S. trochoideus* *Hippeutis cantori* *H. umbilicalis* *Gyraulus convexiusculus* *G. prashadi* *Indoplanorbis exustus?*	**1** **2** **2, 4, 5** 12 **11** **11** 13 12 12 7
			ANCYLIDAE	*Ferrissia tenuis*	**2**
			LYMNAEIDAE	*Fossaria* spp. *Lymnaea* spp. *Stagnicola bulimoides* *Pseudosuccinia columella*	**9, 10** **9, 10** **9** **9, 10**
		STYLOMMATO-PHORA land snails	HELICIDAE	*Helicella candidula*	13
			ENIDAE	*Zebrina detrita*	13
			CIONELLIDAE	*Cionella lubrica* *Achatina fulica* *Bradybaena similaris* *Subulina octona*	13 * * *
		SYSTELLOMM-ATOPHORA	VERONICELLIDAE	*Veronica leydigi*	*

*Angiostrongylus cantonensis. The land planarian *Geoplana septemlineata* has also been found infected with this nematode. *Achatina fulica* may be kept in non-endemic areas as a 'pet'; care is needed to ensure that infected snails are not imported.

TABLE XIII   THE PROTOZOA (PHYLA CILIOPHORA AND SARCOMASTIGOPHORA) OF MEDICAL IMPORTANCE

Phylum etc.	Subphylum etc.	Order	Genus & Species
APICOMPLEXA (see Table IV)			
CILIOPHORA	RHABDOPHORA	VESTIBULIFERIDA	Balantidium coli
SARCOMASTIGOPHORA	MASTIGOPHORA (see Tables VI, VII, VIII)		
	SARCODINA Superclass RHIZOPODEA	AMOEBIDA	Entamoeba coli E. histolytica* E. gingivalis Endolimax nana Iodamoeba bütschlii Acanthamoeba culbertsoni** Acanthamoeba spp.**
		SCHIZOPYRENIDA	Naegleria fowleri**

*Contains numerous 'zymodemes', most of which are non-pathogenic.
**Pathogenic 'free-living' species. The other species are obligatory parasites.

TABLE XIV   THE CESTODES OF MEDICAL IMPORTANCE AND THEIR PREVALENCE IN MAN*

Order	Family	Genus & Species	Estimated Cases (minimum)
PSEUDOPHYLLIDEA	DIPHYLLOBOTHRIIDAE	Diphyllobothrium latum Spirometra spp. 'Sparganum' spp.	16 million rare rare
CYCLOPHYLLIDEA	ANOPLOCEPHALIDAE	Bertiella spp.	rare
	DAVAINEIDAE	Raillietina spp.	rare
	LINSTOWIIDAE	Inermicapsifer spp.	rare
	MESOCESTOIDIDAE	Mesocestoides spp.	rare
	DILEPIDIDAE	Dipylidium caninum	rare
	HYMENOLEPIDIDAE	Hymenolepis nana H. diminuta	36 million rare
	TAENIIDAE	Taenia solium T. saginata Multiceps multiceps Echinococcus granulosus E. vogeli E. multilocularis	5 million 76 million rare thousands rare rare

*See footnote to Table IX

TABLE XV THE SUPERFICIAL AND THE SYSTEMIC MYCOSES

Group	Clinical Syndrome	Causative Agents
SUPERFICIAL (dermatomycoses)		
Mainly hair affected	Black piedra	*Piedraia hortae*
	White piedra	*Trichosporon beigelii*
	Favus	*Trichophyton schoenleinii*
	Tinea barbae	*Trichophyton* spp.
	Tinea capitis	*Microsporon* spp.
Hair not affected	Tinea cruris	*Epidermophyton* spp.
	Tinea pedis	*Trichophyton* spp.
	Tinea unguium	*Trichophyton* spp.
	Tinea corporis	*Microsporum* spp.
	Pityriasis versicolor	*Malassezia furfur*
	Tinea imbricata	*Trichophyton concentricum*
	Otomycosis	various genera
	Superficial candidiasis	*Candida albicans**
SYSTEMIC	Actinomycosis	*Actinomyces israelii*
	Madura foot (Mycetoma)	wide variety of organisms including *Nocardia* spp., *Streptomyces* spp., *Pseudallescheria* spp., etc
	Chromoblastomycosis	*Phialophora* spp. / *Cladosporium carrionii*
	Keloidal blastomycosis (Lôbo's disease)	*Lôboa lôboi*
	Blastomycosis	*Blastomyces dermatitidis*
	Paracoccidioidomycosis	*Paracoccidioides brasiliensis*
	Coccidioidomycosis	*Coccidioides immitis*
	Cryptococcosis (Torulosis)	*Cryptococcus neoformans**
	Systemic candidiasis	*Candida* spp.*
	Sporotrichosis	*Sporothrix schenckii*
	Histoplasmosis	*Histoplasma capsulatum**
	African histoplasmosis	*H. duboisii*
	Zygomycosis	various genera
	Rhinosporidiosis	*Rhinosporidium seeberi*
	Aspergillosis	*Aspergillus fumigatus*

Mycotic infections can become fulminant in immunocompromised subjects. Those marked * are especially associated with AIDS.

TABLE XVI THE MYIASIS-PRODUCING DIPTERA OF MEDICAL IMPORTANCE

Family	Subfamily	Genus & Species	Other Names
CALLIPHORIDAE	CALLIPHORINAE	'metallic group'	
		Chrysomyia bezziana	Old-world screw-worm
		Callitroga hominovorax	New-world screw-worm
		Lucilia spp.	green bottle
		Calliphora spp.	blue bottles
		'non-metallic group'	
		Auchmeromyia luteola	Congo floor maggot
		Cordylobia anthropophaga	Tumbu or mango fly
	SARCOPHAGINAE	*Wohlfahrtia* spp	flesh flies
		Sarcophaga spp.	
OESTRIDAE		*Dermatobia hominis*	
		Hypoderma spp.	'larva migrans'
		Gasterophilus spp.	

TABLE XVII CLASSIFICATION AND CAUSES OF HAEMORRHAGIC FEVERS*

Virus (Family: genus)		Disease	Vector or reservoir
Togaviridae	*Flavivirus*	Dengue	*Aedes aegypti* and other mosquitoes
		Kyasanur Forest disease	*Haemaphysalis* ticks
		Omsk haemorrhagic fever	*Dermacentor* ticks
		Yellow fever	*Aedes aegypti*
	Alphavirus	Chikungunya fever	*Aedes aegypti*
Bunyaviridae	*Phlebovirus*	Rift Valley fever	*Anopheles*
	Nairovirus	Crimea-Congo haemorrhagic fever	*Hyalomma* spp. ticks
	?	Korean haemorrhagic fever**	? tick-borne
Arenaviridae	*Arenavirus*	Junin (Argentine haemorrhagic fever)	*Calomys laucha*
		Machupo (Bolivian haemorrhagic fever)	*Calomys callosus*
		Lassa fever	*Mastomys natalensis*
Marburg-Ebola group	*Filovirus*	Marburg virus	? *Cercopithecus aethiops*
		Ebola virus	? monkeys

*Adapted from Braude, Davis & Fierer (1981) *Medical microbiology and infectious diseases*, W. B. Saunders, Philadelphia.

**Hantaan virus is also associated with Nephropathia epidemica and other manifestations of 'Haemorrhagic fever with renal syndrome' (HFRS). Various rodents serve as reservoirs and it is now suspected that ticks may serve as vectors.

See also Table II

Bibliography

We have found the following key references of considerable value in preparing the third edition of this Atlas. While the list is by no means exhaustive, many further references will be found in each of these works:

Beaver, P C, Jung, R C and Cupp, E W *Clinical Parasitology, 9th Ed.* (Lea & Febiger, Philadelphia, 1984)

Cheesbrough, M *Medical Laboratory Manual for Tropical Countries. 2nd Ed.* (Tropical Health Technology and Butterworths, London, Boston, Durban, Singapore, Sydney, Toronto, Wellington, 1987)

Edington, G M and Gilles, H M *Pathology in the Tropics, 2nd Ed.* (Edward Arnold Publishers, London, 1976)

Maegraith, B G *Adams & Maegraith: Clinical Tropical Diseases, 7th Ed.* (Blackwell Scientific Publications, Oxford and Edinburgh, 1980)

Manson–Bahr, P E C and Bell, D R *Manson's Tropical Diseases, 19th Ed.* (Baillière Tindall, London, 1987)

Marcial-Rojas, R A *Pathology of Protozoal and Helminthic Diseases with Clinical Correlations* (Williams & Wilkins Company, Baltimore, 1971)

Muller, R *Worms and Disease. A Manual of Medical Helminthology* (William Heinemann Medical Books, London, 1975)

Noble, E R and Noble, G A *Parasitology: The Biology of Animal Parasites, 5th Ed.* (Lea & Febiger, Philadelphia, 1982)

Index

References in **bold** are to captions and picture numbers, those in light type to page numbers and those in Roman numerals to Table numbers (on pages 214-232).

Acanthamoeba spp., **729, 730**
Achatina fulica, **493**
Acquired immune deficiency syndrome (AIDS), 681-683
Actinomycetes, 735
Aedes, 3, 5, 7, 12, 13, 228, 234
African Green monkey, **815**
AIDS *see* Acquired immunodeficiency syndrome
  see also Opportunistic infections
Ainhum, **846, 847**
Aleppo button *see* Cutaneous leishmaniasis
Alveolar hydatidosis, **657, 658**
Amastigotes, **159, 171, 173, 193, 207, 209, 210, 221**
Amblyomma hebraeum, **33**
Amoebae
- *Acanthamoeba* spp., **729, 730**
- *Dientamoeba fragilis*, **528**
- differentiation, **524-532**
- *Entamoeba coli*, **524, 529**
- *Entamoeba histolytica*, **525, 530, 533, 535, 536**
- *Entamoeba nana*, **526, 531**
- *Iodamoeba butschlii*, **527, 532**
- *Naegleria* spp., **731, 732**
Amoebiasis, 535-551
- diagnosis, 535-537, **543-545**
- extraintestinal, 538, **548-550**
- immunity, 551
- liver abscess, 542-547
- pathology, 539-541
Anaemia, 69, 84, 341, 342, 615, 805
Ancylostoma duodenale, **328-331, 334, 335, 340**
Ancylostoma spp., **343, 344**
- *see also* Hookworm
Angiostrongyliasis, 496
Angiostrongylus cantonensis, **491, 492, 494, 495**
Angular stomatitis, 802
Animal reservoirs, 12, 30, 35, 44, 49, 117, 134, 156, 157, 171, 182, 196-198, 204, 213, 215, 338, 343, 480, 568, 584, 601, 616, 620, 647, 657, 659, 667, 683, 810, 815
Anisakiasis, 599, 600
Anisakis spp., **600**
Anopheles, I, 4, 6, 7, 9, 11, 59, 60, 62, 234
Ant eaters, 215
Apicomplexa, V
Arboviruses, II
- *see also* Virus infections
Armadillo, **154**
Armillifer armillatus, **668, 669**
Arthropod vectors
- *see* I, Assassin bugs, *Chrysops*, *Culicoides*,

Ectoparasites, Fleas, Kissing bugs, Lice, Mosquitoes, Reduviid bugs, Sandflies, *Simulium*, Ticks, Triatomid bugs, Trombiculid mites, Tsetse flies
Ascariasis, 364-367
Ascaris lumbricoides, **317, 318, 358, 361-363**
Assassin bugs, **153, 154**
Auchmeromyia luteola, **768**
Avitaminoses *see* Vitamins

Babesidae, V
Babesiosis, **123, 124**
Bacteria
- *Bartonella bacilliformis*, **54**
- *Brucella* spp., **516**
- *Clostridium perfringens*, **519**
- coliforms, 509
- *Donovania granulomatosis*, **714**
- fusiform bacteria, 710
- *Mycobacterium leprae*, **692, 703**
- *Mycobacterium tuberculosis*, **783**
- *Mycobacterium ulcerans*, **709**
- *Neisseria meningitidis*, **781**
- *Pseudomonas pseudomallei*, **521**
- *Vibrio cholerae*, **513**
- *Yersinia pestis*, **37**
Baghdad boil *see* Cutaneous leishmaniasis
Balanitis, 550
Balantidiasis, **581, 582**
Balantidium coli, **581, 582**
Bartonella bacilliformis, **54**
Bartonellosis, 54, 55
Bat, **683**
Bedsonia, **675**
Beef Tapeworm, **641-645**
Bejel, **726**
Beri beri, **800, 801**
Big spleen disease, 120-122
Biomphalaria spp., **395, 396, 435, 436**
Bithynia spp., **454**
Bitot's spots, **793**
Black enamel skin, **790**
Black flies *see Simulium*
Black sickness *see* Visceral leishmaniasis
Black vomit, 15
'Black Widow' spider, **840**
Blackwater fever, 84
Bladder
- calculi, 852
- schistosomiasis, 414-419, 422
- worm, 659
Blastocystis hominis, V, **534**
Blood films in
- African trypanosomiasis, **127**
- babesiosis, **123, 124**
- Bartonellosis, **54**

- Chagas' disease, **152**
- filariasis, **250-256**
- hookworm, **342**
- malaria, 69, **76-81, 94-101, 103-116**
- - *see also Plasmodium*
- preparation, 72-75
- relapsing fever, **48, 51**
Blood pathology in
- diphyllobothriasis, 615
- folic acid deficiency, **805**
- haemoglobinopathies, 69
- kala-azar, **186, 189**
- malaria, 84
- snakebite, **836**
Bone marrow, **192, 193, 806**
Bone scan, **518**
Borrelia burgdorferi, IV, **52**
Borrelia duttoni, IV, **48**
Borrelia recurrentis, IV, **51**
Borrelia vincenti, **710, 712**
Bossing of skull, **797, 798, 832, 833**
Bottle feeding, 509
Bradyzoites, **568**
Brain pathology in
- African trypanosomiasis, 143-147
- amoebiasis, 732
- angiostrongyliasis, **495, 496**
- cysticercosis, **639, 640**
- hydatidosis, 655
- Japanese B encephalitis, 24
- malaria, 85 **87-89**
- meningitis, 732, 781, 786
- paragonimiasis, 489
- rabies, 683-686
- schistosomiasis, 428
- sparganosis, 619
- toxocariasis, 370
- toxoplasmosis, 571-574
- *see also* Nervous system
Brucella spp., **516**
Brucellosis, 516-518
Brugia malayi, **222, 233, 243, 244, 251, 252, 259**
Brugia timori, **222, 259-262**
Buffalo gnats *see Simulium*
Bulinus spp., **412, 437, 438**
Burkitt's tumour, **822-825**
Buruli ulcer, **708, 709**
Bushbuck, **134**

Calabar swelling, **269**
Calliphora, **771**
Cancrum oris, **712**
Candida albicans, **755, 756**
Capillaria hepatica, **596**
Capillaria philippensis, **597, 598**

Capillariasis, 596-598
Carcinomata, 422, 460, 826
Card agglutination test (CATT), 148
Carrion's disease, 54, 55
CAT scan see Computerised tomography
Cats, 568
Cattle, 562, 641, 645, 648
Cercaria, 383, 385, 455, 473
Cercarial dermatitis, 394
Cercocyst, 625
Cercopithecus aethiops, 815
Cerebral malaria, 87-89
Cestodes, XIV
- see also Tapeworms
Chagas' disease, 150-168
- diagnosis, 158, 160, 164, 166-168
- distribution, 150
- epidemiology, 153, 156, 157
- immunology, 161, 167, 168
- pathology, 159-165
Chancre, 135, 722
Cheilomastix mesnili, 558, 559
Cheilosis, 803
Chiclero's ulcer, 214
Chigger flea, 762-764
Chinese liver fluke, 451-460
Chironex fleckeri, 842
Chlamydia, 675, 679
Chloroquine resistance, 92, 93
Cholangiocarcinoma, 460
Cholera, 512-515
Chromoblastomycosis, 742
Chrysomyia, 769
Chrysops spp., I, 268
Chyluria, 247, 248
Ciliophora XIII
Circadian rhythm, 260
Circulatory system, schistosomiasis, 401, 402, 410
Clonorchiasis, 453, 459, 460
Clonorchis sinensis, 327, 441, 452-458, 466
Cobra, 834, 838
Coccidial infections, 560-564
- see also Crytosporidiosis
- see also Isosporosis
- see also Toxoplasmosis
Codworm disease, 599
Coenurus cerebralis, 659, 660
Computerised tomography, 143, 144, 478, 640, 649
Congo floor maggot, 768
Congo-Crimea haemorrhagic fever, 22
Cor pulmonale, 410
Cordylobia anthropophaga, 765-767, 770
Coxiella burnetii, 35
Crab, I, 484, 485
Crawcraw, 286
Crayfish, I, 483
Creeping eruption, 269, 343, 350
Cretin, 845
Crotalinae, 835
Cryptococcus neoformans, 749, 750
Cryptosporidiosis, 565-567
Cryptosporidium spp., 565-567
Ctenopharyngodon idellus, 456
Culex, I, 2, 5, 7, 10, 223, 224, 232, 234
Culicoides, I, 262-264

Cutaneous leishmaniasis, 196-221
- diagnosis, 207-211
- distribution, 196, 212
- epidemiology, 197, 198, 213-215
- immunology, 203, 220
- pathology, 201, 219
- see also Chiclero's ulcer
- see also Diffuse cutaneous leishmaniasis
- see also Espundia
Cyclops spp., I, 602, 606, 613, 616
Cyprinus carpio, 463
Cysticercoid, 623, 626, 628, 632
Cysticercosis, 635-640
Cysticercus cellulosae, 632, 637-639
Cysts, protozoal see Protozoa, Flagellates
Cytomegalovirus, 777

Dactylitis, 830, 831
DDT, 25, 59
Dehydration, 511, 515, 791
Delhi sore see Cutaneous leishmaniasis
Dengue, 18-21
Dengue haemorrhagic fever, 20, 21
Dermatobia hominis, 772, 773
Dichuchwa, 726
Dicrocoelium dendriticum, 468
Dientamoeba fragilis, 528
Diphyllobothriasis, 615
Diphyllobothrium latum, 320, 611-614
Dipylidium caninum, 620-623
Dirofilaria immitis, 257
Dirofilaria repens, 312
Disseminated cutaneous leishmaniasis, 220, 221
Dog, 117, 171, 182, 338, 343, 601, 620-623, 646, 647, 657, 659, 683
Dog tapeworm, 620-623
Donovanosis, 714-716
Dracontiasis, 604-610
- diagnosis, 607
- epidemiology, 604, 605, 610
- pathology, 607-610
Dracunculus medinensis, Frontispiece, 606-610
Dum-dum fever see Visceral leishmaniasis
Dwarf tapeworm, 324, 624-627
Dysentery see Amoebiasis, Cholera, Cryptosporidiosis, Gastroenteritis, Typhoid

Ebola fever, 813, 814
Echinococcus granulosus, 646, 648, 651, 652, 654, 656
Echinococcus multilocularis, 657, 658
Ecology, 133, 153, 181, 227, 232, 268, 278, 280, 281, 336, 359, 360, 380, 384, 413, 424, 453, 461, 469, 509, 510, 512, 645, 647
Ectoparasitic arthropods, 757-773
- *Auchmeromyia luteola*, 768
- *Calliphora*, 771
- *Chrysomyia*, 769
- *Cordylobia anthropophaga*, 765-767, 770

- *Dermatobia hominis*, 772, 773
- lice, 25
- *Lucilia*, 771
- mites, 30, 757-761
- *Sarcoptes scabiei*, 758-761
- ticks, 33, 49
- *Tunga penetrans*, 762-764
- *Xenopsylla* spp., 38-43
- see also Mosquitoes
- see also Sandflies
- see also *Simulium*
Egyptian splenomegaly, 400
Eimeriidae, V
Elapidae, 834, 837
Electron micrographs
- *Aedes*, 228
- *Ascaris lumbricoides*, 362
- *Coxiella burnetii*, 35
- *Cryptosporidium*, 566
- *Culex*, 229, 230
- cytomegalovirus, 777
- Ebola fever virus, 813
- *Enterocytozoon bienusei*, 580
- *Giardia lamblia*, 554
- Hantaan virus, 816
- hepatitis virus, 499, 450
- hookworms, 330-334
- Human immune deficiency virus (HIV, HTLV III, LAV), 681
- Lassa fever virus, 809
- *Leishmania*, 173
- *Mansonia*, 231
- *Plasmodium*, 63, 67, 117
- poliomyelitis virus, 497
- *Rickettsia prowazeki*, 26
- smallpox virus, 673
- *Trypanosoma brucei* group, 128
- yellow fever virus, 17
Elephant skin, 287
Elephantiasis, 241-244, 261, 293
Encephalitis, 23, 24
Endemic syphilis, 726
Endomyocardial fibrosis, 843
Entamoeba coli, 524, 529
Entamoeba histolytica, 525, 530, 533, 536
Entamoeba nana, 526, 531
Enteric fever see Typhoid
Enteritis necroticans, 519, 520
Enterobiasis, 593-595
Enterobius vermicularis, 323, 329, 591-593
Enterocytozoon bienusei, 580
Entropion, 677
Eosinophilia, 269, 310, 311
Eosinophilic lung, 310
Erythema chronicum migrans, 52
Eschars, 31, 34
Espundia, 217-219
Esthiomène, 679, 680
Exoerythrocytic schizonts, 64-66
Eye pathology
- *Acanthamoeba* infection, 730
- avitaminosis A, 792-794
- Chagas' disease, 158
- *Coenurus*, 660
- leprosy, 700
- leptospirosis, 522
- loaiasis, 270, 271
- onchocerciasis, 294-297, 304, 305

235

- pentastomiasis, **671**
- sparganosis, **619**
- toxocariasis, **369**
- toxoplasmosis, **575, 576**
- trachoma, **676-678**
- trichinosis, **589**
- whooping cough, **787**

Faeces, **359, 380, 453**
- helminth eggs in, **313-317**
- helminth larvae in, **347, 492**
- in amoebiasis, **537**
- in capillariasis, **598**
- in sprue, **848**
Faeco-oral transmission, 126
Fasciola gigantica, **469**
Fasciola hepatica, **316, 441, 470, 472-477**
Fascioliasis, **469, 475-478**
Fasciolopsiasis, **442**
Fasciolopsis buski, **441, 443, 444, 446**
Field's stain, **72-75**
Filariasis *see Brugia malayi, Brugia timori, Dirofilaria repens,* Eosinophilic lung, Loaiasis, *Mansonella ozzardi, M. perstans,* Onchocerciasis, *M. streptocerca, Wuchereria bancrofti*
Filariform larvae, **337**
Fish, **450, 456, 461, 463**
Fish tapeworm *see* Diphyllobothriasis
Flagellates
- in genitalia, **557, 727**
- in intestine, **552-554**
Fleas, I, **38-43, 622**
Flies *see* Myiasis
Fogo selvagem, **848**
Foliaceus pemphigus, **848**
Folic acid, **805, 806**
Formol gel test, **190**
Framboesiform yaws, **718**
Frei test, **680**
Frog, **616**
Fungi, XV
- *see also* Mycoses
Fungi imperfecti, **735**
Fusiform bacteria, **710**

Gametes, **61**
Gametocytes, **60**
Gangosa, **720**
Gangrene, **28**
Gastrointestinal tract
- amoebiasis, **535-547, 551**
- anisakiasis, **599, 600**
- ascariasis, **364-367**
- balantidiasis, **581, 582**
- candidiasis, **755, 756**
- capillariasis, **596-598**
- Chagas' disease, **164, 165**
- cholera, **512-515**
- coccidiosis, **561, 564**
- codworm disease, **599**
- cryptosporidiosis, **565-567**
- diphyllobothriasis, **611-615**
- enteritis necroticans, **519, 520**
- enterobiasis, **591-595**

- giardiasis, **552-556**
- herringworm disease, **600**
- hookworm, **339, 340**
- hymenolepiasis, **624-629**
- isosporosis, **564**
- schistosomiasis, **397-408, 425-427, 508**
- sprue, **849-851**
- strongyloidiasis, **349, 351**
- taeniasis, **630-645**
- trichuriasis, **376, 377**
- typhoid, **507**
Gastroenteritis, non-specific, **509-511**
Genitalia, **550, 679, 715-717, 722, 723, 728**
Giant cell pneumonia, **776**
Giardia lamblia, **552-554**
Giardiasis, **555, 556**
Giemsa stain, **72-75**
Gingivitis, **808**
Gingivostomatitis, herpetic, **688**
Gland puncture, **139**
Glossina spp., I, **129**
Glossitis, **804**
Gnathostoma spinigerum, **601, 602**
Gnathostomiasis, **603**
Goat, **516**
Goitre, **844**
Gonorrhoea, **717**
Granuloma inguinale, **714-716**
Guinea worm *see* Dracontiasis
Gynaecomastia, **701**

Haemagogus, **12**
Haematuria, **414**
Haemoglobinopathies, **69, 829-833**
Haemorrhagic fevers, XVII, **21, 22**
Haemorrhagic fever with renal syndrome, **816, 817**
- *see also* Hantaan virus
Hair-on-end, **833**
Halzoun syndrome, **662**
Hanging groin, **292, 293**
Hantaan virus, **816, 817**
Heart pathology
- Chagas' disease, **159-163**
- endomyocardial fibrosis, **843**
- schistosomiasis, **410**
Helminth eggs, differentiation, **313-317, 357, 431, 432**
Helminthiases, IX, X, XI, XII, XIV
Hepatitis, **499-504**
Hepatoma, **826**
Herpes simplex, **688, 690**
Herpes zoster, **683**
Herringworm disease, **599, 600**
Heterophyes heterophyes, **441**
Hexacanth embryos, **624**
HFRS *see* Haemorrhagic fever with renal syndrome, Hantaan virus
Hippeutis sp., **443**
Histoplasma duboisii, **753, 754**
Histoplasmosis, **753, 754**
HIV *see* Acquired immune deficiency syndrome (AIDS)
Hoeppli reaction, **398, 408**
Hookworm
- diagnosis, **321**

- distribution, **328**
- epidemiology, **336**
- identification, **321, 330-334**
- life cycle, **335, 337-340**
- pathology, **341-344**
- *see also Ancylostoma, Necator*
HTLV III *see* Acquired immune deficiency syndrome (AIDS)
Hydatid sand, **652**
Hydatidosis, **647, 649, 650, 653-656**
Hydrocele, **240**
Hydronephrosis, **421**
Hymenolepis diminuta, **325, 628, 629**
Hymenolepis nana see Vampirolepis nana
Hyperkeratosis, **719**
Hyperreactive malarial splenomegaly, **120-122**
Hypnozoite, **65, 66, 102**
Hyrax spp., **204**

Immune response in
- acquired immune deficiency syndrome (AIDS), **9**
- African trypanosomiasis, **148**
- amoebiasis, **551**
- Chagas' disease, **167, 168**
- filariasis, **257, 258**
- hydatidosis, **656**
- infective hepatitis, **504**
- leishmaniasis, **190, 191**
- leprosy, **693, 707**
- lymphogranuloma venereum, **680**
- malaria, **71, 119-122**
- meningitis, **782**
- mycoses, **738**
- schistosomiasis, **429**
- smallpox, **674**
- toxocariasis, **372**
- toxoplasmosis, **578**
- trichinosis, **590**
Immunoglobulins *see* Immune response
Infant mortality, **509**
Infantile kala-azar, **185**
Infective hepatitis, **499-504**
Insects, hosts of helminths, **624-626, 628, 629**
Intestinal flukes, **442-450**
Iodamoeba butschlii, **527, 532**
Isoenzymes, **172, 535**
Isospora belli, **563**
Isosporosis, **564**

Japanese B encephalitis, **23, 24**
Jaundice, **501, 522**
Jelly fish, **842**
Jigger flea, **762-764**

Kala-azar, **180-195**
- diagnosis, **183, 184, 192-195**
- distribution, **180**
- epidemiology, **180-182**
- immunology, **189-191**
- infantile, **185**
- pathology, **186, 828**

- post kala-azar dermal leishmaniasis (PKDL), 187, 188
Kaposi's sarcoma, 682, 827, 828
Keratomalacia, 794
Kerteszia, 59
Kidney pathology in
- Burkitt's tumour, 825
- malaria, 84, 85, 118, 119
- schistosomiasis, 414, 420, 421
- toxocariasis, 371
Kissing bugs *see* Reduviid bugs
Koplik's spots, 774
Kwashiorkor, 788-790

Larva migrans, 269, 270, 343, 350, 369-372
Lassa fever, 809-812
Latex agglutination test, 782
Latrodectus mactans, 840
LAV *see* HIV
Leishman stain, 72-75
Leishman-Donovan bodies *see* Amastigotes
Leishmania
- *aethiopica*, 196, 220
- *amazonensis*, 213, 220
- *braziliensis*, 217, 219
- *chagasi*, 180
- classification VIII
- *donovani*, 180
- *guyanensis*, 215, 216
- *infantum*, 180, 205, 828
- life cycle, 170
- *major*, 197-201
- *mexicana*, 214, 220
- *panamensis*, 215
- *tropica*, 202, 203
Leishmaniasis
- concomitant infection in AIDS, 183, 828
- disseminated cutaneous, 220, 221
- epidemiology, 174, 181, 182, 213-215
- immunology, 189-191, 197, 198, 206, 210, 211, 213-215
- mucocutaneous *see* Espundia
- New World cutaneous, 212-216
- Old World cutaneous, 196-211
- post kala-azar dermal, 187, 188
- visceral *see* Kala-azar, 180-195, 828
- *see also* Cutaneous leishmaniasis
Leonine facies, 699
Leopard skin, 290
Lepromin test, 707
Leprosy, 691-707
- diagnosis, 692
- distribution, 691
- epidemiology, 691
- immunology, 693
- indeterminate, 693, 694
- lepromatous, 699-702, 705
- pathology, 703-706
- tuberculoid, 694-698, 704
Leptospira spp., IV, 523
Leptospirosis, IV, 522
Leptotrombidium, 30
Lice, I
Life cycles
- African trypanosomiasis, 126
- ascariasis, 358
- Chagas' disease, 151

- clonorchiasis, 452
- filariasis, 233, 235, 236, 267, 274
- hookworm, 335
- leishmaniasis, 170
- malaria, 57, 76-79, 94-101
- schistosomiasis, 378
- strongyloidiasis, 346
- taeniasis, 630
- trichinosis, 583
- trichuriasis, 373
Linguatula serrata, 661, 663
Liver flukes, 451-478
Liver pathology in
- amoebiasis, 545-547
- ascariasis, 366
- clonorchiasis, 459, 460, 467
- fascioliasis, 475-478
- hepatoma, 826
- *Herpes simplex*, 689
- hydatidosis, 649-652, 657, 658
- infective hepatitis, 503
- kala-azar, 184, 185, 195
- Lassa fever, 812
- leptospirosis, 522
- malaria, 70, 90, 122
- pentastomiasis, 669
- plague, 37
- schistosomiasis, 397-402, 425, 426
- toxocariasis, 96
- yellow fever, 16
Loa loa, 253, 254, 266
Loaiasis, 269-271
- diagnosis, 253, 254, 265, 269, 270, 272
- distribution, 266
- epidemiology, 268
Lôbo's disease, 744
Lôboa lôboi, 745
Louse, 25
Loxosceles laeta, 841
Lucilia, 771
Lumbar puncture, 142
Lung, 86, 409, 410, 486, 487, 548, 653, 654, 776
Lung flukes, 481-483
Lungworm, 667
Lutzomyia spp., I, 55, 175-177
Lyme disease, 52, 53
Lymnaea spp., 440, 471
Lymphadenopathy, 138, 245-247, 488, 577, 679
Lymphangitis, 239
Lymphogranuloma venereum, 679, 680

Machado-Guerreiro reaction, 167
Madura foot, 735-737
Madurella mycetomae, 739
Maduromycosis, 735-741
Main de prédicateur, 696
Malaria, 59-122
- *see also Plasmodium*
Malassezia furfur, 734
Mansonella ozzardi, 255, 309
Mansonella perstans, 256, 262, 265
Mansonella streptocerca, 307, 308
Mansonia, 225-227, 231
Maps of distribution
- African trypanosomiasis, 125

- Burkitt's tumour, 822
- Chagas' disease, 150
- chloroquine resistance, 93
- clonorchiasis, 451
- cutaneous leishmaniasis, 196, 212
- dengue haemorrhagic fever, 20
- espundia, 212
- fasciolopsiasis, 442
- filariasis, 222, 266, 273
- haemoglobin S, 829
- haemoglobinopathies, 829
- hookworm, 328
- kala-azar, 180
- leprosy, 691
- loaiasis, 266
- malaria, 59
- meningitis, 778
- onchocerciasis, 273
- opisthorciasis, 451
- paragonimiasis, 479
- plague, 36
- schistosomiasis, 379, 411
- scrub typhus, 29
- strongyloidiasis, 345
- trachoma, 675
- yellow fever virus, 1
Marasmus, 791
Marburg disease, 815
Marmoset, 215
Mastomys natalensis, 810
Maurer's dots, 77
Measles, 774-776
Mega syndrome, 161, 163, 164
Melioidosis, 521
Meningitis, 690, 781, 786
Meningococcal meningitis, 778-782
Metacercaria, 444, 457, 462, 484
Metacyclic forms, 130, 131, 155
Metagonimus yokagawai, 448
Microfilaria, X
- counts, 249
- differentiation, 250-256, 259, 265, 302, 303, 307, 308
- life cycle, 233, 235, 236, 267, 274
Microsporidia, 579, 580
Milk, 509
'Minocolumn', 149
Miracidia, 381, 470
Mites, I
Mitsuda reaction, 707
Molluscan intermediate hosts, XII
- of schistosomes, 383, 395, 412, 423
- of other trematodes, 433-440
Monkeys, 215, 815
Montenegro test, 211
Morula cell, 146, 147
Mosquitoes
- *Aedes*, 3, 5, 7, 12, 13, 228, 234
- *Anopheles*, I, 4, 6, 7, 9, 11, 59, 60, 62, 234
- *Culex*, I, 2, 5, 7, 10, 224, 232, 234
- *Haemagogus*, 12
- *Kerteszia*, 59
- *Mansonia*, 225-227, 231
- *Stegomyia*, 12, 234
Mott cell, 146, 147
Mucocutaneous leishmaniasis *see* Espundia
Multiceps multiceps, 659
Murine typhus, 35
Muscles, 159, 163, 560, 562, 588, 632, 641

237

Mycobacterium leprae, 692, 703
Mycobacterium ulcerans, 708, 709
Mycoses, XV
- superficial, 733, 734
- systemic, 735-756
Myiasis, XVI
Myocardium *see* Heart
Myoglobinuria, 836

Naegleria spp., 731, 732
Naja naja, 834
Necator americanus, 328, 329, 333, 335, 340, 341
- *see also* Hookworm
Negri bodies, 683
Neisseria meningitidis, 781
Nematodes, IX
- *see also* Angiostrongyliasis, Anisakiasis, Capillariasis, Dracontiasis, Enterobiasis, Filariasis, Gnathostomiasis, Soil-mediated helminthiases, Strongyloidiasis, Trichinosis
Neoplasia, 422, 460, 822-828
Nephrosis, 118
Nervous system in
- beri-beri, 801
- leprosy, 696-698, 706
- poliomyelitis, 498
- rabies, 683
- snake bite, 837, 839
Nicotinic acid, 807
Njovera, 726
NNN medium, 194
Nodules
- bladder, 417, 418
- colon, 403-408
- subcutaneous, 282-284, 306
Nutritional diseases
- avitaminoses, 792-808
- epidemiology, 195
- kwashiorkor, 788-790
- marasmus, 791
- *see also* Vitamins

Onchocerca volvulus, 274, 283, 285, 301-303
Onchocerciasis, 273-306
- diagnosis, 299-304, 306
- distribution, 273
- epidemiology, 278-281, 298
- eye lesions, 294-297, 304, 305
- pathology, 283-285
- skin changes, 286-293
Oncomelania spp., 423, 433
Oncosphere, 624
Oöcysts, 624
Oökinetes, 61
Opisthorciasis, 461-463, 467
Opisthorcis felineus, 327, 441, 451, 464
Opisthorcis viverrini, 451, 461, 465
Opportunistic infections
- candidiasis, 755, 756
- cryptococcosis, 750
- *Cryptosporidium*, 566
- cytomegalovirus, 777
- herpes simplex, 690
- herpes zoster, 683

- histoplasmosis, 753
- isosporosis, 564
- kala-azar, 183, 828
- Kaposi's sarcoma, 682, 827, 828
- *Naegleria fowleri*, 732
- *Pneumocystis carinii*, 818-821
- toxoplasmosis, 574
- tuberculosis, 783
Optic atrophy, 297
Oriental liver fluke, 327, 441, 452-458, 466
Oriental sore *see* Cutaneous leishmaniasis
Ornithodorus moubata, 49
Oroya fever, 54, 55
Osteitis, 711, 721, 785
Osteomalacia, 799

Palm civet, 480
Panstrongylus spp., 154
Paracoccidioides brasiliensis, 746, 747
Paradoxurus hermaphroditus, 480
Paragonimiasis, 483, 486-490
- distribution, 479
Paragonimus africanus, 479
Paragonimus heterotremus, 479
Paragonimus uterobilateralis, 479
Paragonimus westermani, 319, 441, 479, 481-484, 489
Pasteurella pestis, 37
Pathology *see* individual diseases and tissues
Pediculus humanus, 25
Pellagra, 807
Pentastomiasis, 662, 670, 671
Periodic filariasis, 222
Periportal fibrosis, 399
Peyer's patches, 507
Phagedaenic ulcer, 710, 711
Phlebotomus spp., I, 174-177
Physopsis, 438
Pian bois, 215, 216
Pig, 561, 581, 584, 632
Pigbel, 519, 520
Pinta, 725
Pinworm *see Enterobius vermicularis*
Pipestem fibrosis, 399
Pirenella, 448
Pistia, 227
Pit viper, 835
Pityriasis versicolor, 734
PKDL *see* Post kala-azar dermal leishmaniasis
Placenta in malaria, 91
Plague, 36-47
Planarians, 493
Plasmodiidae, V
Plasmodium cynomolgi, 65, 66
Plasmodium falciparum, 67, 76-81
- clinical complications, 83-87
- life cycle, 76-81
Plasmodium malariae, 64, 117-122
- life cycle, 108-115
Plasmodium ovale, 103-107, 116
Plasmodium vivax, 94-102
- hypnozoite, 102
- life cycle, 94-101
Plerocercoid, 614
Pneumococcus, 782
Pneumocystis carinii, 818, 819, 821

Pneumonia, 776, 777, 820
Poliomyelitis, 497, 498
Polyposis
- of bladder, 417, 418
- of colon, 403-408
Pork tapeworm, 630-640
Porocephalus crotali, 664-667
Post kala-azar dermal leishmaniasis, 187, 188
Potamon rathbuni, 485
Primary amoebic meningoencephalitis, 731, 732
Procercoid, 613, 616, 622
Proechimys guyanensis, 213
Proglottids, 612, 617, 621, 627, 643, 644
Promastigotes, 178, 194
Protozoa V VI VII VIII XIII
- in CNS, 731, 732
- in faeces, 524-537, 540, 541, 550, 552-554, 558, 559, 561, 563, 567, 569
- in genitalia, 557, 727, 728
- *see also* Plasmodium
Psammomys obesus, 198
Pseudoterranova decipiens, 599
Ptosis in snakebite, 837
Purpura, 186
Pus, 545

Q fever, 35

Rabbit, 661
Rabies, 684-687
Radio-isotope scan, 425, 543
Rashes, skin eruptions
- African trypanosomiasis, 137
- bartonellosis, 55
- Congo-Crimea haemorrhagic fever, 22
- dengue, 19
- dengue haemorrhagic fever, 21
- Ebola fever, 814
- haemorrhagic fever with renal syndrome, 817
- *Herpes simplex*, 688, 690
- *Herpes zoster*, 683
- hookworm, 343
- kwashiorkor, 788-790
- leishmaniasis, 179, 186
- louse-borne typhus, 27
- Lyme disease, 52
- measles, 774
- meningococcal meningitis, 779, 780
- pellagra, 807
- scabies, 760, 761
- schistosomiasis, 394
- scrub typhus, 32
- smallpox, 672
- tick typhus, 343
- trepanematoses, 725, 726
- typhoid, 505
- *see also* Cutaneous leishmaniasis
- *see also* Leprosy
- *see also* Onchocerciasis
Rat, 45
Rat tapeworm, 628, 629
Redia, 472

Reduviid bugs I, **151**, 153-156
Relapsing fever IV, **48-51**
Rhabditiform larvae, **347**
Rhodnius spp., **154**
Riboflavine, **802-804**
Rickets, **795-798**
Rickettsia
- *conori*, **33**
- *prowazeki*, **26**
- *tsutsugamushi*, **29**
Rickettsioses I III, **25-35**
- epidemiology, **25**
- louse-borne typhus, **25-28**
- murine typhus, **35**
- Q fever, **35**
- scrub typhus, **29-32**
- tick typhus, **33, 34**
Rickety rosary, **795**
Rodents, **45, 195, 197, 198, 213, 810**
Romaña's sign, **158**
Romanowsky stains, **72-75**
Rose spots, **505**

Sabre tibia, **721**
Salmonellosis, **508**
Sandflies, **174-179, 181**
Sarcocystidae V
Sarcocystis hominis, **561, 562**
'*Sarcocystis lindemanni*', **560**
Sarcodina XIII
Sarcoptes scabiei, **758-761**
Schistosoma haematobium, **313, 378, 388, 391, 412**
Schistosoma intercalatum, **431**
Schistosoma japonicum, **315, 378, 390, 393, 411, 423-428, 432**
Schistosoma mansoni, **314, 381-383, 385-387, 389, 392, 395, 441**
Schistosoma mattheei, **431**
Schistosoma mekongi, **411, 423, 424, 432**
Schistosomal dermatitis, **394**
Schistosomiasis, ectopic, **409, 428**
Schistosomiasis, intestinal
- diagnosis, **403-407, 410, 429, 430**
- distribution, **379**
- epidemiology, **380, 384, 396**
- immunology, **429**
- life cycle, **378, 395**
- pathology, **394, 397-410**
- with salmonellosis, **508**
Schistosomiasis, vesical
- diagnosis, **414, 415, 417, 419-421, 429**
- distribution, **411**
- epidemiology, **413, 415**
- life cycle, **378, 412**
- pathology, **414, 416-422**
Schistosomule, **386**
Schüffner's dots, **94-98, 101**
Sclerosing keratitis, **295**
Scolex, **620, 633, 634**
Scotch tape swab, **594, 595**
Scrotum, **240, 242, 293**
Scrub typhus, **29-32**
Scurvy, **808**
Sea snake, **836**
Sea wasp, **842**

Segmentina, **439, 445**
Semisulcospira spp., **448, 483**
Sheep, **469, 648**
Sickle cell disease, **829-833**
Simulium spp., I, **275-281**
Siti, **726**
Skerlievo, **726**
Skin
- amoebiasis, **549, 550**
- biopsy, **208, 299, 300, 702**
- herpes simplex, **690**
- herpes zoster, **683**
- scabies, **760, 761**
- sea wasp sting, **842**
- snakebite, **838, 839**
- spider bite, **841**
- tests, **211, 680, 707**
- yaws, **718, 719**
- *see also* Cutaneous leishmaniasis, Ectoparasitic arthropods, Mycoses, Onchocerciasis, Rashes, Venereal diseases
Sleeping sickness, **125-149**
'Slim disease', **682**
Sloth, **215**
Slugs, **493**
Smallpox, **672-674**
Snails *see* Molluscs
Snakes, **667, 834-839**
Soil-mediated helminthiases
Snowflake opacities, **294**
South American blastomycosis *see* Chromoblastomycosis
SE Asian haemorrhagic fever *see* Dengue haemorrhagic fever
Sowda, **289**
Sparganosis, **616-619**
Sparganum spp., **617-619**
Spider bites, **840, 841**
Spirillum minus, IV
Spirometra spp., **616**
Spleen pathology
- kala-azar, **184, 185**
- malaria, **70, 120, 121**
- schistosomiasis, **400**
Sporocysts, **382**
Sporotrichosis, **751, 752**
Sporozoites, **63**
Sprue, **849-851**
Sputum, **483**
Stegomyia, **12, 234**
Streptomyces pellietieri, **740**
Streptomyces somaliensis, **741**
Strongyloides fülleborni, **352**
Strongyloides stercoralis, **346-350, 357**
Strongyloidiasis, **345, 349-351**
Subperiodic filariasis, **222**
Sushi, **150**
'Swollen belly sickness', **352**
Syphilis, **722-724**

Tachyzoites, **570**
Taenia saginata, **326, 641, 642, 644**
Taenia solium, **326, 631-635, 637-639**
Taeniasis, **632, 635-641, 645**
Tapeworms XIV
- *Diphyllobothrium latum*, **611-614**
- *Dipylidium caninum*, **620-623**
- *Echinococcus granulosus*, **646-656**

- *Echinococcus multilocularis*, **657, 658**
- *Hymenolepis diminuta*, **628, 629**
- *Hymenolepis nana* = *Vampirolepis nana*
- *Multiceps multiceps*, **659, 660**
- *Spirometra* spp., **616**
- *Taenia saginata*, **641-644**
- *Taenia solium*, **630-640**
- *Vampirolepis nana*, **624-627**
Temperature charts
- African trypanosomiasis, **136**
- amoebiasis, **542**
- brucellosis, **517**
- dengue, **18**
- kala-azar, **183**
- malaria, **68, 82**
- relapsing fever, **50**
- typhoid, **506**
- yellow fever, **14**
Ternidens deminutus, **353, 354**
Terranova spp., *see Pseudoterranova decipiens*
Tetanus, **713**
Thalassaemia, **69, 829-833**
Thiamine, **800, 801**
Thiara granifera, **434, 483**
Tick, I, **33, 49**
Tick typhus, **33, 34**
Tinea imbricata, **733, 791**
Tissue paper skin, **291**
Tongue worm, **661-663**
Toxocara canis, **368**
Toxocara cati, **368**
Toxocariasis, **369-372**
Toxoplasma gondii, **568-570**
Toxoplasmosis, **571-578**
Trachoma, **675-678**
Tragelaphus scriptus, **134**
Trematodes XI XII
- *see also* Intestinal flukes, Liver flukes, Paragonimiasis, Schistosomiasis
Treponema carateum, **725**
Treponema pallidum, **724**
Treponema pertenue, **718**
Treponematoses IV
- *see also* Endemic syphilis, Leptospirosis, Pinta, Syphilis, Yaws
Triatomid bugs, **153, 154**
Tribolium spp., **629**
TRIC virus, **676**
Trichiasis, **677, 678**
Trichinella spiralis, **329, 583, 585-588**
Trichinosis, **583-590**
Trichomonas vaginalis, **557, 727, 728**
Trichophyton concentricum, **733**
Trichostrongylus spp., **355-357**
Trichuriasis, **359, 377**
Trichuris trichiura, **322, 329, 336, 374-376**
Tricula aperta, **423**
Trombiculid mites, **30, 757**
Tropical splenomegaly syndrome, **120-122**
Tropical ulcer, **710, 711**
Trypanosoma, VII
- *brucei*, **125**
- *cruzi*, **150, 152, 155, 159, 168**
- *gambiense*, **128, 133**
- life cycles, **126, 131, 151**
- *rangeli*, **169**
- *rhodesiense*, **127, 134, 142-144**

239

Trypanosomiasis
- African, *see* Sleeping sickness
- American, *see* Chagas' disease
- CAT scan, **143, 144**
- diagnosis, **135-142, 148, 149, 158, 160, 164, 166-168**
- distribution, **125, 150**
- epidemiology, **133, 153**
- immunology, **148, 167, 168**
- pathology, **135, 143-147, 159-165**
Tsetse fly, **129, 131, 132**
Tsutsugamushi disease, **29-32**
Tuberculosis, **783-786**
Tumbu fly, **765-767**
Tunga penetrans, **762, 763**
Tungiasis, **764**
'Turista', **510**
Typhoid, **505-507**
Typhus, III
- epidemic, **25-28**
- epidemiology, **25, 30, 35**
- louse-borne, **25-28**
- scrub, **29-32**

Ulcers
- Buruli, **708, 709**
- cancrum oris, **712**
- kwashiorkor, **790**
- *Mycobacterium ulcerans,* **708, 709**
- mycoses, **735, 736, 741, 743, 746, 751, 753**
- phagedaenic, **710**
- tropical, **710**
- *see also* Chancre, Cutaneous leishmaniasis, Espundia
Ultrasound, **650**
Ureters, **420, 421**
Urine
- blackwater fever, **84**
- filariasis, **248**
- helminth eggs, **315**
- hepatitis, **502**
- schistosomiasis, **315, 414, 415**
- snake bite, **836**
Uta, **212**

Vaccination, **519, 674, 687, 778**
Vaginitis, **728**
Vahlkampfidae, **731**
Vampire bat, **683**
Vampirolepis nana, **324, 624-627**
Venereal disease, **679-682, 714-717, 722-724, 728**
- *see also* Acquired immune deficiency syndrome (AIDS)
Venomous animals, **834-842**

Verrucous dermatitis, **743**
Verruga Peruviana, **55**
Vervet monkey, **815**
Vibrio cholerae, **513**
Vincent's organisms, **710, 712**
Viperidae, **835, 839**
Virus infections
- acquired immune deficiency syndrome (AIDS), **681, 682**
Congo-Crimea haemorrhagic fever, **22**
- cytomegalovirus, **777**
- dengue, **18, 19**
- dengue haemorrhagic fever, **20, 21**
- Ebola fever, **813, 814**
- haemorrhagic fever with renal syndrome, **816, 817**
- Hantaan virus, **816**
- hepatitis, **499-504**
- *Herpes simplex,* **688-690**
- *Herpes zoster,* **683**
- HIV (HTLV III, **LAV**), **681, 682**
- Japanese B encephalitis, **23, 24**
- Lassa fever, **809-812**
- lymphogranuloma venereum, **679, 680**
- Marburg disease, **815**
- measles, **774-776**
- poliomyelitis, **497, 498**
- rabies, **684-687**
- smallpox, **672-674**
- SE Asian haemorrhagic fever *see* Dengue haemorrhagic fever
- trachoma, **675-678**
- yellow fever, **1, 14-17**
- *see also* I, II, XVII
Visceral larva migrans *see* Larva migrans
Visceral leishmaniasis *see* Kala-azar
Vitamins
- A, **792-794**
- B1, **800, 801**
- B2, **802-804**
- C, **808**
- D, **795-799**
- folic acid, **805, 806**
- PP, **807**
Vitiligo, **734**
Vomitus, **15**

Water caltrop, **447**
Water chestnut, **463**
Water fleas, I, **602, 606, 613, 616**
Whitmore's bacillus, **521**
Whooping cough, **787**
Winterbottom's sign, **138**
Wuchereria bancrofti
- diagnosis, **249, 250, 257-259**
- distribution, **222**
- epidemiology, **232, 234**
- immunology, **257, 258**

- life cycle, **233, 235-238**
- pathology, **239-242, 244-248**

Xenodiagnosis, **166**
Xenopsylla
- *astia,* **40, 41**
- *brasiliensis,* **42, 43**
- *cheopis,* **38, 39, 44**
Xerophthalmia, **792**
X-rays
- amoebic liver abscess, **544**
- ascariasis, **364**
- Chagas' disease, **164**
- clonorchiasis, **467**
- cysticercosis, **636**
- dracontiasis, **607**
- filariasis, **246, 247**
- hydatid cyst, **653**
- Madura foot, **737**
- melioidosis, **521**
- paracoccidioidomycosis, **747**
- paragonimiasis, **487**
- pentastomiasis, **670**
- pneumonic plague, **47**
- pneumocystosis, **820**
- rickets, **797, 799**
- schistosomiasis, **402, 403, 410, 417, 419-421**
- sickle cell disease, **831**
- sprue, **850, 851**
- thalassaemia, **833**
- toxoplasmosis, **572**
- tuberculosis, **783, 785**
- yaws osteitis, **721**

Yaws, **718-721**
Yellow fever, **1, 12, 14-17**
Yersinia pestis, **37**

Ziehl-Neelsen stain, **692, 709**
Ziemann's dots, **110**
Zoonoses, XVIII
- arthropod, **662, 668**
- bacterial, **32, 34, 35, 36, 55, 516, 522**
- helminth, **243, 261, 262, 266, 307, 309, 311, 312, 343, 353, 368, 394, 424 431, 432, 442, 448, 449, 452, 461, 469, 479, 491, 590, 597, 599-601 611, 616, 620, 624, 628, 646, 657, 660**
- protozoal, **48, 52, 123, 125, 150, 170, 560, 565, 568, 581, 583**
- viral, **1, 23, 809-817**
- *see also* Animal reservoirs